Springer-Verlag Berlin Heidelberg GmbH

W. Becker
J. Meller · H. Zappel
A. Leenen · F. Seseke

Imaging in Paediatric Urology

With 245 Figures in 439 Separate Illustrations

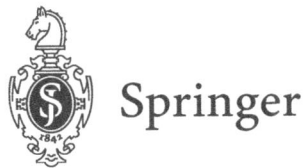

Springer

Prof. Dr. med. W. Becker (†)
Abteilung Nuklearmedizin, Zentrum Radiologie

Dr. med. J. Meller
Abteilung Nuklearmedizin, Zentrum Radiologie

Dr. med. H. Zappel
Kinderklinik und Poliklinik

Dr. med. A. Leenen
Abteilung Röntgendiagnostik I

Dr. med. F. Seseke
Klinik und Poliklinik für Urologie

Georg-August-Universität Göttingen
Robert-Koch-Strasse 40, 37075 Göttingen, Germany

ISBN 978-3-540-43348-4   ISBN 978-3-642-55785-9 (eBook)
DOI 10.1007/978-3-642-55785-9

Library of Congress Cataloging-in-Publication Data
Imaging in paediatric urology/W. Becker... [et al.]. p.; cm. Includes bibliogaphical references and index.
ISBN 3540433481 (alk. paper)
1. Paediatric urology. 2. Paediatric diagnostic imaging. 3. Diagnostic imaging. 4. Urinay organs-Imaging. 5. Children-Diseases-Diagnosis. I. Becker, W.
[DNLM: 1. Urologic Diseases-diagnosis-child. 2. Diagnostic Imaging. 3. Urologic Diseases-therapy-Child. WJ 141 I305 2003] RJ469.I4I434 2003 618.92'60754-dc21
2002021848

http://www.springer.de

© Springer-Verlag Berlin Heidelberg 2003

Originally published by Springer-Verlag Berlin Heidelberg New York in 2003

Cover-Design: Erich Kirchner, Springer-Verlag, Heidelberg
Typesetting: Fotosatz-Service Köhler GmbH, Würzburg

Printed on acid-free paper.   SPIN 10786763   21/3150 ih - 5 4 3 2 1 0

Dedication

Professor Wolfgang Becker, the initiator of this book project, died on 18 May 2002 at the age of 49. For years he fought a serious disease. Until his final days he actively coordinated the contributions of the authors. This book owes much to his inspiring input and his unflagging efforts to drive the project forward. Imaging in Paediatric Urology is dedicated to his memory.

R.-H. Ringert, E. Grabbe and the authors

Preface

Conferences between doctors of different specialties are becoming more and more important as a decision-making tool in diagnosis and treatment of diseases. The benefit of these conferences is that questions from the clinician to the radiologist or the nuclear medicine specialist are discussed in the context of all available imaging results. Written documents and reports for one imaging modality can be reviewed in light of the clinical symptoms and compared with other imaging modalities. Immediate decision-making is possible because specialists from all disciplines are present.

The publication of a urologic – paediatric – radiologic – nuclear medicine atlas from the University Hospital of Göttingen indicates that such conferences have matured over the years. They are now routine monthly events that form the basis of clinical and surgical decisions. The learning benefit for students and participating physicians is high. Responsible for this success and development is the urologist of the hospital, one of whose main interests is paediatric urology.

Formal training in paediatric nuclear medicine is limited for most nuclear medicine practitioners. As a consequence, paediatric urologic and nephrologic diseases are familiar only to those who see children on a daily basis.

Since many children, if not the majority, are studied in non-paediatric imaging centers, a book on paediatric urology, nephrology, radiology and nuclear medicine featuring case reports is valuable as a handy reference. Examples of pathologic conditions, both common and rare, define the technique required for appropriate imaging and assist the interpretation of unfamiliar disorders. Furthermore, these case illustrations concentrate a wealth of information into one easily accessed volume to help busy practitioners to localize and recognize its clinical significance of their patients' findings.

- The topics presented in this atlas include all the common and rare urologic conditions encountered in children who need further imaging.
- The information assembled here is based on years of experience in both the obtaining and the interpretation of images in children with kidney diseases.
- Regular use of this book will repay the users in time saved, knowledge gained and improved quality of their practice for years to come.

W. Becker, MD FRCP   Professor of Nuclear Medicine
E. Grabbe, MD   Professor of Radiology
R.-H. Ringert, MD   Professor of Urology

Contents

1   **Clinical Aspects of Paediatric Urology**   1
         F. Seseke

1.1   Embryology   1
1.1.1   Development of the Kidney   1
1.1.2   Development of the Ureter   3
1.1.3   Development of the Bladder   3
1.1.4   Development of the Sinus Urogenitalis   3
1.1.5   Development of the Genital Ducts   4
1.1.6   Development of the Male Genitalia   4
1.1.7   Development of the Female Genitalia   5

1.2   Anomalies of the Upper Urinary Tract   6
1.2.1   Renal Dysgenesis   6
1.2.2   Cystic Disease of the Kidney   8
1.2.3   Renal Anomalies of Ascent, Fusion and Rotation   10
1.2.4   Anomalies of the Collecting System and Ureter   14

1.3   Anomalies of the Lower Urinary Tract   20
1.3.1   Bladder Exstrophy   20
1.3.2   Other Congenital Anomalies of the Bladder   22
1.3.3   Anomalies of the Urachus   23
1.3.4   Neurogenic Disorder of the Lower Urinary Tract   23
1.3.5   Posterior Urethral Valves   25
1.3.6   Other Congenital Anomalies of the Urethra   27

1.4   Prune-belly Syndrome   28
1.4.1   Aetiology and Pathogenesis   28
1.4.2   Clinical Presentation and Evaluation   28
1.4.3   Therapy and Prognosis   29

1.5   Urinary Tract Infections   30
1.5.1   Aetiology and Pathogenesis   30
1.5.2   Clinical Presentation   31
1.5.3   Clinical Evaluation   32
1.5.4   Therapy   33
1.5.5   Genitourinary Tract Infection   33

1.6   Urolithiasis   34
1.6.1   General Pathophysiology of Stone Formation   34
1.6.2   Specific Pathophysiology of Stone Formation   34
1.6.3   Clinical Presentation and Evaluation   36
1.6.4   Therapy   37

1.7   Vesico-ureteral Reflux   40
1.7.1   Aetiology and Pathogenesis   40
1.7.2   Clinical Presentation   40
1.7.3   Clinical Evaluation   41

1.7.4   Grading   42
1.7.5   Therapy   42

1.8   Megaureter   48
1.8.1   Definition   48
1.8.2   Pathophysiology   48
1.8.3   Clinical Presentation and Evaluation   49
1.8.4   Therapy   50
1.8.5   Operative Techniques   51

1.9   Obstructive Uropathy   51
1.9.1   Pathophysiology   51
1.9.2   Clinical Presentation   52
1.9.3   Clinical Evaluation   52
1.9.4   Clinical Management   53
1.9.5   Ureteropelvic Junction Obstruction   54
1.9.6   Ureterovesical Junction Obstruction   56

1.10   Paediatric Oncology   57
1.10.1   Wilms' Tumour   57
1.10.2   Neuroblastoma   59
1.10.3   Testicular Tumours in Children   61
1.10.4   Rhabdomyosarcoma of the Pelvis   63

         References   64

2   Diagnostic Procedures in Paediatric Uroradiology   69
         A. Leenen

2.1   Introduction   69

2.2   Ultrasonography   69
2.2.1   Grey-scale US   69
2.2.2   Doppler US   74
2.2.3   Contrast-enhanced Voiding US   75

2.3   Voiding Cysto-urethrography   76
2.3.1   Technique   76
2.3.2   Clinical Applications   77

2.4   Intravenous Urography   78
2.4.1   Technique   78
2.4.2   Clinical Applications   78

2.5   Computed Tomography   79
2.5.1   Technique   79
2.5.2   Clinical Applications   80

2.6   Magnetic Resonance Imaging   81
2.6.1   Technique   81
2.6.2   Clinical Applications   82

2.7   Conclusions   82

         References   83

3　　**Nuclear Medicine Imaging and Therapy
in Paediatric Urology** 89
J. Meller and W. Becker

3.1　　Radiopharmaceuticals for Dynamic Renal Scintigraphy . . . 89
3.1.1　Iodine-123 o-Iodohippurate 89
3.1.2　Technetium-99m-diethylene Triamine Pentaacetic Acid . . . 89
3.1.3　Technetium-99m-mercaptoacetyltriglycine 90

3.2　　Radiopharmaceuticals for Static Renal Scintigraphy 90
3.2.1　Technetium 99m-dimercaptosuccinic Acid 90
3.2.2　Technetium 99m-glucoheptonate 91

3.3　　Dose Schedules and Radiation Burden 91

3.4　　Renal Imaging 91
3.4.1　Planar Scintigraphy 91
3.4.2　Single Photon Emission Computed Tomography 91
3.4.3　Dynamic Renal Scintigraphy 92

3.5　　Renal Clearance 95

3.6　　Diuresis Scintigraphy 96

3.7　　Renal Cortical Scintigraphy 103
3.7.1　^{99m}Tc-DMSA in the Diagnosis of Renal Malformation 103
3.7.2　^{99m}Tc-DMSA in the Diagnosis
of Upper Urinary Tract Infection 104
3.7.3　^{99m}Tc-DMSA in the Diagnosis of Renal Scarring 106
3.7.4　Cortical Scintigraphy: Conclusion 108

3.8　　Radionuclide Cystography 108
3.8.1　Direct Radionuclide Cystography 108
3.8.2　Indirect Radionuclide Cystography 110
3.8.3　Clinical Studies in Reflux 110
3.8.4　Radiation Burden 112

3.9　　Meta-iodobenzylguanidine in Neuroblastoma 112
3.9.1　Pharmacology 112
3.9.2　Scintigraphy with ^{131}I-Meta-iodobenzylguanidine 113
3.9.3　Scintigraphy with ^{123}I-Meta-iodobenzylguanidine 113
3.9.4　The ^{123}I-MIBG Scan in Neuroblastoma 113
3.9.5　^{131}I-MIBG Therapy in Neuroblastoma 115
3.9.6　Radiation Burden of MIBG Scintigraphy and Therapy . . . 116

　　　References 116

4　　**Case Reports** 123
H. Zappel and J. Meller

　　　Introduction 123

Case 1:　Bilateral Renal Hypoplasia 124
Case 2:　Unilateral Renal Agenesis Combined with VUR
on the Contralateral Side 126
Case 3:　Pancake Kidney 129
Case 4:　Unilateral Renal Dysplasia
with Contralateral Subpelvic Obstruction 130
Case 5:　Horseshoe Kidney and Symptomatic Urinary Tract Infections　134

Case 6: Horseshoe Kidney with a Megaureter on the Right Side . . . 136
Case 7: Upper Urinary Tract Infection Combined
with Reversible Renal Lesions Seen on ^{99m}Tc-DMSA Scan
and Ectopic Position of One Kidney 140
Case 8: Renal Damage Following Multifocal Pyelonephritis 143
Case 9: Subpelvic Obstruction During Early Childhood 147
Case 10: Recurrent Renal Colics Caused
by an Extrinsic Subpelvic Stenosis 152
Case 11: Dilatation of the Renal Pelvis Without Obstruction 156
Case 12: Prenatally Diagnosed Unilateral Dilation of the Renal Pelvis 159
Case 13: Intermittent Colics with Macrohaematuria
Due to Extrinsic Subpelvic Stenosis 163
Case 14: Prune Belly Syndrome (Unilateral Manifestation) 167
Case 15: Obstructive Megaureter 171
Case 16: Congenital Bilateral Megaureter 176
Case 17: Incontinence Caused by an Ectopic Ureter 181
Case 18: Bilateral Single Ectopic Ureter 183
Case 19: Duplex System with Ectopic and Obstructive Megaureter . . 187
Case 20: Renal Duplication with Dysplastic Upper Pole
and Ureterocele 190
Case 21: Bilateral Renal Duplication and VUR 194
Case 22: Duplex-System with Dysplastic-Lower Pole
and Reflux Nephropathy 196
Case 23: Dysplastic Kidney with Severe VUR 200
Case 24: Reflux Nephropathy After Two Episodes
of Pyelonephritis Caused by Secondary Reflux
and a Meatal Stenosis 202
Case 25: High-grade Bilateral VUR and Reflux Nephropathy 206
Case 26: Functional Disturbance of Micturition
with Secondary Bilateral VUR 209
Case 27: Left-sided Dysplastic Multicystic Kidney
and Testicular Dysplasia Combined
with Contralateral High-grade VUR 212
Case 28: Polycystic Kidney (Autosomal Dominant Type) 214
Case 29: Tuberous Sclerosis – Cystic Renal Disease 216
Case 30: Urethral Valve – Severe Secondary Reflux 217
Case 31: Terminal Renal Insufficiency Due to Obstructive Uropathy
Caused by a Urethral Valve: Renal Transplantation
at $2^{1}/_{2}$ Years of Age 221
Case 32: Bladder Exstrophy and Uretero-enterostomy
(Mainz Pouch I) 223
Case 33: Neonatal Renal Vein Thrombosis 228
Case 34: Nephrolithiasis, Cystinuria 231
Case 35: Hereditary Nephrolithiasis
Due to Hyperresorptive Hypercalciuria 235
Case 36: Renal Bruise on the Right Side 237
Case 37: Wilms' Tumour – Aniridia Syndrome with Deletion of 11p12 239
Case 38: Neuroblastoma 241

Subject Index 245

Clinical Aspects of Paediatric Urology

F. Seseke

1.1
Embryology

An understanding of the normal embryological development of the human genitourinary tract eases recognition, evaluation and treatment of the majority of specifically congenital urological diseases in paediatric patients. The earlier the disturbance of the normal development takes place the more complex is the extent of the disease, contributing to rather heavier demands on the paediatric urologist. However, the exact aetiology of most congenital diseases is still unclear. This section is intended to give a short overview of the normal embryological development of the genitourinary tract and serve as a basis for better understanding of the urological diseases described later in the chapter. The pathoembryology of each disorder is described within the section devoted to that disorder.

1.1.1
Development of the Kidney

The development of the human kidney starts in the 4th week of gestation, when the pronephros appears adjacent to the primitive somites between segments 2 and 6. The mesodermal cells differentiate into tubular structures connected by a primitive duct extending caudally and forming the later mesonephric or "wolffian" duct. The pronephros disappears completely after a short time. The tubules have no secretory function.

At the end of the 4th week the mesonephric duct, after further caudal elongation, connects with the primitive cloaca. In the meantime, the contact of the duct with the surrounding intermediate mesoderm has initiated the development of new tubular structures differentiating to primitive nephrons (mesonephroi) to create the mesonephros (Fig. 1a). At the time of connecting with the cloaca about 40 pairs of mesonephroi are apparent and already show a secretory function. After 10 weeks of gestation the caudal

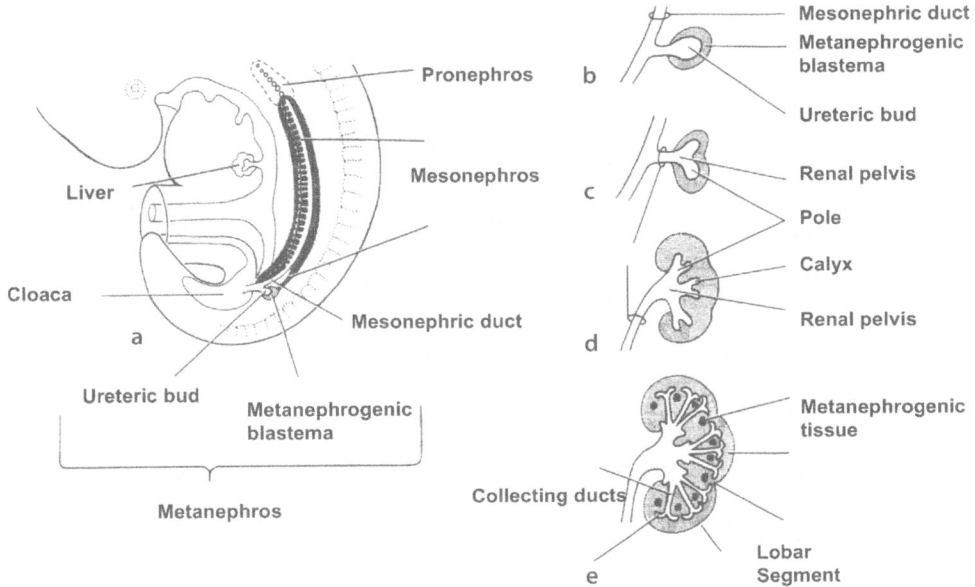

Fig. 1. **a** Five-week-old embryo. Pronephros and mesonephros. **b**–**e** Development of the metanephros. Appearance of the ureteric bud, dichotomous branching and determination of the renal pelvis, calyces and collecting ducts. (From [97])

tubules of the mesonephros degenerate and the cranial tubules are incorporated into the primitive gonadal anlage.

As the mesonephric duct comes in contact with the cloaca a diverticulum appears at the posteromedial aspect of the cloaca, the ureteric bud. The bud bulges into the metanephrogenic blastema. The interaction of the ureteric bud and the metanephrogenic blastema causes development of the human kidney (metanephros) during the 5th to 36th weeks of gestation.

The ureteric bud starts dichotomous branching. The first branching defines the two poles of the later kidney, while the subsequent branchings create the renal pelvis and the calyces (Fig. 1b–d). Branching occurs faster at the periphery of the kidney than at its centre, contributing to the characteristic shape of the organ.

Subsequent generations of branches define the collecting ducts (Fig. 1e). After the 7th week of gestation the first nephrons develop by way of tight connections of the branches of the ureteric bud to the metanephrogenic blastema. First a vesicle appear in the metanephrogenic blastema, which is covered by a primitive epithelium that has differentiated from mesenchymal cells. The vesicle elongates and coils, and connects to the collecting ducts. Simultaneously, the vascularization of the nephrons develops by successive enclosure of the nephric vesicle by mesenchymal cells, which later differentiate to endothelial cells.

The next phase of nephrogenesis is characterized by asymmetrical branching of the ureteric bud. About eight nephrons develop from each branch of the ureteric bud, contributing to increased centrifugal extension of the organ. This results in the typical appearance of the kidney, with the medullary position

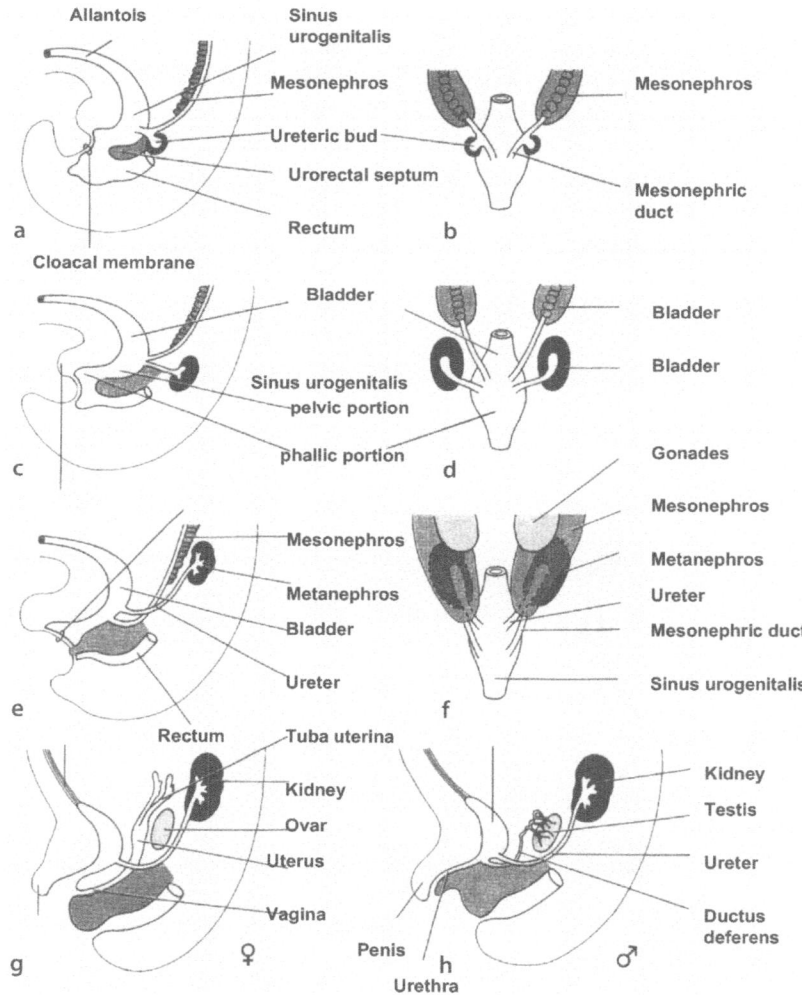

Fig. 2a–h. Fifth to twelfth weeks of gestation. Separation of the cloaca by the urorectal septum into sinus urogenitalis and rectum. Degeneration of the mesonephros. Development of the kidney and renal ascent. Development of the bladder and proximal urethra. Topographical change of ureter and mesonephric duct. **a, c, e, g, h** Lateral views. **b, d, f** Dorsal views. (From [97])

of the collecting ducts and the cortical location of the nephron structures. At the 36th week of gestation the branching of the ureteric bud stops spontaneously, followed only by modification of the spatial arrangement of the nephron structures. With this, the morphological development of the kidney is complete.

The primary position of the developing metanephros is near the upper sacral somites. The final position near the upper lumbar vertebrae results from an accumulation of different mechanisms subsumed under the term "ascensus renalis". As the kidney is fixed in the retroperitoneal cavity, the caudal longitudinal growth of the fetus leads to a passive ascent of the kidney supported by the active longitudinal growth of the ureter. Simultaneous rotation around a longitudinal axis causes the final arrangement of the kidney, with the medially positioned renal pelvis and the laterally positioned calyces (Fig. 2 a – h).

1.1.2
Development of the Ureter

After the induction of the ureteric bud the primitive ureter develops, initially as a patent tube. The connection to the sinus urogenitalis is closed by Chwalla's membrane. The lumen of the primitive ureter is filled with secretion from the mesonephros. The increase in hydrostatic pressure in the ureter leads to the rupture of this membrane.

The ensuing period is characterized by near-complete obliteration of the ureteral lumen, most probably caused by the rapid longitudinal growth of the ureter. The subsequent recanalization of the lumen starts in the middle of the organ and migrates to the pyeloureteral and ureterovesical junctions. This explains, in part, the predisposition of these areas to congenital stenosis. Then, after complete recanalization at the 9th week of gestation, the first urine drained from the metanephros initiates the development of the ureteral musculature.

The longitudinal growth of the ureter is faster than that of the fetus overall, contributing to a interim kinking of the ureter with the consequent appearance of ureteral folds. Only after birth does the relation of the growing speeds change so that the ureter is stretched.

1.1.3
Development of the Bladder

At the end of the 4th week the mesonephric duct connects with the primitive cloaca, which is simultaneously divided by the urorectal septum into the rectum and the sinus urogenitalis (Fig. 2 a – d). The later bladder develops from the part of the sinus urogenitalis that is cranial to the point of insertion. The mesonephric duct, after initiating the ureteric bud, migrates distally, whereas the surrounding mesenchyme migrates from its lateral position into the sinus urogenitalis towards the midline and fuses, forming the primitive trigone.

In the meantime, the mesonephric duct has separated from the primitive ureter, moved caudally and rotated ventrally, connecting with the paramesonephric duct (müllerian duct) to form the later verumontanum (colliculus seminalis).

At the 10th week of gestation the primitive bladder is a tube surrounded by connecting tissue connecting cranially to the vesicoallantoic canal, the later urachus. After a further 3 weeks muscular fibres are differentiated from the surrounding mesenchyme, forming three layers on the bladder surface. One layer with longitudinally aligned fibres lies between two layers of fibres with circular alignment. The development of musculature concerns mainly the region of the trigone. The subsequent restriction of the lumen in this area initiates the development of the bladder neck and the later continence mechanism by successively surrounding the urethral part of the sinus urogenitalis with muscular fibres. Around the 16th week of gestation, which is about 5 weeks before completion of the muscularization of the bladder trigone, the primitive bladder is continent. The extent of muscularization depends on the mechanical distension of the bladder wall and thus on the bladder capacity. The interaction of regular filling and emptying of the primitive bladder contributes to its normal development.

A further condition for undisturbed development of the bladder is normal development of the caudal abdominal wall, which is brought about by migration of the mesenchyme structures to the midline cranial to the cloacal membrane.

1.1.4
Development of the Sinus Urogenitalis

After insertion of the mesonephric duct the primitive bladder is separated from the sinus urogenitalis, which develops further into parts of the external genitalia and the urethra. This is sexually indifferent during the first 10 weeks of gestation. Distal to the insertion point of the mesonephric duct the sinus urogenitalis narrows and forms the pelvic urethra. The more distal part expands towards the cloacal membrane and forms the phallic urethra (Fig. 2 a – h).

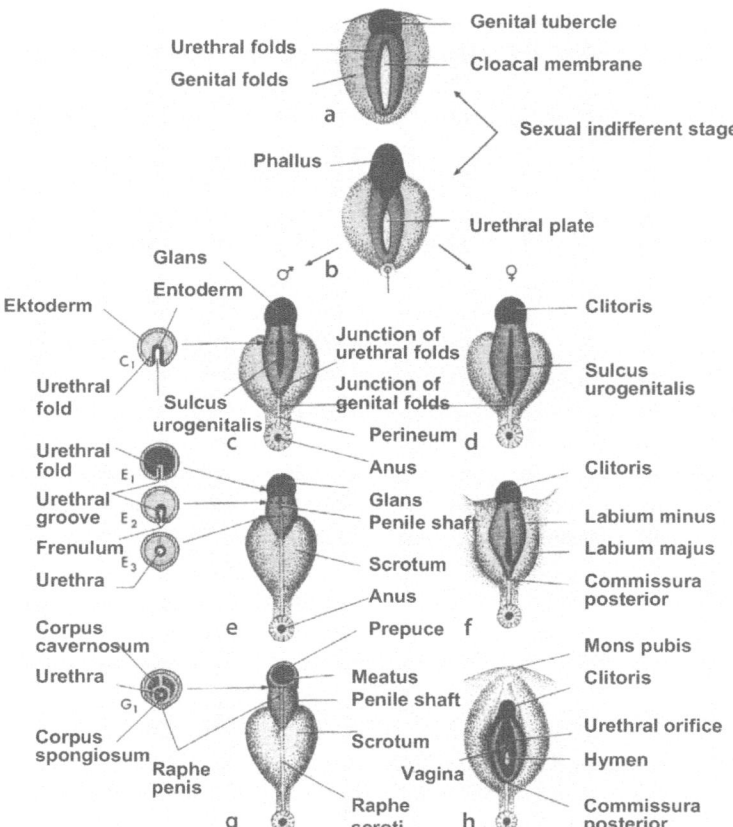

Fig. 3 a–h. Fourth to twelfth weeks of gestation. Development of the external genitalia in dependence on the sexual differentiation. **a, b** Sexually indifferent stage. **c, e, g** Seventh to twelfth weeks of gestation: development of the male extern genitalia. **e** Cross sections of the penis. **d, f, h** Seventh to twelfth weeks: development of the female external genitalia. (From [98])

Along the lateral margins of the phallic portion of the sinus urogenitalis the mesenchyme condenses and raises the adjacent ectoderm, forming the urethral groove. After the disintegration of the urogenital membrane the endoderm of the sinus urogenitalis migrates towards the urethral groove to create the urethral plate. Further mesenchymal growth along the margins of the urethral plate creates the urethral folds (Fig. 3 a). The further development of the sinus urogenitalis is dependent on the sexual differentiation.

1.1.5
Development of the Genital Ducts

The genital ducts arise between the 5th and 6th weeks of gestation. Until the 10th week their development, like that of the sinus urogenitalis, proceeds in a sexually indifferent mode. From the 6th week onward the müllerian duct descends at the dorsolateral side of the mesonephric duct to the cloaca. The distal part fuses with the contralateral duct, forming the utero-

vaginal primordium, which connects with the dorsal wall of the sinus urogenitalis forming the müllerian tubercle mediocranial to the inserting mesonephric ducts. Between the 4th and 8th weeks of gestation the cranial parts of the mesonephros degenerate and the caudal parts fuse with the indifferent primitive gonadal anlage, where the appearance of endocrine active cells induces further development of the genitalia dependent on the sexual differentiation of the embryo.

1.1.6
Development of the Male Genitalia

The ectodermal portion of the genital tubercle proliferates. The elongation results in the appearance of the primitive phallus. Distal to the tip of the genital tubercle an oblique groove appears, separating the glans from the later penile shaft (Fig. 3 c). Along the shaft condensed mesenchymes form the corpora cavernosa. At the end of the 12th week the primitive penis is complete (Fig. 3 e, g). At the ventral side of the glans a groove appears, defining the later fossa navicularis. Then, especially at the dorsal side of the penis, the skin grows over the glans, finally fusing on the ventral side and forming the prepuce. The point of the midline fusion represents the later frenulum.

Simultaneously with the development of the penis the bulbar and penile urethra is created. First the lateral margins of the urethral groove fuse in the midline, forming a tube. The fusion begins proximally, extending towards the fossa navicularis. After reaching the fossa the development of the glandular urethral part is induced. For this the lateral margins of the ventral glandular groove fuse in the midline, bringing the urethral meatus to the tip of the glans.

The distal portion of the sinus urogenitalis forms the prostatic and membranous urethra. From the 8th week of gestation onward, fibroblasts differentiate from the mesenchymal cells surrounding the pelvic urethra. At the 10th week the fibroblasts migrate towards the sinus urogenitalis and separate into five groups. By the 12th week these cells have formed tubular structures defining the primitive lobes of the prostate gland.

Group 1 is located dorsally between the bladder and the orifices of the ejaculatory ducts and determines the middle lobe. Group 2 and 3 originate from the lateral urethral wall and determine the later lateral lobes of the prostate. Group 4 cells migrate from distal to the ejaculatory ducts in a dorsal direction to behind the lateral lobes, from which they are separated by a thin membrane, and determine the prostate capsule. Group 5 cells originate on the ventral side of the prostatic urethra, forming an anterior prostatic lobe that degenerates completely after the 21st week of gestation. Its function is not known.

In the 12th week of gestation the Cowper's glands (glandulae bulbourethrales) develop from the sinus urogenitalis at the region of the membranous urethra as an endothelial evagination. They are lined by epithelial cells by the 18th week.

Between the distal and the membranous parts of the prostatic urethra, muscle fibres with a circular orientation proliferate. In addition, muscle fibres from the anterior wall of the rectum migrate ventrally. Together they create the external sphincter mechanism of the pelvic floor.

The primitive testicle develops from the gonadal anlage under the influence of increased androgen levels. At the 12th week of gestation the testicular tubules fuse the tubules of the distal part of the mesonephros and form the rete testis and the vas efferens. In this way, the mesonephric duct becomes the primitive vas deferens. The cranial portion of the mesonephric duct coils, creating the epididymis. The caudal part elongates towards the sinus urogenitalis and separates into the primitive seminal vesicle and the ejaculatory duct. The remaining parts of the mesonephric duct degenerate.

The testicle descends to its final position in the scrotum in three different phases. The first phase is characterized by a passive approach towards the internal inguinal ring effected by the longitudinal growth of the fetus. The second phase is represented by an increase in the volume of the gubernaculum testis, a jelly-like substance at the caudal testicular pole. The gubernaculum actively pulls the testicle through the inguinal canal. The exact mechanism is unclear. The testicle is accompanied by a ventrally positioned evagination of the peritoneum, the processus vaginalis peritonei. In the third phase, the gubernaculum shrinks, thereby pulling the testicle to its final position in the scrotum. Normal testicular descent is completed around the 32nd week of gestation.

Simultaneously with the testicular development, beginning at the 8th week the first Sertoli cells produce a substance leading to degeneration of the müllerian duct. The cranial parts of the müllerian duct may persist, facultatively, as a testicular appendix. After 16 weeks the caudal müllerian duct has degenerated to the level of the ejaculatory duct. The uterovaginal primordium becomes the verumontanum, with the utriculus prostaticus in the distal part of the prostatic urethra.

1.1.7
Development of the Female Genitalia

The pelvic part of the sinus urogenitalis of a female fetus develops into the distal portion of the urethra and the distal vagina (Fig. 2g). At the 11th week of gestation, in a manner reminiscent of male prostatic development, tubular structures develop from the mesenchyme surrounding the distal sinus urogenitalis, connecting the primitive distal urethra and forming Skene's glands (glandulae paraurethrales). The absence of androgens or deficiency of sensitivity to the hormone lead to feminization of the external genitalia. The primitive phallus coils ventrally and becomes the clitoris (Fig. 3d). Furthermore, the lateral margins of the urethral groove stay unfused. The phallic region of the sinus urogenitalis becomes the vaginal vestibulum (Fig. 3h). Caudal to the genital tubercle an evagination of the sinus urogenitalis induces the development of Bartholinis glands, the female analogue of Cowper's glands in males.

The genital folds fuse dorsally and form the posterior commissura of the later introitus. The genital folds form the labia majora, while the labia minora develop from the unfused urethral folds (Fig. 3 f, h).

In the absence of androgens, the uterus, the fallopian tubes and the cranial part of the vagina develop from the müllerian ducts. The distal portions of the müllerian ducts fuse and form the müllerian vagina and the uterus, while the cranial parts stay unfused and become the fallopian tubes. The müllerian vagina contacts with the urogenital sinus, forming the müllerian tubercle. In the meantime, the tubular mesonephric ducts have degenerated to connecting tissue running at the lateral margins of uterus and vagina, the Gartner's ducts. The epithelium of the sinus urogenitalis condenses around the müllerian tubercle, fuses the müllerian vagina, and form the solid vaginal plate. Whilst the plate extends cranially, it becomes recanalized from distal. After the 24th week of gestation the sinus vaginae and the müllerian vagina form a connecting tube separated from the vaginal vestibulum distally by the hymen, a thin membrane which ruptures in the course of further development.

In the absence of androgens the indifferent gonadal anlage develops into the ovary.

1.2
Anomalies of the Upper Urinary Tract

1.2.1
Renal Dysgenesis

Maldevelopment of the kidney that affects its size, structure or shape is called renal dysgenesis. Very early impairment results in complete agenesis of the kidney, while later developmental damage causes the three different principal types of dysgenesis: dysplasia, hypoplasia and cystic disease. Renal dysplasia is always associated with hypoplasia of the organ, whereas renal hypoplasia can occur in isolation. In the sections below the different forms of renal dysgenesis are clearly defined; it is associated with many nephro-urological diseases in childhood.

1.2.1.1
Renal Agenesis

Absent kidney development leads to renal agenesis. This may be due to impairment of the mesonephric duct, the ureteric bud or the metanephrogenic blastema. Bilateral agenesis of the kidney is a lethal malformation, because of consecutive pulmonary hypoplasia resulting from oligohydramnios [113]. It occurs in 1 of 4000 births and there is a male pre-

dominance. In many cases bilateral agenesis is associated with other congenital anomalies, not all of the urogenital tract.

Unilateral renal agenesis is more common. It occurs in 0.1–0.5% of births [7]. Because of the normally matured contralateral kidney, the prognosis in terms of renal function and pulmonary development is good. If the agenesis is caused by a defect of the mesonephric duct, the neighbouring müllerian duct may also be affected. Therefore, unilateral renal agenesis can be associated with anomalies or agenesis of the internal female genitalia as well as the unilateral testicle, vas deferens or epididymidis in males (Chap. 4, Case 2).

1.2.1.2
Renal Dysplasia

'Renal dysplasia' is a histological and not a clinical diagnosis, even though some radiographic dysmorphisms are diagnosed as dysplastic kidneys. The dysplasia can affect the whole kidney or only parts of the organ. There are various alterations in size, from normal to small, and different degrees of organ deformation. Cysts are not mandatory for this diagnosis but may be present, when they cause cystic dysplasia. When there is a preponderance of cystic areas this condition is referred to as polycystic dysplastic kidney. When a kidney is nonfunctioning because of dysplastic alterations this is called renal aplasia. Renal dysplasia may be accompanied by several anomalies of the collecting system.

The aetiology of renal dysplasia is not clear. Mackie and Stephens, in their "bud theory", suggest a correlation between ectopia of the ureteral orifice and the development of renal dysplasia. This is supported by the observation that in duplex systems the part of the kidney that inserts into the bladder in an ectopic location more often shows dysplastic alterations. One possible explanation is inappropriate penetration into the metanephrogenic blastema because of the ectopic insertion of the ureteric bud [86].

Furthermore, renal obstruction seems to have a major influence on the development of renal dysplasia [10]. However, there is evidence to show that impaired interaction between epithelial and mesenchymal structures during nephrogenesis results in renal dysplasia with or without the presence of renal obstruction [137]. As obstruction could only affect draining kidneys, the development of multicystic dysplasia must begin before urine formation. In these cases Potter suggests teratogenic effects [114].

There are few histological findings that seem to confirm renal dysplasia. These are alterations that could only be caused by aberrant embryonic organ development. The suggestion was put forward earlier that the presence of primitive ducts and cartilage in the kidney was an unequivocal sign of dysplasia [40]. This definition has meanwhile been revised, because in addition to kidneys affected by chronic inflammation normally matured kidneys can also show small areas of cartilage.

Dysplastic kidneys are frequently smaller than normal organs and are therefore also called hypodysplastic kidneys or renal hypodysplasia. This condition must be clearly differentiated from renal hypoplasia.

1.2.1.3
Renal Hypoplasia

In contrast to renal (hypo)dysplasia, renal 'hypoplasia' means a kidney with fewer nephrons and calyces than normal, resulting in a generally smaller organ. Furthermore, the decreased number of nephrons leads to impaired renal function. The exact incidence of the anomaly is unknown, as many patients remain asymptomatic. The clinical relevance of renal hypoplasia depends on the degree of renal insufficiency, which is dependent on the shape of the contralateral organ. Bilateral renal hypoplasia, or hypoplasia combined with unilateral agenesis, results in oligohydramnios with impaired pulmonary maturity or in early end-stage renal insufficiency in childhood. In addition, renal hypoplasia can be associated with vesico-ureteral reflux with consequent urinary tract infections. Hypertension can be caused by renal hypoplasia.

Hypoplastic kidney can only be suspected on clinical evaluation. The diagnosis cannot be confirmed except by histomorphological investigation. Ultrasound shows a small kidney. Intravenous pyelography might show a small kidney and collecting system, but might also fail to detect the kidney at all if the renal function is too poor for contrast medium to be excreted. Alternatively, MRI urography or retrograde pyelography could be used to image the ureter, which generally has a normal calibre, and the hypoplastic collecting system. The differential diagnosis is atrophy of a prior normal kidney caused by chronic pyelo- or glomerulonephritis.

Special forms of renal hypoplasia are oligomeganephronia and Ask-Upmark kidney. The latter is a small kidney with at least one typical furrow on the lateral convexity of the organ, resulting from a hypoplastic segment of the kidney. The anomaly is not congenital but rather derives from chronic vesico-ureteral reflux, so that it is classified as a special form of reflux nephropathy [129].

The majority of patients present with recurrent urinary tract infection (UTI) or hypertension. In cases of bilateral involvement different degrees of renal insufficiency may be present. The treatment of choice is nephrectomy to control hypertension, as correcting the reflux in isolation may prevent further renal damage but does not influence the hypertension.

'Oligomeganephronia' means a small kidney with nephrons that are reduced in number hypertrophic [119]. The anomaly is bilateral in most cases and affects boys three times as frequently as girls. It is commonly associated with multiple other malformations of the skeletal, ocular and auditory systems.

The clinical relevance depends on the degree of renal insufficiency. The hypertrophic nephrons have only an impaired capability for urinary concentration, resulting in dehydration and loss of electrolytes and protein as the first clinical symptoms in the majority of patients. Even if adequate therapy means that the renal function stays stable at a lower level for a long time, the majority of patients end up needing dialysis or a renal transplant (Chap. 4, Case 1).

1.2.1.4
Multicystic Renal Dysplasia

Multicystic dysplastic kidney is the most severe form of renal dysplasia. The affected organ lacks normally functioning parenchymatous structures and a calyceal collecting system. In some cases the renal pelvis is present. The organ consists of a high number of cysts adjacent to a fibrous stroma. The multicystic kidneys can reach excessive sizes and occupy almost the whole of the abdomen.

The aetiology of multicystic renal dysplasia is still unclear. Two principal theories have been suggested. Felson and Cussen argue that very early extreme obstruction in fetal development of the kidney results in multicystic dysplasia [42]. However, many attempts to reproduce multicystic renal dysplasia in animal models have failed. Early obstruction did produce renal dysplasia, but not multicystic dysplasia. This supports the explanations proposed by other authors, who suggest an impaired connection of the ureteric bud with the metanephrogenic blastema, resulting in multicystic dysplasia. Nevertheless, the frequent association of multicystic dysplasia with atresia of the ureter supports both obstruction and disconnection of the ureteric bud from the metanephric blastema as explanations.

Bilateral multicystic dysplasia, the association of multicystic renal dysplasia and contralateral renal agenesis, is not compatible with survival, because of the severe pulmonary immaturity resulting from oligohydramnios. Other patients, if the condition has not been detected by antenatal ultrasound, present with an abdominal mass, abdominal pain or flank pain. Furthermore, multicystic dysplasia is frequently associated with contralateral vesico-ureteral reflux or ureteral obstruction with its specific symptoms. Older children may present with hypertension.

The majority of patients with multicystic renal dysplasia are now detected by antenatal or neonatal ultrasound. The sonomorphological differentiation between severe hydronephrosis and multicystic disease may be particularly problematic. Usually, hydronephrosis shows a more systematic arrangement of the liquid structures in the kidney, and areas of parenchyma may be observed. However, in these cases a CT scan or MRI urography, probably with a 3D reconstruction of the upper urinary tract, may be helpful to allow better differentiation. Intravenous pyelography fails to visualize a multicystic dysplastic kidney. A ^{99m}Tc-DMSA scan could also help to discriminate between the two anomalies, because even a severely hydronephrotic kidney generally has some residual renal function that is detectable by radionuclear renography. Voiding cysto-urethrography is recommended if multicystic dysplasia is suspected, because of the high incidence of contralateral reflux (Chap. 4, Case 27).

There is still controversy about whether or not nephrectomy of the multicystic dysplastic kidneys is necessary. Its advocates argue that there is a possible risk of malignancy or hypertension in patients who still have kidneys. Nevertheless, neither a higher risk of malignancy nor a higher risk of hypertension has yet been confirmed. Therefore, removal of the multicystic kidney is not advisable as a routine measure. A different attitude is needed in cases with progressive enlargement of the affected kidney or symptoms arising from the enlarged organ itself. Furthermore, the therapeutic concept of multicystic dysplasia has to concentrate on effective treatment of likely contralateral anomalies, such as reflux or renal obstruction. It is recommended that asymptomatic multicystic dysplastic kidneys be followed up by regular sonography. Some of these kidneys may shrink in size or completely involute as a result of progressive resorption of the fluid from the cysts.

1.2.2
Cystic Disease of the Kidney

The kidney is frequently affected by cystic disease, which can be congenital, sporadic or acquired. There are heritable and nonheritable cystic lesions of the kidney. However, even though they can be rather similar in their histopathological form of presentation despite their different pathogenesis, their clinical implications and outcome vary considerably, and they range from asymptomatic to lethal. The terms 'polycystic' and 'multicystic', while both meaning the presence of many cysts, define completely different entities of cystic disease. Multicystic kidney is a specific form of renal dysplasia and is described elsewhere, whereas polycystic disease is a heritable form of renal cystic disease. Furthermore, there are several multiple malformation syndromes associated with renal cysts. In particular, Bourneville-Pringle syndrome and von Hippel-Lindau syndrome are common in paediatric urology.

1.2.2.1
Infantile Polycystic Kidney Disease

Infantile polycystic kidney disease is a genetically determined renal malformation with an autosomal recessive pattern of inheritance. The time of its first appearance varies between the neonatal period and early adolescence, with the frequency decreasing with increasing age. Earlier clinical manifestation is associated with a poorer prognosis of the patient. The malformation affects both kidneys and is combined with progressive hepatic fibrosis with consequent portal hypertension. The incidence of infantile polycystic disease is unclear to say the least, but is estimated at between 1:40000 and 1:5000 [13]. About 50% of the affected patients die within their first days of life, and only half the survivors reach their 10th birthday [61].

The usually enormously enlarged kidneys show multiple morphologically subcapsular cysts deriving from dilated collecting ducts with otherwise normal nephron architecture. The cyst can increase in size with age. The renal collecting system is displaced, but the renal pelvis and the ureter appear to be normal.

The children usually present with huge masses in both flank areas. Neonates have pulmonary distress because of severe pulmonary hypoplasia resulting from oligohydramnios and show progressive uraemia after cessation of the placental dialysis. Older children more commonly show symptoms of liver involvement, such as portal hypertension with hepatosplenomegaly, but can also present with vascular hypertension.

The majority of patients with infantile polycystic kidney disease are diagnosed by antenatal ultrasound investigation. The kidneys seem to be enlarged and are homogeneously hyperechogenic. Different degrees of oligohydramnios may be present. Huge cysts are rare in newborns, but their incidence increases with age.

The treatment concentrates on acute treatment of the pulmonary distress and, for those who survive the first months, management of end-stage renal failure, hypertension and the consequences of hepatic fibrosis.

1.2.2.2
Adult Polycystic Kidney Disease

Adult polycystic kidney disease is a renal malformation with an autosomal dominant mode of inheritance, which usually leads to end-stage renal failure after the fourth decade of life. The kidneys show multiple cysts that vary extremely in size, which are widely distributed over the whole of the parenchymatous structures. The cysts are surrounded by a partly hyperplastic epithelium with a suggested tendency to malignant degeneration. However, the risk of developing renal cell carcinoma is no higher in patients with adult polycystic disease than in the general population. The collecting system is partly displaced by but not directly involved in the cystic alterations.

Two genes on chromosomes 16 and 4 have been identified as causal in this disease, with a penetrance of 100% [110, 116]. Its incidence is about 1:1000 at least. Although the majority of patients develop symptoms as adults, newborns with symptomatic adult polycystic kidney disease have also been observed. Cystic disease of the liver, spleen, pancreas and lung is commonly associated. Furthermore, cardiovascular anomalies, such as prolapse of the mitral valve and aneurysms of the cerebral arteries, are frequently observed in patients with adult polycystic kidney disease.

The majority of patients present with abdominal or retroperitoneal masses because of their enormously enlarged polycystic kidneys. It is not unusual for a polycystic kidney in an adult to have a weight of several kilograms. Even in newborns renal cystic enlargement is usually present, but only in severe cases does intrauterine renal excretory insufficiency result in oligohydramnios with consequent pulmonary hypoplasia. These patients are usually stillborn or die within their 1st year of life. A marked number of patients with adult polycystic disease are asymptomatic for a long time and attract medical attention later because they have arterial hypertension, gross haematuria or decreasing kidney function. Others present with symptoms caused by subarachnoid haemorrhage due to intracranial aneurysms.

Ultrasound investigations of patients with adult polycystic kidney disease reveal massively enlarged kidneys with multiple cysts of different sizes between sections of parenchyma that have a normal appearance. CT scan or MRI can help to identify cystic involvement of other organs, but ultrasound is usually enough. Involvement of both kidneys combined with cysts of the liver, pancreas or spleen or intracranial aneurysm makes this diagnosis extremely probable. However, only evidence of affected other family members over at least three generations can confirm the diagnosis of adult polycystic kidney disease if a cytogenic investigation is not available (mutations in the *PKD1* and *PKD2* genes cause 85% of cases of this disease).

The treatment of adult polycystic kidney disease concentrates on the management of hypertension and renal insufficiency. Treatment of symptomatic liver cysts may be necessary. Furthermore, if the diagnosis is clear, screening for intracranial aneurysms is recommended, with elective treatment when they are found. Besides these features it may be necessary to remove one or both polycystic kidneys if they are causing pain or displacement is impairing the function of other organs, such as the intestine, or compressing the central vessels. Furthermore, nephrectomy may improve hypertension.

The autosomal pattern of inheritance causes a 50% risk for every child of an affected patient. This means that after the condition is diagnosed in a parent, any children he or she has should by screened, by cytogenic techniques if these are available or at least by ultrasonography. The risk of adult polycystic kidney disease in offspring of an affected person declines with time if ultrasound fails to detect renal cysts before the age of 35 years (Chap. 4, Cases 28 and 29).

1.2.2.3
Simple Renal Cyst

Simple renal cysts are singular or multiple liquid renal lesions completely separated from the normal nephron structures and enclosed by a thin wall consisting of a one-layer cuboidal epithelium. The inner fluid is usually a clear, straw-coloured transudate. Simple renal cysts can be unilateral or bilateral.

McHugh et al. postulate an average incidence of about 1:500 for simple renal cysts in age groups from newborn to adult [91]. The incidence then increases as age advances further.

Simple renal cysts are usually asymptomatic and are frequently diagnosed incidentally. But especially huge cysts could cause an asymptomatic, or also a painful, abdominal mass, particularly if they increase in size. Displacing other renal structures, renal cysts could also cause segmental ischaemia, resulting in potential hypertension, or provoke calyceal or pelvic obstruction. Spontaneous rupture of a simple cyst could cause acute flank pain or haematuria if the cyst opens into the collecting system. Furthermore, rupture into another adjacent cyst may be associated with bleeding into the other cyst, which could later be mistaken for a renal tumour.

Simple renal cysts are easily diagnosed and evaluated by ultrasonography. There are clearly defined criteria characterizing such a cyst in ultrasonography [83]. These cysts have a spherical or slightly oval liquid formation without internal echoes, enclosed by walls giving thin, sharp margins; behind the formation is an acoustic enhancement caused by completely unimpaired sound transmission through the liquid parts of the cyst. If any of these criteria is not satisfied further evaluation of the formation is strongly recommended to investigate the possibility of a cystic neoplasm.

The method of choice in these cases is CT scan after intravenous injection of contrast medium. The CT characteristics of a simple renal cyst are similar to its ultrasound characteristics. Enhancement of contrast medium should be observed neither in its wall nor in the liquid area. If any of these criteria is not satisfied, the cystic lesion is at least classified as a complicated renal cyst, or a neoplasm is suspected. In such cases open surgical exploration and biopsy are usually unavoidable.

Asymptomatic simple renal cysts do not need treatment and can merely be kept under regular observation, e.g. by ultrasonographic investigation. In any that progressively increase in size surgical resection may be indicated. Percutaneous puncture and aspiration of the fluid is possible, but generally not very effective as the cyst commonly fills up again. Other indications for resection of a simple renal cyst are hypertension if no other possible explanation can be found for it, symptomatic calyceal or pelvic obstruction, and displacement of adjacent structures by an asymptomatic or symptomatic abdominal mass. Open surgical techniques and laparoscopic techniques are of equal value if the suspicion of a neoplasm has been ruled out preoperatively. When a malignancy is suspected preoperatively a radical nephrectomy is required. After therapy or without treatment, the prognosis of simple renal cyst is excellent.

1.2.3
Renal Anomalies of Ascent, Fusion and Rotation

1.2.3.1
Renal Ectopia

Renal ectopia consists in the failure of a complete ascent of a otherwise normally matured kidney to the renal fossa. In such patients the kidney is never located in its physiological position. This condition therefore has to be differentiated from renal ptosis, in which the kidney falls from its normal position to a lower one, depending on the body posture.

The general incidence of renal ectopia is 1:500 to 1:1000 as disclosed by autopsies [1]. About 10% of patients affected have bilateral involvement. Single ectopic kidneys are also very rare. There is no constant ratio reflecting a sex- or side-related incidence.

Ectopic kidneys may be located along the path of renal ascent from the pelvis to the renal fossa on the ipsilateral side, but can also cross over to the contralateral side, where fusion with the contralateral organ may take place. A pelvic kidney lies below the aortic bifurcation, while the iliac or lumbar kidney lies near the promontory in front of the iliac vessels. The abdominal kidney is located adjacent to the second lumbar vertebra. These ectopic positions of the kidney are found with approximately the same frequency.

Ectopic kidneys are mostly smaller in size and are malrotated. This means that the renal pelvis lies anterior to the kidney, as against the medial position of normally rotated kidneys. Malrotation could provoke dilatation of the renal collecting system. However, renal ectopia combined with ureteropelvic junction obstruction or vesico-ureteral reflux is not uncommon [48]. The ureteral orifice is generally orthotopically positioned in the bladder neck.

Several other, specifically genital, defects are often associated with renal ectopia. In females anomalies of the uterus or vagina may be present. In males the associated anomalies observed have mostly affected the urethra and testes [144].

The development of renal ectopia is no longer possible after the period of normal renal ascent between the 5th and 9th weeks of embryogenesis. Several theories have been suggested. As ectopic kidneys are frequently associated with other malformations, both genetic and teratogenic causes affecting the ureteric bud and the metanephric blastema have been discussed [89]. Another suggestion is an isolated defect in the metanephric blastema, disturbing normal upward migration of the kidney [149]. Campbell assumes a defect of the ureteric bud [22]. However, a definitive explanation for renal ectopia is still lacking.

An ectopic kidney itself normally does not cause clinical symptoms. It is frequently the evaluation of associated anomalies that leads to the diagnosis of renal ectopia. Common symptoms are recurrent UTI, stone formation causing renal colic or haematuria, abdominal pain and hypertension (Chap. 4, Case 7).

As ultrasonography in newborns has become a routine investigation, asymptomatic ectopic kidneys have been diagnosed more frequently. In symptomatic patients without evidence of a kidney in the normal position, the diagnosis of renal ectopia is made by IV pyelography or MRI urography. In particular, IV pyelography bears a risk of misinterpretation if the collecting system of the ectopic kidney is covered by bony structures of the pelvis. Furthermore, if the function of the ectopic kidney is poor the collecting system will not be seen because of a lack of contrast medium excretion. In these cases malposition of other abdominal organs, such as the colon or bladder, is an indirect sign of an unrecognized mass that can lead to the finding of renal ectopia. In addition, static radionuclear renography using ^{99}Tc-DMSA is a sensitive method of detecting even poorly functioning renal tissue in an ectopic position.

In some cases, especially those with a single ectopic kidney that has to be operated on, precise preoperative imaging of the renal vascular supply by angiography is strongly recommended.

As the majority of ectopic kidneys are asymptomatic, any treatment depends on the particular symptoms. The prognosis of renal ectopia is excellent (Chap. 4, Case 3).

THORACIC RENAL ECTOPIA ▶ About 5% of all patients with renal ectopia present with a thoracic kidney. The exact incidence is unclear. Males are twice as often affected as females. In thoracic ectopia, in contrast to "normal" renal ectopia, the kidney is positioned too high. The organ lies in the posterior mediastinum separated from the retroperitoneum by the diaphragm, but also separated from the pleural space by a thin membrane surrounding the intrathoracic parts of the kidney. The adjacent lower pulmonary lobe may be hypoplastic. The rotation process of the collecting system during renal ascent is generally completed. Bilateral thoracic kidneys have been described [80].

The exact development of the thoracic ectopia is unclear. The question is whether the normal separation of the pleural from the peritoneal space in embryogenesis is delayed, or whether the renal ascent is faster than the development of the diaphragm.

Thoracic kidneys are generally asymptomatic. The majority of symptoms are pulmonary. The diagnosis is mostly made following the incidental findings of a chest X-ray investigation revealing an intrathoracic mass. If renal ectopia is suspected IV pyelography or nuclear renography is recommended. Alternatively, a CT scan with intravenous contrast medium can lead to the diagnosis. Once the diagnosis is made no further therapy is necessary.

1.2.3.2
Crossed Renal Ectopia With or Without Fusion

Ectopic kidneys can also be positioned at the contralateral side of their ureteral insertion point and are mainly fused to their contralateral fellow. This is called crossed ectopia with or without fusion. The incidence of crossed ectopia varies for its different forms. The overall incidence has been estimated at 1:1000 to 1:2000. Crossed ectopia without fusion is very rare. Unilateral ectopia with contralateral renal agenesis and bilateral crossover have both been reported anecdotally. The majority of cases without fusion are of crossed ectopia inferior to the normal contralateral kidney.

The known types of crossed ectopia with fusion are, in declining order of frequency, unilateral inferior fusion, sigmoid or S-shaped kidney, lump kidney, L-shaped kidney, disc kidney and unilateral superior fusion (Fig. 4b: 1–6).

The exact mechanism leading to crossed ectopia of the kidney is unknown. It was suggested that the ureteric bud migrates accidentally to the opposite side and fuses with the contralateral metanephric blastema [112]. Others have supposed that the caudal part of the fetus malrotates, displacing the cloaca and the structures inserting to one side of the vertebral column, allowing the ureteric bud to contact its contralateral metanephric blastema [88].

Crossed renal ectopia may be associated with other anomalies mainly affecting the bones and genital organs. Particularly patients with crossed ectopia of a solitary kidney are affected.

Crossed renal ectopia has more symptomatic significance than the normal renal ectopia. Nevertheless, the majority of patients are asymptomatic. Frequent symptoms are recurrent UTI, stone formation and renal obstruction. As the insertion of the ureter

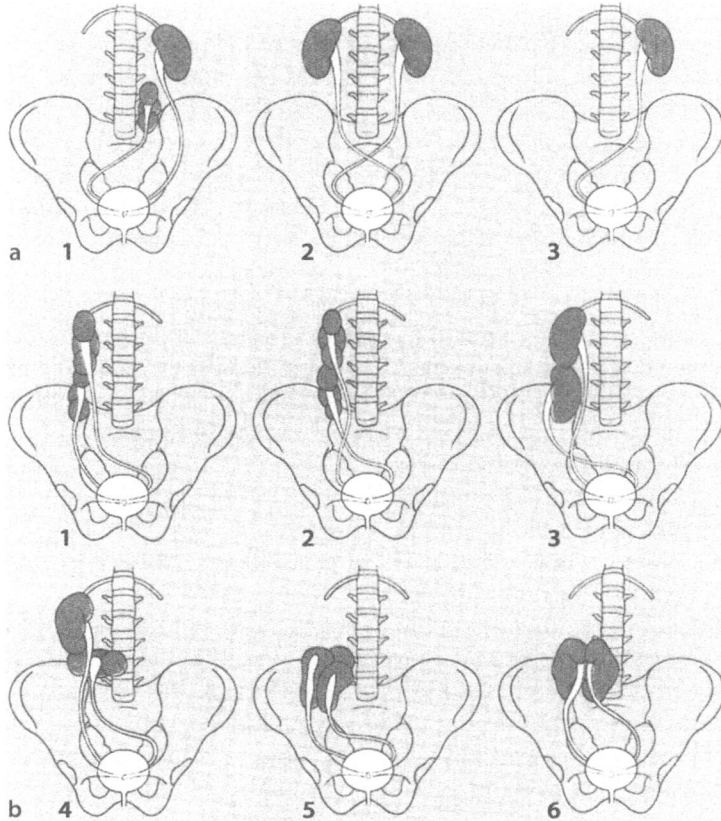

Fig. 4a, b. Variants of crossed renal ectopia. **a** Unfused variants. **b** Fused variants: *1* unilateral superior fusion; *2* unilateral inferior fusion; *3* sigmoid or S-shaped kidney; *4* L-shaped kidney; *5* lump kidney; *6* disc kidney. [130]

in the bladder is generally orthotopic, vesico-ureteral reflux is rather rare in these patients.

The diagnosis is made by ultrasound, IV pyelography, MRI urography, nuclear renography or CT scan. If a surgical approach is planned, precise evaluation of the blood supply of the fused kidneys is strongly recommended.

The treatment depends on the symptoms. Especially in cases with stone formation, the usual treatment strategies with ESWL are less effective because of impaired radiographic exposure of the stone owing to its location in the ectopic kidney. In these patients, therefore, open stone surgery is exceptionally strongly indicated.

1.2.3.3
Horseshoe Kidney

The most common renal fusion anomaly is the so-called horseshoe kidney. This means a fusion of two paravertebrally located vertically aligned kidneys connecting at their lower poles by a parenchymatous or fibrous isthmus (Fig. 5). The renal ascent is in-

complete as the kidney's position is markedly lower than normal. The blood supply to horseshoe kidneys varies, especially that to the isthmus area, which has a separate supply direct from the aorta or the inferior mesenteric artery. The incidence of horseshoe anomaly is 1:400. Males are affected twice as frequently as females. A genetic disposition with low penetrance has been postulated [78]. Patients with Turner's syndrome have a predisposition to horseshoe kidney.

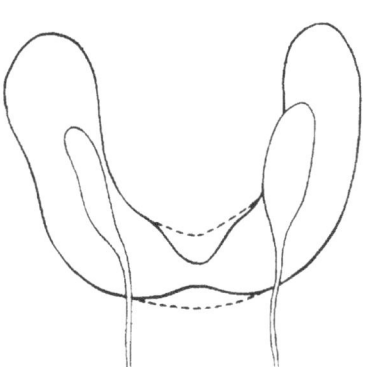

Fig. 5. Schematic of a horseshoe kidney

The exact pattern of the development of horseshoe kidneys is unknown. The initial step is terminated before the beginning of normal rotation of the renal anlage, as in horseshoe kidney the renal pelvis and proximal ureter are anteriorly positioned and the calyces point posteriorly and partly medially. It has been suggested that between the 4th and 6th weeks of gestation a distinct change in the normal course of the early iliac vessels could alter the vertical arrangement of the early kidney to a more oblique position. This brings the lower poles closer to each other and may result in fusion [16]. Others have postulated an accidental migration of metanephric cells to the midline initiating ectopic development of the renal parenchyma. This comes in contact with the lower poles of the early kidneys and may fuse with them [35].

Patients with horseshoe kidneys frequently have other congenital anomalies. Thus, a very high frequency of association with severe congenital malformations, especially of the cardiovascular system, was noted, as in autopsy series children are more commonly found to be affected than adults. However, the survivors also show associated malformation of the uterus or vagina in females, and undescended testis or hypospadias in males. It is worth mentioning the presence of vesico-ureteral reflux in over 50% of the patients, and ureteral obstruction is also not uncommon with horseshoe kidneys. Renal cancer can also develop in horseshoe kidneys. Interestingly, a disproportionate number of tumours arise from the isthmus area, suggesting that teratogenic effects are responsible for its accidental development. Furthermore, the risk of developing nephroblastoma is twice as high in patients with the horseshoe anomaly as in the normal population [95].

Compared with the other fusion anomalies of the kidney, symptomatic disorder is much more frequent. Only 30% of the patients remain asymptomatic. Most of the others present with recurrent urinary tract infection, hydronephrosis or stone formation, which has been observed in up to 80% of affected patients [128].

Antenatal ultrasonography may disclose horseshoe kidneys even before birth, but usually the diagnosis is made after evaluation of often unspecific symptoms. Ultrasonography shows kidneys located in abnormally low positions on both sides. The fibrous isthmus is particularly often overlooked. Other findings, such as hydronephrosis or intrarenal calculi, may be observed. Particularly on IV pyelography, there are very characteristic findings, such as a high-inserting ureter in an anteriorly placed renal pelvis and the posteriorly pointing calyces with caudal and medial orientation of the lower calyx (Chap. 4, Cases 5 and 6).

As a horseshoe kidney itself does not usually cause symptoms, the treatment is concentrated on the associated diseases. Especially in patients with stone disease, the conventional noninvasive therapeutic strategies are less effective, which results in a higher rate of more aggressive approaches, such as open or percutaneous stone surgery in these patients.

1.2.3.4
Malrotation of the Kidney

Malrotation of the kidney is present if the rotation round the longitudinal axis during the normal renal ascent is incomplete. Unimpaired rotation of the kidney leads to ventral insertion of the supplying blood vessels, a dorsal position of the renal pelvis and laterally pointing calyces. The rotation is most probably caused by asymmetrical growth of the renal structures out of the ureteric branches. Normally the ventral parenchymatous development is faster than the dorsal, which results in medial rotation of the renal pelvis. If the ureteric bud inserts into the metanephrogenic blastema too late, the kidney will develop from an atypical segment of it. It has been suggested that this leads to impaired ureteral branching, resulting in malrotation [151].

The degree of renal malrotation varies and is affected by the position of the renal pelvis. In the most common form the renal pelvis has a ventral position with posteriorly pointing calyces. Other forms, with a lateral or dorsal pelvic position, are much rarer.

As the atypical position of the renal pelvis is associated with an atypical blood supply to the kidney, extrinsic obstruction of the ureteropelvic junction obstruction by aberrant vessels is the most frequent symptom of renal malrotation. UTI or stone formation with consequent specific symptoms are also common attendant phenomena. Nevertheless, the majority of malrotated kidneys are asymptomatic.

The diagnosis is frequently made incidentally during the evaluation of hydronephrosis, UTI or haematuria. Ultrasound is usually not capable of detecting renal malrotation. The typical alteration of orientation of the renal pelvis and calyces can be imaged by IV pyelography, MRI urography or retrograde pyelography. The treatment of renal malrotation depends on the particular symptoms; the malrotation itself does not need any therapy.

1.2.4
Anomalies of the Collecting System and Ureter

1.2.4.1
Anomalies of the Calyces and Renal Pelvis

CALYCEAL DIVERTICULUM ▶ Diverticula of the renal calyces are cystic formations surrounded by renal parenchyma. There is a narrow connection between the calyx and the diverticulum. The anomaly most frequently affects the upper calyceal group. Another, generally larger, variant of calyceal diverticula is connected directly to the renal pelvis. The incidence of the anomaly is approximately 1:2000 newborns. The aetiology is not clear. Persistence of an isolated branch from the ureteric bud in the fetal development of the kidney has been suggested [81].

Calyceal diverticula are generally asymptomatic and are frequently incidental findings during routine examinations of the kidney. However, there is a tendency to progressive growth in some cases, which become symptomatic. Increasing or especially acute urinary outflow obstruction from the diverticulum to the calyx may lead to flank pain, stone formation with consequent haematuria or recurrent infections. Progressive obstruction of an infected diverticulum can cause a renal abscess. Interestingly, calyceal diverticula are frequently associated with vesico-ureteral reflux [3]. Furthermore, Timones and co-workers found stone formation in 39% of their observed patients with calyceal diverticula [145].

The anomaly is diagnosed via ultrasound investigation, which shows a cystic formation located more centrally than a normal cortical renal cyst. The ultrasonographic result should be checked by IV pyelography, retrograde pyelography, MRI urography or CT scan.

Asymptomatic calyceal diverticula do not need any therapy. The therapy of the symptomatic anomaly is operative removal of the affected part of the kidney, mostly via partial nephrectomy.

HYDROCALYCOSIS ▶ Hydrocalycosis is a rare cystic dilatation of a complete major calyx owing to functionally relevant obstruction during normal fetal development of the collecting system of the kidney. There is always a small narrow link to the renal pelvis. The anomaly is frequently asymptomatic. A really huge dilatation could cause flank pain and even a palpable abdominal mass. Obstruction of the hydrocalyx fosters UTI.

The diagnosis is made via ultrasound, IV pyelography, retrograde pyelography, CT scan or MRI urography.

Therapy is only necessary in symptomatic cases. In these cases an endoscopic incision of the stenotic area between the dilated calyx and the renal pelvis could relieve the obstruction and result in sufficient drainage of the calyx. Otherwise a partial nephrectomy of the affected region of the kidney is indicated.

MEGACALYCOSIS ▶ Megacalycosis is an anomaly of the collecting system of the kidney, involving dilatation and malformation of the renal calyces, which in addition are frequently increased in number. The renal pelvis is not involved in the anomaly. The renal parenchyma is also unaffected, which indicates the generally normal function of the affected kidneys.

The reasons for the malformation are not understood, or at least not completely. Impaired development of the renal papillae has been suggested. There is a male-to-female ratio of 6:1. The majority of cases are bilateral. As unilateral megacalycosis is observed only in females, an X-chromosome-linked pattern of heredity has been suggested [47].

The majority of patients with megacalycosis are asymptomatic, but the prolonged urinary stasis in the dilated system supports infection and calculus formation with consequent symptoms, such as flank pain and haematuria.

Ultrasound investigation shows the dilated calyces without a dilated renal pelvis and a normal appearance of the renal parenchyma. IV, retrograde or MRI urography demonstrates the calyceal architecture and the number more precisely than ultrasonography alone. Even if the renal pelvis is not dilated more sensitive differentiation from renal obstruction, for example ureteropelvic junction obstruction, by radionuclear diuretic renography is recommended.

Megacalycosis itself generally does not need any therapy, but such secondary effects as infection, increasing secondary renal obstruction or stone formation need the specific treatment.

ANOMALIES OF THE RENAL PELVIS ▶ Anomalies of the renal pelvis are almost always observed as asymptomatic variants of the normal. The most frequent alterations are extrarenalization of the renal pelvis, which may lead an investigator to the mistaken suspicion of renal dilatation or even renal obstruction. The renal pelvis is located completely outside the kidney. The urinary drainage from the pelvis to the upper ureter is unimpaired. No therapy is necessary.

Another common variant of the normal is a bifid renal pelvis. The pelvis divides very early into two major calyces. The anomaly is completely asymptomatic and does not require treatment.

1.2.4.2
Ureteral Duplication

Ureteral duplication is the existence of two separate ureters draining at least one renal but generally two renal collecting systems and inserting into the bladder via one orifice (bifid ureter) or two different orifices (complete ureteral duplication). This has to be differentiated from much rarer cases with two ureters draining two complete separate kidneys on the ipsilateral side (supernumerary kidney) (Fig. 6).

Early branching of the ureteric bud leads to the development of two ureters draining two different renal collecting system, but joining before their insertion into the bladder. If the orifice of this bifid ureter lies in an orthotopic position, pathology of the ipsilateral upper urinary tract is not expected.

If two ureteric buds accidentally derive from the mesonephric duct and contact the metanephrogenic blastema, a complete duplication of the collecting system of one organ develops. Only in cases with a additional division of the metanephrogenic anlage will a supernumerary kidney be created. The probability of pathology of the affected upper urinary tract is dependent on the degree of deviation from a normotopic position of the ureteral orifice. The more ectopically the ureter inserts into the bladder the more pathology of the upper urinary tract is expected.

The incidence of ureteral duplication in autopsy series is 0.7 % [23]. It has been suggested that females are more frequently affected than males, but a reliable sex ratio has not yet been confirmed. The incidence of unilateral ureteral duplication is about sixfold that of bilateral duplication. The frequency of a bifid ureter is equal to that of complete duplication. A combination of ipsilateral bifid ureter and contralateral complete ureteral duplication in the same patient is possible.

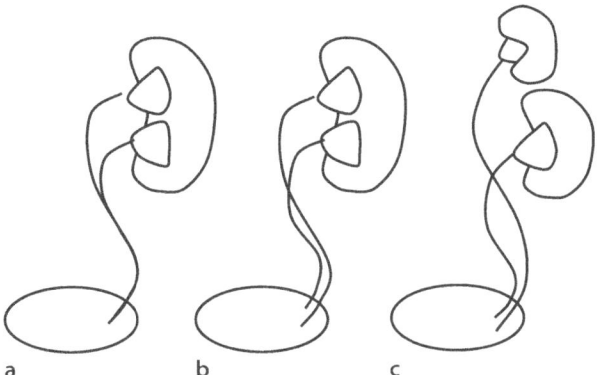

Fig. 6a–c. Variants of renal duplication. **a** Bifid ureter. **b** Complete ureteral duplication. **c** Supernumerary kidney

There is evidence of an autosomal dominant pattern of inheritance, as children of parents with ureteral duplication have about 20-fold the normal risk of having this anomaly [30].

In cases with complete ureteral duplication the positions of the two orifices show a characteristic arrangement described in what is called the Meyer-Weigert law. This means that the ureter draining the upper collecting system inserts in the bladder caudally from the one draining the lower system. Only sporadic cases that deviate from this law have been reported. During normal embryological development of the urinary tract the insertion of the mesonephric duct into the sinus urogenitalis initiate the development of the trigonum of the bladder. The ureter separates from the mesonephric duct, which migrates more caudally. This procedure and the simultaneous progressive dorsal spreading of the trigonum provoke rotation of the primitive bladder neck. In cases with two separate ureters this rotation switches their inserting positions (Fig. 7).

Ureteral duplication itself is an anomaly that does not automatically lead us to expect a disorder of the affected upper urinary tract. Nonetheless there are a lot of pathologic conditions that can be associated with it. The most frequent coexistent disorder is vesico-ureteral reflux, which is strictly correlated with an ectopic position of the orifice of the affected ureter. Deviation to a more lateral and cranial position of the upper orifice is associated with reflux into the lower collecting system (Chap. 4, Case 22). This dislocation of the orifice in patients with a bifid ureter will be followed by reflux into both systems (Chap. 4, Case 21). A more caudal and medial position of the lower orifice may lead to reflux into the upper tract. A combination of both anomalies also results in reflux into both systems, with a correspondingly higher morbidity.

Besides reflux, ureteral duplication can also be associated with renal obstruction or renal dysplasia. The majority of the patients have other anomalies of the distal upper urinary tract, such as ureteroceles or ectopic insertion of the ureter (Chap. 4, Cases 19 and 20). Nevertheless, renal obstruction due to ureteropelvic junction obstruction mainly of the lower collecting system is not uncommon.

The clinical evaluation of ureteral duplication includes ultrasound and fluoroscopic investigations. Ultrasound shows a division of the kidney into two areas separated by a parenchymal margin. Furthermore, hydronephrosis or ureteral dilatation may be detected, but a reliable differentiation between bifid ureter and complete ureteral duplication by ultrasound is nearly impossible. This is one of the remain-

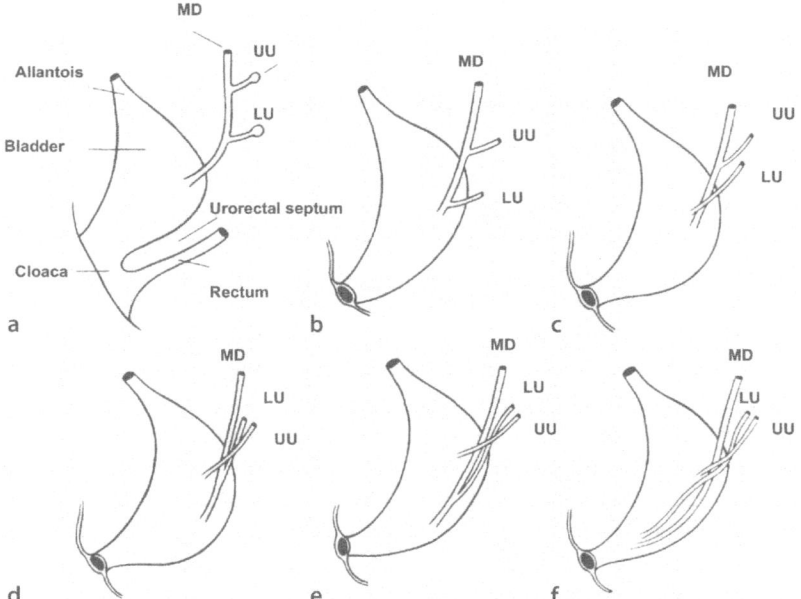

Fig. 7a–f. Fourth to twelfth weeks of gestation. Embryological development of ureteral duplication. Change of topographical relation between the two ureters and the mesonephric duct (*MD*) The ureter draining the upper renal pole (*UU*) crosses the lower one (*LU*) and inserts caudally into the bladder or ectopically (Meyer-Weigert's law). **a** Appearance of two ureteric buds from MD. **b, c** Longitudinal growth of both ureters and separation of the distal ureter from MD, with subsequent rotation of MD to an insertion point lying further dorsal and distal. **d, e** Further distal orientation of the insertion of MD. **f** Separation of the UU from MD, with subsequent distal ectopic insertion into the sinus urogenitalis

ing important possibilities of IV pyelography, which provides detailed information of the morphology of the urinary tract. Nevertheless, direct imaging by IV pyelography is dependent on adequate renal function. That surely is one reason why it will be successively replaced by MRI urography.

Whether or not any treatment is necessary in patients with ureteral duplication depends on the clinical presentation. Asymptomatic patients do not need therapy, whereas the treatment of symptomatic patients must be tailored to its specific causality and is described elsewhere in the sections concerned with the particular diseases concerned.

1.2.4.3
Ectopic Ureter

The term 'ectopic ureter' is used for a false insertion of the ureter more distally or outside the trigonum of the bladder, into structures developing from the prior mesonephric duct. Lateralization or cranialization of the ureteral orifice, although it does mean an ectopic location, is generally not included under this term.

An ectopic ureter is found in 1:2000 births. Females are affected three times as often as males [38]. Bilateral involvement is found in about 15% of cases. In 80% of the patients a duplication of the collecting system is found, with ectopic insertion of the upper pole ureter [23]. The majority of male patients with ectopic ureters have only single systems. The places of insertion of ectopic ureters are, in declining order of frequency, the posterior urethra, utriculus prostaticus, the seminal vesicle or ductus deferens in males and the posterior urethra, introitus vaginae, vagina or internal genitalia in females [38]. Ectopic insertion of the ureter is often associated with other congenital anomalies, such as imperforate anus or oesophageal atresia.

Ectopic ureters are frequently combined with some renal malformation and dysfunction, namely dysplasia. The severity of renal dysplasia is directly linked with the degree of ectopia. The more markedly ectopic the insertion of the ureter is, the more badly impaired will be the normal development of the affected renal unit [123]. Furthermore, the ectopic ureter itself is malformed in structure and function. However, it is not clear whether these malformations are primary or are secondary (to impaired urinary drainage, for example).

CLINICAL PRESENTATION AND EVALUATION ▶ Symptoms arising from ectopic insertion of a ureter are mainly dependent on its localization. In females only, the point of insertion may be located inside or outside the external sphincter, which determines whether the patient will be continent or incontinent. Persistent incontinence in a girl with otherwise normal voiding patterns after exclusion of neurogenic bladder disorder is the most frequent picture in the case of an ectopic ureteral insertion outside the external sphincter (Chap. 4, Case 17). Other frequent symptoms of ectopic ureters are recurrent UTI, stone formation, vesico-ureteral reflux and hydronephrosis resulting from ureteral obstruction. More and more patients with ectopic ureters are diagnosed while asymptomatic by perinatal ultrasound screening investigations.

In male patients recurrent epididymitis may be the first symptom of ectopic insertion into the seminal tract. More common symptoms in boys are urgency and frequency. A possible late symptom of an ectopic insertion is infertility.

Clinical evaluation when the diagnosis of ectopic ureter is suspected may be problematic. In a minority of cases at least the diagnosis is possible by operative exploration. In other cases a simple clinical inspection of the female external genitalia may disclose the ectopic ureteral orifice in the vestibule.

Ultrasonography of the urinary tract in patients with ectopic ureter may show a duplicated collecting system, hydronephrosis and megaureter with a dilated distal ureter behind a normal bladder. The renal parenchyma may show different degrees of damage from recurrent infections or chronic pressure elevation.

Fluoroscopic investigations provide more anatomical detail. IV pyelography may show an adequately functioning renal unit, a probable duplication of the collecting system, hydronephrosis and, ideally, the course of the ectopic ureter and its insertion point. More commonly, the renal unit with the ectopic ureter shows different degrees of renal dysfunction, which results in a lack of contrast of the affected collecting system. In these cases, indirect signs lead to the diagnosis. Mostly the medial and caudal dislocation of a collecting system or the entire lower kidney pole is due to hydronephrosis of an upper pole system. Nevertheless, this alterations are not specific for ectopic insertion of the ureter. More sensitive even in cases with severe renal dysfunction, MRI urography provides highly detailed anatomical information on the ectopic system.

A voiding cysto-urethrography (VCUG) may show different degrees of reflux in ectopic systems, which also indicate the insertion position of the ureter. It is important to keep in mind that VCUG is not able to detect existing reflux in a ureter inserting into the direct area of the external sphincter. ^{99m}Tc-DMSA provides sensitive information on the function of the affected renal units, which is important for planning of the therapeutic approach. Furthermore, urethro-cystoscopy and vaginoscopy may disclose the ureteral orifice of the ectopic system.

THERAPY ▶ The treatment of ectopic ureter includes relieving the clinical symptoms and preserving as much of the kidney function as possible. The majority of renal units drained by ectopic ureters are seriously impaired in function. In these cases hemi- or nephrectomy of the affected kidney is indicated. Especially in single systems, this decision must be made carefully. If a nephrectomy is necessary, the decision for a complete ureterectomy is dependent on the clinical presentation of the ectopic insertion. Especially for patients with high-grade reflux in the ectopic ureter, complete excision is recommended. In these cases a second incision is generally necessary. During this procedure in male patients the surgeon has to be particularly aware of the danger of damaging the seminal structures, so as to avoid later infertility.

In cases with salvageable kidney function, ureteropyelostomy is the treatment of choice in double systems and ureterocystoneostomy, in single systems.

A special challenge is the therapeutic management of bilateral single ectopic ureters. As orthotopic insertion of the ureter into the sinus urogenitalis is necessary for the normal fetal development especially of the bladder trigonum, but also of the bladder itself, bilateral ectopia results in insufficiency of the bladder neck and marked maldevelopment of the bladder. Besides having the expected restriction of the kidney function and a high incidence of high-grade reflux, these patients are completely incontinent and have a markedly restricted bladder capacity.

The therapy of bilateral single ectopic ureters, therefore, includes ureterocystoneostomy for reflux, construction of a continence mechanism by bladder neck reconstruction or implantation of a artificial sphincter and, if the bladder capacity fails to increase adequately after gaining continence, augmentation of the bladder, e.g. by ileocystoplasty (Chap. 4, Case 18).

1.2.4.4
Ureteral Stenosis and Ureteral Valves

Congenital ureteral stenosis is a rare cause of ureteral obstruction. It can affect any part of the ureter and can be present in more than one segment of the ipsilateral ureter. The main locations affected are, in declining order of frequency, the prevesical part of the ureter, the ureteropelvic junction and the mid-ureter crossing the iliac vessels.

The morphological studies of the narrow areas show rarefaction of normal smooth muscle cells without evidence of fibrosis. This suggests impaired mesenchyme surrounding the ureter in this area during embryological development, resulting in impaired muscular development [2].

Another rare alteration of the ureteral wall that may result in ureteral obstruction is the formation of ureteral valves. These may be annular mucosal folds containing a submucosal smooth muscle layer. There is a central narrow opening in the middle of the valve [148]. Other forms of ureteral valves have been described by Cussen [34]. These valves are not annular, but have an eccentric configuration. It was suggested that they are left behind by impaired straightening of the fetal ureter, which frequently shows kinks and folds resulting from a faster longitudinal growth of the ureter than of the entire fetus [87].

The clinical significance of both ureteral stenosis and ureteral valves is dependent on the degree of obstruction. Antenatal hydronephrosis in ultrasonographic studies is often the first sign of ureteral obstruction. Other symptoms are flank pain, recurrent UTI, stone formation or simply failure to thrive. MRI urography, IV pyelography and retrograde pyelography provide excellent detailed morphology of the cause of ureteral obstruction. Radionuclear renography documents the obstruction and gives sensitive information about disturbance of the renal function.

The treatment of choice is operative resection of the stenosis or the obstructive area of the ureter and, depending on the location, pyeloplasty, ureteroureterostomy or ureterocystoneostomy.

1.2.4.5
Ureterocele

The ureterocele is an anomaly of the distal ureter, whose clinical presence is highly heterogeneous. Its clinical importance varies, as the picture ranges between asymptomatic and renal failure. The clinical management of ureteroceles, therefore, requires individual decisions on each case, to ensure diagnosis-adapted treatment.

A ureterocele is a cystic dilatation of the distal ureter. The aetiology is unknown. Several theories have been suggested, but none of them is backed by solid evidence. As the ureteral orifice in general is very narrow, the hypothesis of incomplete persistence of Chwalle's membrane dividing the ureteric bud from the urogenital sinus in the early development of the upper urinary tract is very popular.

Ureteroceles are bilateral in 10% of cases. The female-to-male ratio is 4:1. Ureteroceles are frequently associated with other anomalies of the upper urinary tract, such as duplication of the collecting system (Chap. 4, Case 20), which is present in almost 80% of cases of clinically relevant ureteroceles or ureteral ectopia.

CLINICAL PRESENTATION AND EVALUATION ▶ The main clinical symptom of ureteroceles is infection of the upper urinary tract, but acute renal failure or urosepsis are not uncommon primary symptoms. Unspecific symptoms, such as a palpable mass caused by hydronephrosis, abdominal pain or failure to thrive, have been observed. Furthermore, urinary stasis caused by renal obstruction or recurrent infections may result in stone formation.

Depending on their size, ectopic ureteroceles in particular may prolapse into the vaginal introitus and appear there as a mass. These masses must be differentiated from other vaginal masses, such as urethral prolapse, periurethral cyst and rhabdomyosarcoma of the bladder. Very large intravesical ureteroceles can restrict urinary drainage from the contralateral ureteral orifice and provoke renal obstruction. They can also irritate the normal function of the bladder neck, resulting in voiding disorder and incontinence. However, an increasing proportion of patients are diagnosed while asymptomatic, by prenatal or perinatal ultrasonographic screening investigations.

Once a ureterocele is suspected, its influence on the upper part of the urinary tract must be evaluated. In general, ureteroceles obstruct the upper part of the collecting system. Vesico-ureteral reflux (VUR) is observed only infrequently. In cases with a duplicated collecting system the ureterocele obstructs the upper part, while the lower part frequently shows VUR. However, a large ureterocele could affect the normal trigonal architecture and also result in VUR into the contralateral collecting system. Sen et al., in a series of 127 patients, reported VUR of the ipsilateral lower pole systems in 54% and VUR into the contralateral unit in 28% [125].

The basic tool in the evaluation of ureteroceles is ultrasonography. An increasing number of patients are detected already in the prenatal period, showing hydronephrosis in the antenatal ultrasound investigation. After birth, direct investigation of the child may reveal duplication of the hydronephrotic collecting system, especially of the upper pole but probably also of the lower pole. Ultrasound of the kidneys should include assessment of the status of the renal parenchyma, which if reduced could indicate impaired renal function of this area. Hydronephrosis, furthermore, must lead to evaluation of the lower urinary tract. Intravesical ureteroceles are perceived as cystic structures at the lateral trigonum, separated from the normal bladder by a thin wall. The filling grade of the bladder has to be considered, because both a maximally filled and an empty bladder can conceal a ureterocele. Frequently, the dilated distal ureter can be shown behind the bladder. However, the absence of a widely dilated ureter or dilatation of the collecting system does not exclude the presence of a significant ureterocele [127]. Ultrasound cannot differentiate reliably between orthotopic and ectopic ureteroceles.

A VCUG is necessary in all cases of symptomatic ureterocele. The fluoroscopic, in contrast to the radionuclear, method allows visualization of the ureterocele as well as classification of an accompanying ipsi- or contralateral VUR. IV pyelography can show the anatomical details of the collecting system, especially the ectopic position, and gives some preliminary information on renal function. But in cases with heavily impaired function of the affected part of the kidney, which are frequent, none of the collecting system can be directly revealed. In these cases, indirect radiographic signs could help with the diagnosis. An extremely tortuous, laterally positioned, ureter from an inferiorly and laterally relocated lower pole indicates hydro-ureteronephrosis of the upper system. Furthermore, the ureterocele may be identified as a noncontrasted area in the bladder. Otherwise, in cases with intravesical single-system ureteroceles the so-called cobra head phenomenon can be observed. This is an area of high contrast density in the bladder, which has the form of a cobra's head surrounded by a small margin of lower contrast.

Although it is not yet a routine investigation, MRI urography provides advantages over conventional IV pyelography. This method also allows an anatomically detailed visualization of nonfunctioning normal or dilated renal collecting systems, which is very important for conscientious planning of an operative correction.

Furthermore, a sensitive analysis of the differential function of the particular renal units of the duplicated system is necessary to enable decisions on whether the obstructed, generally upper, part of the kidney can be preserved or not. A static radionuclear scan of the kidney using ^{99}Tc-labelled DMSA is the most sensitive method if the areas of interest are chosen carefully. Another alternative is a ^{99m}Tc-MAG$_3$ clearance, which could show the obstruction of the upper kidney pole by the ureterocele, but this is less competent in detecting the function of the different kidney parts.

A cystoscopy provides information of the intravesical or ectopic extent of the ureterocele and should be performed at least preoperatively. Furthermore, endoscopy is an option for therapeutic decompression of the ureterocele.

THERAPY ▶ The form of treatment of ureteroceles depends on its clinical significance. Asymptomatic ureteroceles with no effect on kidney function do not need any therapy. Careful evaluation of the disease is therefore mandatory. The main therapeutic principles are preservation of the kidney function, mainly by relief of the obstruction, and avoidance of UTI by management of VUR. Furthermore, unimpaired and controlled bladder emptying should be maintained after any therapeutic approach.

There are two general opinions about operating on ureteroceles, the so-called upper tract approach and the combined upper and lower tract approach. In addition, there is the option of operating endoscopically. The upper tract approach includes upper pole nephrectomy with partial ureterectomy in cases with no or very poor renal function of the upper unit. If there is significant function a ureteropyelostomy or uretero-ureterostomy to the lower collecting system combined with partial ureterectomy of the upper part is recommended. The operation should lead to decompression of the ureterocele, which should also normalize the trigonal architecture resulting in resolution of bilateral VUR and unimpaired micturition. Particularly in cases with high-grade reflux to the lower pole and huge ectopic ureteroceles the method carries up to 47 % risk of reoperation because of persisting reflux, recurrent UTI or persistent bladder outlet obstruction [121]. Interestingly, there is a significant risk of reflux in a preoperatively uninvolved contralateral system. Furthermore, the persisting ureterocele and its remaining ureter stump could remain refluxive or filled, which could result in recurrent UTI or pyo-ureter.

A combined upper and lower tract approach includes upper pole nephrectomy or ureteropyelostomy to the lower system, ureterectomy of the upper ureter, resection of the ureterocele from the bladder and ureteral reimplantation of the lower part of the ureter via two incisions. Scherz and co-workers compared the two approaches and found a significantly lower rate of reoperation (14 %) for the combined approach [121]. The main risk of this method is injury of the musculature and nerves, especially of the bladder neck, with consequent incontinence.

Endoscopic decompression of ureteroceles has been performed for many years. Initially, the ureteroceles were widely "unroofed" by transurethral resection of their anterior wall. As high-grade reflux resulted in the majority of cases [142], this method is only indicated in cases with therapy-resistant urosepsis, for rapid drainage of a pyonephrosis of the obstructed collecting system. Blythe et al. found a 27% reoperation rate after endoscopic incision of the anterior wall of the ureterocele [15]. The incision has to be made during minimal bladder filling to obtain optimal drainage of the ureterocele even with an empty bladder. The main problem of endoscopic incision of ureteroceles too is VUR. Especially in cases with ectopic ureteroceles, the results of endoscopic decompression are poor relative to those obtained with intravesical ureteroceles. The reoperation rate in these cases was 50%, as against 7% for intravesical ureteroceles. Nevertheless, the minimal invasiveness of this procedure, which may be possible as day surgery, supports this approach especially in patients with intravesical ureteroceles without or with only low-grade reflux into the lower system.

In conclusion, the decision on the therapeutic approach has to be made individually for each patient, as no one surgical method is appropriate in every case. Besides any perioperative risk and morbidity, the decision depends on the location of the ureterocele, renal function, degree of obstruction, degree of reflux and the surgeon's experience and preferences.

1.3
Anomalies of the Lower Urinary Tract

1.3.1
Bladder Exstrophy

Bladder exstrophy is a complex congenital anomaly of the ventral abdominal wall with consequent severe urogenital malformations. The incidence is 1:30000–35000 live births, with a marked male predominance. The risk of recurrence of bladder exstrophy in an affected family is about 1:100 [55]. The risk of bladder exstrophy in the offspring of affected people is about 500-fold that in the general population [126].

The major influence of bladder exstrophy on the physical, psychic and sexual development and the resulting problems for the affected patients and their families make heavy demands on the physician and should be coordinated by centres with a concentration of relevant experience. Without adequate surgical treatment, the mortality of bladder exstrophy is about 75% up to the age of 15 years. The main problem is progressive renal insufficiency due to recurrent UTI and bilateral renal obstruction.

1.3.1.1
Aetiology

The cause of the defect in the ventral abdominal wall originates during the early embryonic development of the urogenitalia. Between the 4th and 7th weeks of gestation, the primitive cloaca is divided by the urorectal septum into sinus urogenitalis and rectum. The cloaca is demarcated ventrally from the amniotic cavity by the cloacal membrane, which is also divided into an anal and a urogenital membrane. Simultaneously, the lateral tubercular genitalia fuse in the midline, displacing the cloacal membrane in a caudal direction. This leads to mesodermal stabilization of the ventral abdominal wall by initiating the development of supporting tissues.

Muecke postulated overdevelopment of the cloacal membrane as a contributory factor in the absence of a normal midline fusion of the mesenchymal structures of the lower abdomen [98]. The genital tubercles fuse caudal to the cloacal membrane. The region of the cloacal membrane, therefore, stays uncovered by supporting tissue, and the membrane ruptures with ongoing longitudinal growth of the embryo. The time of the rupture determines the extent of affected organ systems (rectum, bladder, urethra, abdominal wall) by the exstrophy. The later the rupture, the less severe the resultant defect.

Another, less popular, explanation for the development of bladder exstrophy was postulated by Patten and Barry. They suggest that the rather caudal fusion of the genital tubercles is due to their primarily abnormal caudal position [106]. The persistence of the cloacal membrane, therefore, is a result of the malpositioned tubercles, and not the opposite. Nevertheless, the consequence for the development of the abdominal wall is similar.

1.3.1.2
Clinical Presentation and Evaluation

The clinical presentation of bladder exstrophy is rather characteristic, and the diagnosis can easily be made. The defect of the abdominal wall leads to a symphyseal separation, a caudally positioned umbilicus and, in between, the uncovered bladder plate, which varies widely in size. The bladder plate herniates externally with elevation of the abdominal pressure when the child cries. The bladder mucosa appears quite normal at birth, but can also show oedematous or hyperplastic alterations. The trigonum may be widened with lateralization of the usually gaping refluxive ureteral orifices. An isolated bowel loop may appear in addition. Males have a shortened flat penis with complete epispadia, whereas females present with a bifid clitoris and gaping labia minora and majora. The anus is positioned rather ventrally.

In addition to the characteristic clinical presentation of bladder exstrophy, evaluation of the upper urinary tract is recommended to assess the overall extent of the disease. Dilatation of the collecting system by VUR can easily be detected by ultrasound, whereas IV pyelography has lost its importance. In cases with suspected severe restriction of the renal function, precise evaluation can be performed by radionuclear renography, if necessary even in newborns. The precise assessment of an impaired renal function is important for the therapeutic strategy chosen later (Chap. 4, Case 32).

1.3.1.3
Therapy

There is no standard procedure for the treatment of bladder exstrophy, but there are basic principles. The purposes of any contemporary therapy are approximation of the symphysis, closure of the abdominal wall defect, creation of urinary storage and continence, and protection of the renal function. To ensure undisturbed sexual development, if at all possible, plastic reconstruction of the external genitalia, especially in males, has a very important role in the treatment of bladder exstrophy.

Urinary diversion was the first successful approach to the treatment of bladder exstrophy. But resection of the bladder plate with consecutive antirefluxive ureterosigmoidostomy, which was formerly very popular [28], has been abandoned because of severe complications from recurrent infections, stone formation and acidosis in spite of several techniques of improved antirefluxive ureteral implantation. Besides the risk of primary malignancy of the left bladder plate in 4–7.5% [39], nitrosamines also cause an increased risk of carcinogenesis in the area of the ureterosigmoidal anastomosis [158].

Therefore, primary functional closure of the bladder should be achieved if possible. This includes closure of the bladder itself, approximation of the ventral pelvis, reconstruction of a continent bladder neck and reconstruction of the external genitalia. There is controversy about the timing of the single steps of the procedure. The popular so-called staged approach involves three steps:

1. Primary closure of the bladder and anterior pelvic ring by bilateral iliac osteotomy, or during the first 48 hours without osteotomy, because of the malleability of the pelvic ring [5] at the age of 72 hours or earlier. This leads to an approximation of the levator and puborectal sling, with inclusion of the bladder neck into the pelvic ring, resulting in better later continence rates [46].
2. Continent reconstruction of the bladder neck (Young-Dees-Leadbetter technique) combined with a simultaneous antirefluxive ureteral reimplantation at the age of 3–5 years.
3. The last step is the plastic reconstruction of the clitoris or penis with correction of the epispadias a the age of 5 years.

Another successful approach to the functional closure of bladder exstrophy by a single-stage procedure was postulated by Schrott and Sigel [122]. They combined the closure of the bladder, reconstruction of the bladder neck, prophylactic antirefluxive ureteral reimplantation, penile elongation, urethroplasty and glanduloplasty with a simultaneous closure of the pelvic ring in a single operation at the age of 6–8 weeks at the earliest. The main advantages of this strategy are better operative conditions without scars from prior operations, quicker acquisition of bladder capacity because of the increased bladder outlet resistance and decreased psychic stress because of repeated operations. The main disadvantage is that one complication could jeopardize the entire repair.

Nevertheless, the results of both strategies are rather satisfactory. The primary functional closure of the bladder is successful in over 70% of the patients in terms of renal function and continence rates. Education, employment and family life are not seriously affected, erectile function, sexuality and sexual function are well preserved and female patients, especially, show normal fertility [12].

In children with bladder exstrophy, primary urinary diversion is indicated only in cases with bladder plates smaller than 5 cm^2 or extreme dilatation of the upper urinary tract with consequent restriction of the renal function. These cases should be diverted primarily by a conduit that can be converted later into a continent form of urinary diversion. Indications for a secondary urinary diversion are failed primary bladder closure and repeated failure of continent bladder neck reconstruction. Inadequate bladder capacity could be improved by bladder augmentation by different bowel segments.

1.3.1.4
Cloacal Exstrophy

Cloacal exstrophy is the most severe defect of the formation of the anterior abdominal wall. It occurs in 1 : 300 000 births, and there is a male predominance. As in classic bladder exstrophy, again the persistence of the cloacal membrane prevents the midline fusion of the mesenchymal structures of the primitive abdominal wall, but at a time when the urorectal septum has not yet separated the cloaca into rectum and sinus urogenitalis.

This leads to an exstrophied foreshortened hindgut or caecum between two hemibladders, two hemiphalluses and a bifid scrotum in males. Clinically an omphalocele is present cranially. The bony pelvic ring is open anteriorly. The anomaly is frequently combined with spina bifida and meningoceles.

The therapeutic aims include primarily resection of the omphalocele, separation of the exstrophied bowel segments from the bladder halves, terminal ileostomy or colostomy, joining and closure of the bladder halves and anterior closure of the pelvic ring. Ureteral reimplantation and continent bladder neck reconstruction and reconstruction of mostly female genitalia independently of genotype should be performed later. Although the perioperative mortality of patients with cloacal exstrophy has significantly decreased during recent decades, the general mortality of these patients is dependent on other, mainly septic, complications during the newborn period. Nevertheless, the results of the reconstructive surgical approaches are promising, but the complexity of the anomaly limits the therapeutic approaches.

1.3.2
Other Congenital Anomalies of the Bladder

Most congenital anomalies of the bladder are so extremely rare that only a few cases have been reported in the literature.

1.3.2.1
Agenesis and Hypoplasia of the Bladder

Agenesis of the bladder is a severe defect that is only compatible with life if the upper urinary tract is drained by way of a patent urachus, persisting cloaca, or ectopic insertion of the ureter to structures of the müllerian ducts. Campbell reported on 7 cases with bladder agenesis out of nearly 20 000 autopsies [23]. The anomaly is associated with other severe anomalies of the urinary tract, such as renal uni- or bilateral agenesis or absence of the prostate or seminal vesicles. The aetiology of bladder agenesis is not known. As in each reported case the hindgut was normal, the problem must occur after the cloacal is separated by the urorectal septum. Absence of a normal insertion of the mesonephric ducts in the cloaca has been suggested as the initiator of the anomaly. The main components of treatment are urinary diversion and protection of the remaining renal function.

Congenital hypoplasia of the bladder is associated mainly with impaired storage function of the bladder, which can be caused, for example, by bilateral single, ectopically inserting, ureters.

1.3.2.2
Duplication of the Bladder

Complete duplication of the bladder has so far been described in the literature in only 45 cases [64]. The anomaly is more frequent in boys. It involves two complete bladders, each with a unilateral ureter and its own urethra. The anomaly is frequently associated with anomalies of other organ systems, especially duplication of the external genitalia, the spine or the lower gastrointestinal tract. Incomplete bladder duplication, as opposed to the complete anomaly, is characterized by two bladders draining into one urethra.

1.3.2.3
Diverticulum of the Bladder

Congenital diverticulum of the bladder wall is a rare anomaly affecting almost exclusively boys. It occurs without evidence of subvesical obstruction and has to be differentiated of the more frequent pseudodiverticula secondary to bladder outlet obstruction. The complete bladder wall is evaginated. Nevertheless, the bladder wall of the diverticulum is mostly thinner and contains hypoplastic muscle fibres. The diverticula originate near the ureteral orifice at the area where the trigone joins the detrusor muscle. If a diverticulum includes the ureteral orifice, VUR occurs as the transmural course of the distal ureter is shortened. Furthermore, huge diverticula can cause ureteral obstruction as well as bladder outlet obstruction. Residual urine is an uncommon problem in children compared with adults. The treatment of congenital diverticula of the bladder depends on the symptoms they cause. If symptoms appear resection of the diverticulum and ureteral reimplantation is necessary.

1.3.3
Anomalies of the Urachus

The urachus connects the anterior bladder dome with the umbilicus and is located between the peritoneum and the fascia transversalis. During embryogenesis the cranial part of the primitive bladder tube narrows but maintains continuity with the allantoic duct, becoming the urachus. During later fetal development the urachus is obliterated. After birth the persisting fibrotic urachal cord fuses the obliterated umbilical arteries and forms the medial umbilical ligament or the chorda urachii. Anomalies of the urachus affect boys about twice as frequently as girls. Malignancy may occur in adults.

A patent urachus is a rare anomaly with an unknown aetiology. It may appear typically as persistence of the urachal lumen with a rather normally configured bladder or as a vesico-umbilical fistula from an undescended bladder. It appears clinically as a wet umbilicus and has to be differentiated from a persistent omphalo-enteric duct. The evaluation includes catheterization of the urachus, VCUG, cystoscopy and abdominal ultrasonography.

Other anomalies of the urachus are the urachal cyst, the external urachal sinus and the urachal diverticulum. In contrast to the patent urachus the urachal sinus represents a connection between umbilicus and urachus without affecting the bladder. In turn, the connection between the bladder and the urachus results in a urachal diverticulum. The urachal cyst is located between the bladder and the umbilicus, but may connect the two structures.

Urachal cysts and external urachal sinus can cause various problems if they become infected. The clinical symptoms are lower abdominal pain, fever and, occasionally, peritonitis after intraperitoneal perforation. The diagnosis is unproblematic, being made by abdominal ultrasound. The treatment includes resection of the complete remaining urachal structures (Fig. 8a–c).

1.3.4
Neurogenic Disorder of the Lower Urinary Tract

Neurogenic dysfunction of the lower urinary tract is a frequent challenge for the paediatric urologist. The reason for neurogenic bladder disorder may be congenital (neurospinal dysraphism), or more uncommonly acquired (spinal tumours, trauma, infections). The consequences for the bladder are dependent on the location of the neurogenic involvement. In general, the neurogenic disorder may affect the storage and/or voiding function of the lower urinary tract, leading to incontinence or urinary retention as the primary symptoms. However, the secondary effects in particular, such as VUR, ureteral obstruction and urinary tract infection, frequently complicate the situation and are responsible for the high morbidity of the disease.

Whereas in the past the majority of patients with neurogenic dysfunction of the lower urinary tract ultimately underwent urinary diversion, the establishment of sterile intermittent (self)-catheterization (CIC) at the beginning of the early 1970s has completely changed the management of this disease. Furthermore, technical progress has led to earlier and much more precise evaluation of individual disorders of the lower urinary tract, contributing to much earlier onset of the therapy, and thereby to better outcome and prognosis for the affected patients.

The innervations of the lower urinary tract involves parasympathetic, sympathetic and mixed nerves. The parasympathetic centre representing the lower motoneuron is located in segments S1–4. The upper motoneuron consists of sympathetic fibres originating in T11 to L3. The pudendal nerve contains parasympathetic and sympathetic nerve fibres and innervates the pelvic floor and the external sphincter (Fig. 9).

Involvement of the different nervous structures leads to characteristic patterns of disturbance of the bladder function, which may appear in isolation or

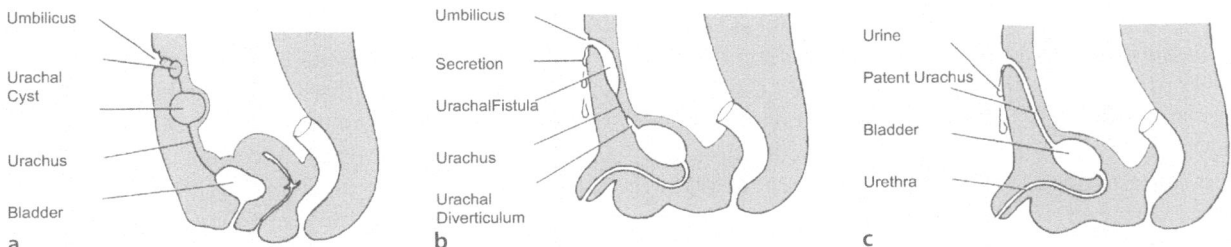

Fig. 8a–c. Anomalies of the urachus. **a** Urachal cyst. **b** Urachal fistula and urachal diverticulum. **c** Patent urachus. (From [97])

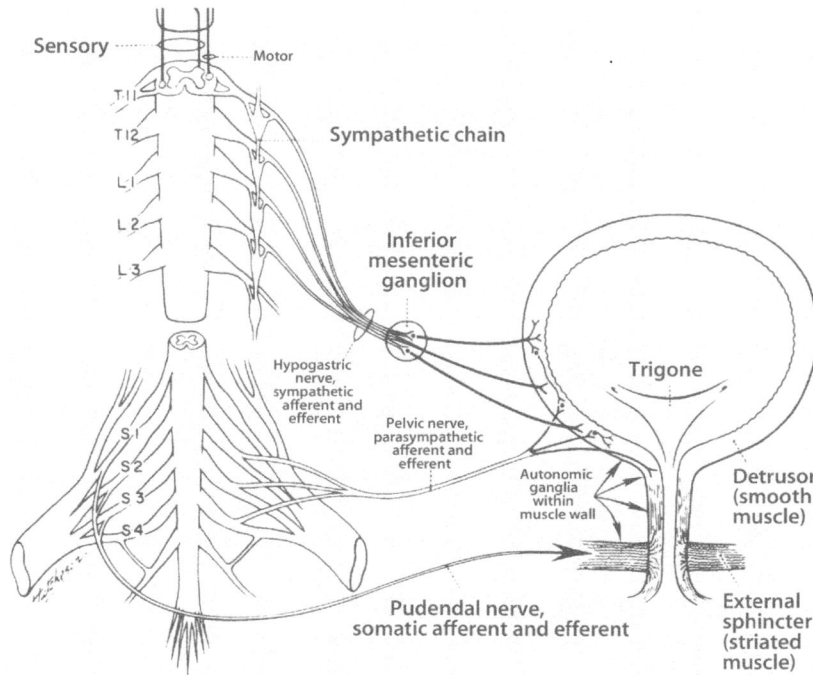

Fig. 9. Schematic of the parasympathetic, sympathetic and mixed innervation of the bladder, bladder neck and pelvic floor. (From [131])

combined. The basic forms of neurogenic bladder disorder are:

- Hyperreflexia of the detrusor muscle: incontinence, decreased capacity, increased intravesical pressure
- Hyperreflexia of the sphincter mechanism: obstructive hypercontinence, residual urine
- Arreflexia of the detrusor muscle: weak bladder with hypercontinence, residual urine
- Arreflexia of the sphincter mechanism: complete incontinence, absence of functional capacity.

The most important tool in the evaluation of neurogenic bladder disorder is urodynamic evaluation in combination with VCUG (video-urodynamic evaluation). The morphological condition of the urinary tract may be imaged by ultrasonography. IV pyelography has lost its importance. Evaluation of the renal function should be performed by renal scintigraphy.

The treatment concentrates on the protection of the upper urinary tract by avoiding recurrent UTI (long-term antibiotic prophylaxis, antireflux surgery) and facilitating the emptying of the bladder, thereby simultaneously reducing the elevated intravesical pressure by CIC and/or anticholinergic medication and also contributing to improved management of VUR.

Nevertheless, the treatment of neurogenic bladder disorder is frequently only one part of a complex therapeutic strategy in patients with further nonuro-

logical neurogenic disorders. Therefore, sufficient interdisciplinary care with professional coordination of the different therapies is absolutely mandatory for these patients and contributes to the improved prognosis of the disease.

Urodynamic evaluation is an extremely valuable tool when combined with VCUG, representing the most important technique in the evaluation of functional, neurogenic or organic bladder dysfunction in both paediatric and adult patients.

During the investigation the bladder is filled artificially under controlled conditions. Simultaneously, the intravesical and intraabdominal pressure and also the myogenic activity of the pelvic floor are evaluated, and during voiding the urinary flow. The investigation allows assessment of the storage and voiding functions of the bladder. The results of the study allow conclusions on neurogenic or functional bladder disturbances with due consideration for the innervation status of the lower urinary tract, thereby leading to an adequate therapy.

Nevertheless, besides its exceptional value in the evaluation of bladder disorder, the reliability is extremely vulnerable to external influences. Lack of experience on the part of the investigator and disregard of the mandatory need for the child to cooperate are particularly likely to lead to misinterpretation. The investigator must coordinate and correlate the results of the examination with the general appearance and reaction of the patient. Usually isolated interpretation of the pressure, myogenic and flow results recorded is not sufficient.

1.3.5
Posterior Urethral Valves

The presence of posterior urethral valves with consequent obstruction of the upper urinary tract is a rare but serious congenital malformation of the proximal urethra. The incidence is between 1:5000 and 1:8000. The time of clinical manifestation varies with the degree of renal obstruction. One third each of the patients present during the 1st year of life, between 1 and 5 years of age and after 5 years. Bilateral dilatation of the upper urinary tract can be detected prenatally by antenatal ultrasound screening investigations. Affected boys can then be diagnosed at the latest at birth, and the treatment can be started early, contributing to an improvement of the prognosis. Thus, neonatal mortality occurs in only 2–3% of these cases [27]. However, the mortality rate among children with primary pulmonary hypoplasia is still 50% [99].

As early as 1919, H. Hampton Young suggested the classification of the posterior urethral valves that is still currently used with a division into three different types [157]. A type-1 valve is a circular membrane arising from the verumontanum and inserting at the beginning of the ventral part of the membranous urethra. The membrane is perforated by a narrow opening near the verumontanum, allowing partial urinary drainage. Almost 95% of all patients have type-1 valves. Type-2 valves arise from the verumontanum and insert cranially at the dorsolateral bladder neck. There is now general agreement that type-2 valves, if they really exist in this form, are not obstructive, and they have therefore been disregarded below. A type-3 valve is a circular membrane in the membranous urethra, with a tight central opening (Fig. 10).

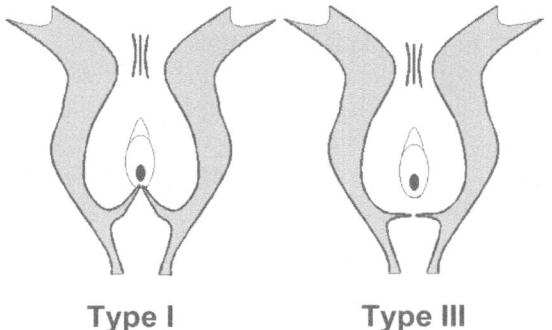

Type I   **Type III**

Fig. 10. Variants of posterior urethral valves

1.3.5.1
Aetiology

The exact aetiology of posterior urethral valves is not known. Several theories on the embryological development of the male urethra have been suggested. Anomalous insertion of the mesonephric ducts into the cloaca has been implicated in the development of type-1 valves. Normally the mesonephric ducts insert in the cloaca laterally, inducing generation of the primitive bladder neck. The openings of the ducts then migrate cranially and medially while remaining at the verumontanum. If the mesonephric ducts insert in the cloaca more anteriorly, the dorsal and cranial migration of their orifices is impaired, resulting in fusion at the anterior wall of the sinus urogenitalis. Analogous to the plicae colliculi in normal development of the proximal urethra, the movement of the wrongly inserting mesonephric ducts also causes slight plicae, but from the lateral to the anterior wall, and these form the later valves [141].

In normal development of urogenitalia the primitive cloaca is successively subdivided by the urorectal septum into the rectum and the sinus urogenitalis. The cloacal membrane that separates the cloaca from the amniotic space is also subdivided, into the urogenital membrane and the anal membrane. Both membranes later dissolve to allow the normal passage of urine and faeces. Incomplete dissolution of the urogenital membrane correlates with type-3 posterior urethral valves. These valves may prolapse into the bulbar part of the urethra and give the impression of a bulbar urethral obstruction [43].

1.3.5.2
Clinical Presentation

The timing and severity of clinical presentation of patients with posterior urethral valves depends heavily on the degree of bilateral renal obstruction. The more severe the obstruction, the earlier the symptoms appear and the more serious they are. Newborns present at clinical examination with a palpable, massively full bladder and severe hypertrophy of the bladder wall. The kidneys show different degrees of dilatation owing to secondary VUR. In addition, the abdomen may be distended by gas in the intestine and bulging with urinary ascites. Interestingly, patients with severe obstructive uropathy and the presence of urinary ascites have a better outcome than patients without [118]. In severe cases in which renal obstruction has been present during intrauterine life, pulmonary distress may have resulted from immaturity of the lung caused by oligohydramnios, complicating the situation further (Chap. 4, Case 31). Older children with quite a normal upper urinary tract at birth attract attention because of failure to thrive, exsiccosis, electrolyte abnormalities or recurrent UTI caused by voiding disorder and secondary VUR. The first symptom of posterior urethral valve, therefore, may be urosepsis (Chap. 4, Case 30). Mild variants of valves may cause only few and/or mild symptoms, such as those of primary enuresis diurna et nocturna. Nevertheless, the majority of patients with posterior urethral valves, regardless of the time of clinical presentation, show some degree of urinary incontinence caused by functional disorder of the detrusor muscle.

Besides the pulmonary problems responsible for the perinatal mortality, the main problem of patients with posterior urethral valves even after sufficient deobstructive treatment is progressive renal insufficiency due to different degrees of renal dysplasia caused by an intrauterine renal obstruction. Furthermore, recurrent infections of the upper urinary tract can also damage the renal parenchyma and cause a decline in renal function. The outcome of renal function has been found to be related to the serum concentration of creatinine at a defined date. The cut-off seems to be a serum creatinine of 1.0 mg/dl after the 1st year of life. Higher values are correlated with a high risk of end-stage renal failure.

1.3.5.3
Clinical Evaluation

The majority of patients with severe renal obstruction by posterior urethral valves are now detected by antenatal ultrasound investigations. These show bilaterally dilated kidneys and ureters and an overfull bladder with a hypertrophied bladder wall. In some cases the prostatic part of the urethra is observed to be dilated. Some degree of oligohydramnios may also be present. Postnatal ultrasound shows similar alterations, sometimes associated with ascites. However, the most important diagnostic tool in the evaluation of posterior urethral valves is still fluoroscopic VCUG, which shows a massively dilated prostatic section of the urethra proximal to a pronounced stenosis of the membranous part of the urethra. The distal urethra is normally calibrated. In addition, different degrees of VUR to both kidneys may be observed. Urethroscopy is not usually necessary to diagnose the valves and is performed as a therapeutic approach.

1.3.5.4
Treatment and Prognosis

The treatment of posterior urethral valves depends on the age of the patient at the time of the first clinical presentation and, in terms of extent, on the degree of renal insufficiency. In older children with only mild symptoms, endoscopic destruction of the valves is usually an adequate treatment, but perinatally detected patients, especially, need more than this.

At the time of presentation, newborns show different degrees of pulmonary distress, which may make assisted respiration necessary. Furthermore, the renal function usually is markedly impaired. The first step, therefore, is transurethral or suprapubic catheterization of the bladder to decompress the upper urinary tract. However, antibiotic treatment should be given simultaneously, to avoid UTI. In the majority of patients the renal function is significantly improved by these measures, and endoscopic destruction of the valves can then be performed. The valves should be incised at the 12 o'clock, 8 o'clock and 4 o'clock positions.

The patients should then be given long-term antibiotic prophylaxis to protect the urinary tract from infections caused by VUR. With such prophylaxis, maturation or improvement of the reflux can be expected. Otherwise antirefluxive reimplantation or endoscopic treatment of the reflux is necessary.

In patients whose renal function does not respond adequately after decompression of the upper urinary tract by catheterization, endoscopic destruction of the valves in isolation does not seem to be an adequate treatment, but the kind of additional treatment that can improve the prognosis in terms of renal function in these patients is a subject of controversy. Loop ureterostomy, vesicostomy and urinary diversion via ileum or colon conduits have all been postulated as safer ways of achieving decompression of the upper urinary tract and thus providing greater improvement of renal function. However, there is evidence that the outcome for renal function is similar with or without supravesical urinary diversion [117]. Nevertheless, in these conditions, the decision on whether to perform supravesical urinary diversion in patients with severely impaired renal function should be made individually. An imperative indication for diversion is urosepsis with a dilated collecting system, but in these cases a percutaneous nephrostomy is usually sufficient.

Decreased compliance of the bladder and consequent frequency, urgency or incontinence in older toilet-trained children can usually be satisfactorily improved by anticholinergic therapy.

Another therapeutic concept that has been postulated for posterior urethral valves is antenatal surgical intervention to attain much earlier decompression of the upper urinary tract. This can be performed by establishing a vesico-amniotic shunt. However, substantial side effects of the therapy, such as danger to the fetus and the mother from amniotic infection, initiation of premature delivery and miscarriage, have to be weighed against only questionable improvement in outcome in terms of later renal function. Furthermore, antenatal diagnosis of posterior urethral valves is unreliable. The decision on whether an antenatal intervention is indicated therefore has to be carefully considered. Only oligohydramnios has been observed to be improved by vesico-amniotic shunting, and at present this is the only undisputed indication for an antenatal intervention aimed at improving pulmonary maturity by the time of birth.

Although the first treatment of posterior urethral valves is now given at an earlier stage than formerly, a large proportion of the patients show progressive loss of renal function and consequent end-stage renal failure requiring a renal transplant. However, implantation of a transplant ureter into a valve bladder can itself cause new problems and has to be considered in the planning phase for renal transplantation. Nevertheless, in recent decades the prognosis of children with posterior urethral valves has improved successively. The mortality has fallen to 2–3% [27]. The prognosis of the disease depends directly on maintenance or improvement of renal function.

1.3.6
Other Congenital Anomalies of the Urethra

Congenital anomalies of the urethra other than posterior urethral valves are much less common. They include anterior urethral valves (congenital urethral diverticula), valvular obstruction of the fossa navicularis, syringoceles (cysts of Cowper's glands), megalourethra and duplication of the urethra.

Anterior urethral valves have been described in almost all parts of the anterior urethra in both male and female patients. They are diverticula of the urethra, which become filled with urine during voiding and may then prolapse into the urethral lumen, obstructing the urinary flow. As the margins of the entrance of such a diverticulum look like valvular structures, the anomaly is referred to as 'anterior urethral valves'. The aetiology is unknown.

The clinical relevance of this anomaly depends on the degree of subvesical obstruction. If it is suspected, VCUG easily leads to the diagnosis. In severe cases with congenital bilateral hydronephrosis the management is similar to that of posterior urethral valves, with initial decompression of the urinary tract and removal of the valves after stabilization of the patients. This may be performed by open surgical urethroplasty, or more commonly by endoscopic incision of the valve. The further treatment depends on the severity of alterations to the bladder and upper urinary tract. Valvular obstruction of the anterior urethra without a urethral diverticulum is extremely rare. It is not known whether these anomalies are the same entity as diverticula. The treatment includes elimination of the obstruction and protection of the upper urinary tract.

Syringoceles are rare cystic dilatations of the bulbo-urethral (Cowper) glands. They frequently cause no clinical symptoms, but some can cause bladder outlet obstruction. The treatment includes endoscopic unroofing of the cyst, leading to a pseudodiverticulum of the bulbar urethra, which itself can cause an obstruction. In such cases open surgical resection of the syringocele and urethroplasty are indicated.

Congenital megalourethra is a rare nonobstructive dilatation of the distal male urethra caused by abnormal development of the corpus spongiosum (scaphoid variant) and, facultatively, the corpus cavernosum (fusiform variant). Megalourethra is commonly associated with other anomalies of the upper urinary tract. It frequently occurs in patients with the prune-belly syndrome, suggesting an underlying mesenchymal deficiency. The clinical relevance depends on the changes in the upper urinary tract and the degree of damage to the corpora cavernosa. The diagnosis is easily made by VCUG. The urethra may be surgically trimmed by resection of the surplus urethral tissue. Major damage to the corpora cavernosa may result in the need for demasculinization of the patients.

A variant of megalourethra is the megameatus urethrae, which is often misinterpreted as a mild form of hypospadias. The patients show a coronarily positioned and markedly wide meatus but a completely fused prepuce and no ventral chordee.

Urethral duplication is a rare anomaly in males and unknown aetiology. The two urethras may be positioned one above the other or next to each other. Usually there is one normally functioning urethra with a sufficient continence mechanism, while the other is incontinent. Treatment includes resection of the nonfunctioning urethra and, if necessary, reconstruction of the remaining urethra to the tip of the penis.

1.4
Prune-belly Syndrome

The prune-belly syndrome (triad syndrome, Eagle-Barrett syndrome) is a congenital triad of absence, deficiency or hypoplasia of the caudal ventral abdominal wall, hypotonic bladder (Fig. 11) and refluxive hydro-ureteronephrosis combined with bilateral cryptorchidism. Its incidence is 1:35000–50000. Boys are affected in 95% of cases. The syndrome is thought to be hereditary, but the pattern of inheritance is unknown.

1.4.1
Aetiology and Pathogenesis

The exact aetiology of the prune-belly syndrome remains obscure. Several theories had been presented without adequate evidence. Pagon et al. [103] suggest obstruction of the posterior urethra in early development with consecutive enormous bladder distension and fetal ascites: this would impair the normal development of the abdominal wall and hinder the normal testicular descensus, which would explain the predominance of male patients. The problem with the theory is the lack of a similar incidence of cryptorchidism in patients with other forms of congenital subvesical obstruction. Furthermore, severe congenital bladder outlet obstruction, as in patients with posterior urethral valves, leads to hypertrophy of the bladder musculature and is not associated with defects of the ventral abdominal wall.

Smith postulated a fault in the paraxial intermediate and lateral mesodermal plate in early embryonal development contributing to a defect of the caudal abdominal wall and simultaneously of the genitourinary tract [135]. However, the presence of primary renal dysplasia and of renal dysplasia secondary to renal obstruction in different patients with prune-belly syndrome suggest that their effects begin at different times before (primary dysplasia) and after (secondary dysplasia) the 16th week of gestation.

1.4.2
Clinical Presentation and Evaluation

The clinical presentation of the full-blown syndrome is rather characteristic and it would be difficult to overlook it during the first postnatal examination. The deficiency of the abdominal wall leads to the characteristic prune-belly appearance of the lower abdomen. When this is combined with bilateral empty scrotum, the diagnosis has practically made itself even before evaluation of the urinary tract.

Furthermore, the syndrome is commonly associated with other congenital anomalies, which frequently occupy more of the limelight during the first days of life than the mandatory triad itself. Phenomena that can especially complicate the perinatal period are pulmonary hypoplasia due to oligohydramnios and such cardiac anomalies as ventricular and atrial septal defects and Fallot's tetralogy.

Other accompanying anomalies affect the gastrointestinal tract, e.g. intestinal malrotation [132] and constipation resulting from the defective abdominal musculature with consequent megacolon, or orthopaedic problems, such as club feet [84], hip dysplasia and spinal deformities.

Nevertheless, despite the accompanying defects, the triad itself can complicate the perinatal period with urosepsis and progressive functional renal insufficiency. The impaired capability for urinary con-

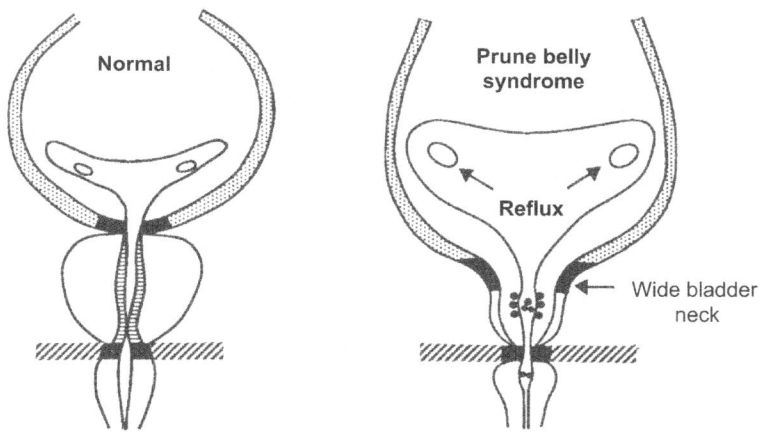

Fig. 11. Schematic of the bladder pathology in prune-belly syndrome

centration leads to a continuous loss of sodium, potassium and water.

The clinical evaluation of patients with prune-belly syndrome is concentrated mainly on the urinary tract. As soon as in the 20th week of gestation, bilateral hydroureteronephrosis, bladder distension and a characteristic alteration of the abdominal circumference on the antenatal ultrasound evaluation may indicate the anomaly. Nevertheless, at this stage of development a clear differentiation from other forms of congenital bilateral dilatation of the urinary tract is impossible.

VCUG may detect VUR. Radionuclear renography should not be used for evaluation of the differential renal function in babies younger than 4–6 weeks. The suspicion of renal obstruction often cannot be ruled out by routine ^{99m}Tc-MAG$_3$ diuretic renography, because the collecting system is too much extended. In these cases obstruction can only be evaluated by pressure flow measurements, such as Whitacker's test. However, studies that require instrumentation should be avoided if they are not needed for decisions on therapy, because of the risk of bacterial contamination (Chap. 4, Case 14).

1.4.3
Therapy and Prognosis

The treatment of prune-belly syndrome depends mainly on the extent of the disease and its accompanying anomalies. After stabilization of the pulmonary and cardiac situation the treatment is concentrated on the urinary tract, and especially on renal function. When the serum creatinine levels, urinary bacteriology and ultrasound of kidneys and bladder are followed up a strategy for clinical management can be elaborated.

1.4.3.1
Urinary Tract

First, the voiding pattern is of major interest. Assisted micturition with manual expression of the bladder should be performed 5–6 times daily at first. If bladder emptying is impaired with consequent increases in the retention parameters, endoscopic evaluation of the urethra and, if necessary, simultaneous removal of obstructing structures such as stenosis, folds or valves, which are present in about 20% of cases, is indicated. Otherwise a suprapubic percutaneous vesicostomy should be performed. If the retention parameters decline or normalize the vesicostomy can be closed, and later removed if voiding without residual urine is possible. If not, an operative cutaneous vesicostomy should be performed. Alternatively, in patients with further deterioration of the renal function bilateral pyelocutaneostomy should be considered for complete decompression of the upper urinary tract.

About 20% of the children with prune-belly syndrome need a reduction cystoplasty to improve bladder emptying by maximizing the contraction effort of the detrusor muscle. Perlmutter postulated that resection of the tube-like bladder dome would yield a more nearly spherical form of the bladder, which would improve intravesical pressure during voiding [108]. Unfortunately there is evidence that after cystoplasty bladder function deteriorates with time in some patients [19].

Cystoplasty is commonly combined with antirefluxive ureteral reimplantation as a single or a staged procedure [156]. This should include shortening and stretching of the ureter by resection of the lower parts, as the upper parts are frequently less markedly dilated and damaged. The implantation techniques are similar to those used in patients with normal VUR.

In about 25% of patients with prune-belly syndrome progressive deterioration of the renal function continues despite whatever therapeutic approach is adopted, and this is an indication for renal transplantation. The transplant ureter can be transplanted into the size-reduced bladder, or alternatively a uterocutaneostomy can be performed. The results of renal transplantation are more promising in these patients than in patients with end-stage renal failure resulting from posterior urethral valves [44].

1.4.3.2
Reconstruction of the Abdominal Wall

Successful reconstruction of the abdominal wall in patients with prune-belly syndrome results in an improved pulmonary status and better bowel and bladder function as well as the cosmetic and psychological effects. It is indicated in nearly all affected patients. If necessary, the procedure can be combined with reconstructive surgery of the urinary tract with no problems. Several surgical techniques have been described, but Monfort's abdominoplasty is one of the most popular [96]. After the excision of redundant skin parts, the technique involves approximation of the central plate of the muscular and fascial abdominal wall to the lateral internal abdomen. This leads to stretching and to improvement in the stability and thickness of the abdominal wall. The results reported are excellent.

1.4.3.3
Cryptorchidism

Although fertility is doubtful in male patients with prune-belly syndrome, testicular hormonal function is more or less normal, resulting in normal puberty. Cryptorchidism involves an elevated risk of testicular malignancy. Orchiopexy is therefore recommended. However, the normal techniques of inguinal orchiopexy are frequently insufficient, and alternative extended techniques are indicated. In patients who need reconstructive surgery on the urinary tract during the first months of life, simultaneous transabdominal mobilization of the testis usually results in undisturbed relocation of the testis to the scrotum with no necessity for cutting the spermatic vessels [155].

In older children the Fowler-Stevens technique is frequently used. This involves dividing the spermatic vessels at the level of the internal inguinal ring before it joins the vas deferens. The testis can then be positioned in the scrotum along with the vas deferens and an accompanying peritoneal flap to preserve the vasculature surrounding the vas, which is intended to maintain a sufficient blood supply to the testes [45]. As an alternative to the Fowler-Stephens procedure, testicular autotransplantation promises good result in patients with prune-belly syndrome.

1.4.3.4
Prognosis

About 25% of patients with prune-belly syndrome are stillborn or die of pulmonary, cardiac or septic complications within the first weeks of life. Another 25% experience progressive deterioration of renal function and require haemodialysis or renal transplantation. The other half of the patients have adequate renal, bladder and sexual function with or without major surgical intervention. Their fertility is severely restricted.

However, the improved medical, surgical and technical care available to these patients has resulted in an improved prognosis in terms of both survival and quality of life. Nevertheless, the variability of the severity of the disease leads to the necessity for individual therapeutic strategies. Each patient has to be carefully evaluated and followed up because the severity of the condition can change with time.

1.5
Urinary Tract Infections

Urinary tract infection (UTI) occurs when there is a significantly increased number of bacteria in the urine. It is one of the most frequent bacterially caused infectious diseases in childhood. About two thirds of the patients presenting with UTI have associated anatomical urinary tract anomalies. The majority of these have VUR or renal obstruction.

Cystitis and pyelonephritis are the two possible pathologic conditions of the urinary tract. The tendency of UTI to renal scarring, even after the first episode but with increasing likelihood in recurrent disease, means it is important clinically as the main reason for renal functional loss in childhood. Early detection and immediate implementation of adequate therapy, therefore, are mandatory to protect the urinary tract from further damage.

The incidence of UTI during the 1st year of life is about 3% in boys and 1% in girls. This ratio changes with advancing age, to the point where girls predominate (3–10%) over boys (1%) [154]. In addition, asymptomatic bacteriuria is observed in about 2% of girls thought to be healthy during screening investigations.

Several classification systems have been suggested for UTI. A commonly used system was presented by Stamey, who categorized UTI into (1) first infection, (2) unresolved bacteriuria with therapy, (3) bacterial resistance at a defined location, and (4) reinfection [138].

1.5.1
Aetiology and Pathogenesis

The bacterial colonization of the urinary tract usually occurs when bacteria ascend from the periurethral region. Only in newborns can a haematogenous pattern of infection be discussed. Bacterial invasion of the bladder does not inevitably result in UTI. Increasing duration of the presence of bacteria in the bladder, with the consequent increase in the probability of bacterial reproduction, is thought to be one of the main reasons for a relevant UTI. This is commonly due to impaired bladder emptying as the result of a neurogenic disorder or subvesical obstruction.

In general, the pathogenesis of UTI is dependent on bacterial virulence, the immune status of the patient, urinary drainage and any anatomical anomalies of the urinary tract.

More than 75% of all UTI are caused by *Escherichia coli* bacteria (*E. coli*), especially the O-serotypes O1, O2, O4, O6, O7, O18, O75. Usually, the bacterial colonization of the urine is similar to faecal colonization in the patient. Other frequently found bacteria are *Klebsiella* in newborn UTI and *Proteus*, which is found especially often in older boys. Problematic bacterial colonization, for example with *Pseudomonas aeruginosa*, is frequently associated with recurrent hospitalization or arises after urogenital surgery performed to correct anatomical anomalies of the urinary tract. Nevertheless, in patients with recurrent UTI combined with urogenital anomalies too, the most common bacteria is *E. coli*.

There is more and more evidence to suggest that specific bacterial properties are responsible for the induction of clinically relevant UTI. Antigens (O-, H-, K-antigens) on the bacterial surface initiate a systemic immune response. Enzymes excreted by the bacteria play an important part in destruction of the urothelium and parenchyma, but probably the most important factor in bacterial virulence is the capability of uroepithelial adherence by fimbria or pili that connect to the urothelium and resist natural urinary washout. As these fimbria bind to the human p-blood-group antigen they are called p-fimbria. About 90% of the *E. coli* strains causing pyelonephritis show the presence of p-fibrin, whereas only a few strains causing cystitis or asymptomatic bacteriuria show this.

There is also evidence showing that the immune response to bacterial colonization of the urinary tract is disturbed in patients with UTI. The urothelium of healthy patients is able to eliminate adherent bacteria, or at least impair their reproduction, but the urothelium of patients with UTI fails to do this [90].

Impaired urinary drainage, especially of the lower urinary tract, involves a high risk of UTI. The obstruction offers conditions that foster bacterial adherence and reproduction. Neurogenic bladder disorder or subvesical obstruction, therefore, is nearly always combined with UTI. Obstruction of the upper urinary tract, on the other hand, can stay sterile for a long period if not complicated by VUR. The risk of infection is increased after surgical manipulation for correction of the obstructive defect. Therefore, an overlapping antimicrobial prophylaxis continued for some weeks after surgery is recommended.

1.5.2
Clinical Presentation

The clinical presentation of UTI is influenced by the age and gender of the patient, the number of prior episodes, anatomical anomalies of the urinary tract, and the localization of the infection. Severe fever usu-

ally indicates involvement of the upper urinary tract, but renal damage can already have occurred in almost asymptomatic patients. However, there is a tendency to less severe symptoms with increasing number of recurrences.

Newborn patients frequently presents with urosepsis, whereas older children often show only unspecific symptoms, with fever, failure to thrive, weight loss, abdominal pain, or nausea and vomiting. With increasing age such local symptoms as flank pain and voiding disorder gain more and more clinical importance. Febrile episodes decline in frequency. Boys usually show milder symptoms than girls, but present more frequently with gross haematuria. A clear clinical differentiation between cystitis and pyelonephritis is frequently lacking, as the clinical symptoms correlate only poorly with the localization of the infection [21].

Recurrent UTI are a common problem in paediatric urology. The risk of having a second episode after a first infection is about 20–25% for children in the 1st year of life, whereas the risk decreases markedly once a patient has been free of recurrence for 12 months. The risk of recurrence is increased to 30–40% if the patients is older at the time of the first infection. This is probably due to the difference in the immune status between newborns and older children, which contributes to changes in the pattern of infection from haematogenous in newborns to ascendant in older patients. The risk of recurrence also decreases, by analogy with that in newborns, in older children after 1 year without evidence of reinfection, but it will never disappear completely. Winberg correlated the risk of reinfection during the following 12 months with the number of previous episodes of UTI. He suggested a risk of nearly 75% in a patient who had a history of three or more prior episodes of UTI [154].

Disturbance of the normal bladder function is frequently associated, especially, with recurrent UTI. The common clinical symptoms are frequency, urgency, and diurnal and nocturnal enuresis. Urodynamic evaluation of these patients shows such pathologic findings as detrusor overactivity and low-compliance hyper-, but also hypotonic, bladders in the majority of patients, as well as detrusor–sphincter dyscoordination even in patients with a normal neurological status. The voiding disorder is frequently combined with constipation and other types of bowel dysfunction.

Some patients have presented with asymptomatic bacteriuria during screening investigations. Nevertheless, a high proportion of these patients had prior symptomatic UTI or more unspecific symptoms such as enuresis or other functional voiding disorder. The majority of these patients show normal morphology of the urinary tract. Nevertheless, renal scarring can occur even in nearly asymptomatic children. Therefore, even asymptomatic bacteriuria may be a indication for treatment, even if a marked number of the patients concerned will acquire symptomatic infection or reinfection in the future [57].

Renal scarring caused by parenchymatous damage resulting from bacterial infection may initiate the development of pyelonephritogenic nephropathy (Chap. 4, Cases 8 and 26). Renal hypertension is a common complication of UTI, particularly in patients who have detectable renal scars. Nevertheless, the degree of renal damage does not directly correlate with the prediction of hypertension. The risk of developing hypertension, however, is up to 20% in patients with pyelonephritogenic nephropathy [56]. Hypertension itself could further complicate the nephropathic disease and initiate further progressive renal functional loss due to glomerular sclerosis. However, end-stage renal failure is rare in patients with UTI, even if it is recurrent.

In contrast to the adult situation, haemorrhagic cystitis is rare in children. This specific form of urinary infection of the lower tract is usually not induced by bacteria, but by different subgroups of adenovirus, and it is, therefore, not susceptible to antimicrobial therapy. The children show only slight fever, gross haematuria, frequency and urgency without bacterial colonization on urinary culture.

1.5.3
Clinical Evaluation

The first measures to be instituted on suspicion of UTI, before the beginning of any therapy, are urinalysis and urinary culture. Particularly in young children who are not yet toilet-trained, it is difficult to obtain reliably uncontaminated urine specimens. The safest method, therefore, is bladder catheterization or suprapubic bladder puncture. A so-called bagged urine specimen, obtained by attaching a plastic bag over the external genitalia, is absolutely unsuitable for the detection of bacteriuria, as it will reveal only the normal perineal and rectal bacterial flora. In older patients a midstream-voided specimen may be acceptable. However, the clinical relevance of the number of bacteria counted depends on the method of urinary sampling. In suprapubically aspirated urine any bacterial colonization is clinically relevant, while at least 10^5 bacteria/ml are required for a similar level of relevance in the case of midstream-voided urine. A lower degree of bacterial concentration requires repetition of the investigation.

Urinalysis allows the detection of leucocyturia, microhaematuria (indicative of bacterial affection of the urothelium), proteinuria (indicative of tubular damage), and urine pH and the urinary nitrite concentration; as an additional marker of bacteriuria, florid UTI can only be suspected by this method. Nevertheless, the most sensitive test of UTI is urinary culture. To avoid false-negative results the specimen has to be taken before the beginning of the antibiotic therapy.

The complete blood count is only irregularly altered during UTI, whereas the C-reactive protein is usually increased. However, increased CRP and leucocytosis indicates involvement of the upper urinary tract. An increase in the renal retention parameters creatinine or BUN is rare and indicates complications of the disease.

Ultrasonography of the kidneys and bladder is indicated at least with the first febrile episode of UTI. It allows sensitive imaging of the renal parenchymatous condition and any urolithiasis present and assessment of the collecting system with detection of several anatomical anomalies. Furthermore, the status of the ureter and bladder wall (thickness of the bladder wall) could indicate functional voiding disorder, subvesical obstruction or VUR. Ultrasonographic follow-up investigations are well suited to the observation of renal growth after UTI, and especially after recurrent UTI (Chap. 4, Case 7).

In cases with symptomatic upper UTI or recurrent infections of the lower urinary tract VCUG is indicated to disclose VUR, subvesical obstruction or functional voiding disorder. The investigation should be performed not earlier than 4 weeks after adequate treatment of the infection, to avoid reinfection by the transurethral manipulation and minimize artificial pathological findings caused by the infection itself. Fluoroscopic VCUG may detect more anatomical details, whereas radionuclear VCUG provides a higher sensitivity of reflux detection. Usually, the first VCUG should be performed by the fluoroscopic technique, and further investigation to follow up a patient should take the form of radionuclear examinations.

The indications for IV pyelography or MRI urography are only facultative if precise anatomical details are required for the planning of a possible operative therapy or the infection is complicated by urolithiasis. Renal scarring can be documented just as well by ultrasound investigations. Nevertheless, the most sensitive method of detecting renal scarring is static renal scintigraphy with ^{99m}Tc-DMSA (Chap. 4, Cases 7 and 8).

1.5.4
Therapy

The goal of therapy for UTI is to treat the existing infection sufficiently and to avoid reinfection so as to prevent any loss of renal function following structural damage of the kidney. The treatment is therefore dependent on the age of the patient, the clinical performance of the therapy, and the severity and location of the infection. The main principle of any form of therapy is to administer a broad-spectrum antimicrobial agent to the patient, which may be adapted to a more specific one after the results of the resistogram conducted on the urinary culture are available. Frequently used broad-spectrum antibiotics of first choice are sulphonamides (cotrimoxazole), aminopenicillins (ampicillin, amoxicillin), third-generation cephalosporins (cefotaxime, cephalexin) and aminoglycosides (gentamicin). In severe cases a combination of some of these substances may be helpful to broaden the antimicrobial spectrum.

The route of administration, parenteral or oral, depends on the severity of the disease and the age of the patients. UTI with high fever, especially in very young children, should be treated with parenteral antimicrobial therapy at least until the fever disappeared. The treatment should be followed by a possibly narrower oral antibiotic medication for at least 10–14 days after the result of the resistogram is known. Adequate fluid substitution at the beginning of the therapy is mandatory.

Simple cystitis without fever should be treated with an oral broad-spectrum antibiotic for 3–5 days. In these cases too, adequate fluid intake is recommended. Recurrent infections, even without fever, require a longer duration of therapy lasting at least 10 days.

The necessity for treating asymptomatic bacteriuria is the subject of some controversy. Even in cases with unspecific symptoms, especially voiding disorder, the symptoms usually persist after antimicrobial therapy. Furthermore, the frequency of reinfection does not vary with the administration or omission of therapy, and the risk of renal damage in these patients is very low [57]. Therefore, whether or not treatment is indicated should be decided individually.

Recurrence of a UTI during a period of 6 months is an indication for long-term antimicrobial prophylaxis, even in cases without anatomical or functional disorders of the urinary tract. Nevertheless, especially in these cases, the susceptibility to UTI remains unaltered after the termination of even long-term treatment with antibiotics at a prophylactic dosage. However, particularly patients with VUR benefit from antimicrobial prophylaxis, as it provides a high spontaneous resolution rate. The most frequently used agents for long-term prophylaxis are trimethoprim (1 mg/kg) and nitrofurantoin (1 mg/kg). In patients with impaired kidney function administration of a third-generation cephalosporin or amino-penicillin is more effective.

In addition to any antimicrobial treatment, any functional or anatomical disorder contributing to UTI must be treated adequately. The urinary tract should be free of stones, unimpaired urinary drainage must be ensured, and VUR should be adequately treated.

1.5.5
Genitourinary Tract Infection

The most frequent infectious disease of the genitourinary tract besides UTI is epididymitis or epididymo-orchitis; orchitis in isolation is rarer. As the clinical correlate is the acute scrotum, differential diagnosis against acute testicular torsion is necessary. The two conditions are comparable in frequency and age distribution. Epididymo-orchitis has two incidence peaks, in boys' first 2 years of life and after puberty.

The route of infection differs from the haematogenous pathway in young boys to an ascendant pathway from the urethra in older boys, who are commonly already sexually active. Furthermore, the incidence of epididymitis, especially in young patients, correlates with functional and anatomical disorders of the lower urinary tract. Isolated orchitis is commonly due to viral infection. It is especially important to be aware of the so-called mumps orchitis appearing after puberty, because of its frequent involvement in male infertility.

Physical examination shows a swollen, inflamed and painful part of the scrotum. Fever is not regular but is common. Preceding urgency, frequency or dysuria is not uncommon. Leucocyturia and/or leucocytosis may be present. Nevertheless, although all these symptoms are possible, they do not allow reliable differentiation from acute testicular torsion. This may be achieved more reliably by modern Doppler ultrasound investigation, which can detect testicular perfusion as well as allowing precise morphologic imaging of the scrotal contents. Reactive hydrocele or increased size of the epididymis are common ultrasonographic findings. Disappearance of the normal homogeneous ultrasonographic aspect of the testis indicates that it is affected by the infection. However, as in a significant number of patients clear differentiation from testicular torsion is not possible even after Doppler ultrasound investigation, operative testicular exploration, even in patients with epididymitis or epididymo-orchitis, is not uncommon.

The treatment of epididymitis or epididymo-orchitis depends on its specific cause and the age of the patient. Usually, treatment with antimicrobial agents, as for UTI, should be performed. The treatment should be continued for at least 10 days. In severe cases intermittent suprapubic urinary diversion is necessary to decrease the risk of urinary influx into the seminal tract, which might foster the infection. Scrotal abscess requires immediate operative drainage. However, the operative exploration involves the risk of irreversible testicular damage requiring orchiectomy for local control of the infectious disease. There is no specific therapy for virally induced orchitis.

After adequate therapy of epididymitis or epididymo-orchitis the possible causes should be precisely evaluated. Evaluation of the bladder function and the urethra is especially important, to minimize the risk of recurrence. The main problem caused by recurrent infections of the epididymis is occlusion of the vas deferens, with consequent infertility.

1.6
Urolithiasis

The appearance of urolithiasis in children fluctuates widely in dependence on regional differences. Whereas in southeast Asia, the Middle East and Africa stone formation is frequent in children, in North America and Scandinavia the incidence is considerably lower. In central Europe the frequency of stone disease in childhood has markedly decreased during the last century, improved diet and hygiene having been contributory factors in this. Furthermore, there has been a change of the affected part of the urinary tract from the lower to the upper part. The general incidence of urinary stones in children in Europe is about 5% [14]. This frequency increases in the second decade of life because of a increased probability of forming calcium oxalate stones. In younger children stones caused by urinary infection and congenital metabolic disorder are more common.

1.6.1
General Pathophysiology of Stone Formation

Every substance contributing to urinary stone formation is normally excreted in a soluble form within the normal urine production. Stone formation is the result of a complex combination of processes involved in crystallization, mediation of salt solution and molecular aggregation. At least 2–10% of every stone, no matter what its exact composition, consists of an organic noncrystalline substance called stone matrix, which exerts a central role in initiating the aggregation of crystallized substances. Although its exact origin is at best unclear, the matrix is known to contain aggregated mucoproteins out of the urine.

The saturation of substances in a fluid is dependent on their thermodynamic solubility product. A decrease in this leads to precipitation of the substance. Precipitation of a salt from a salt solution following a decrease in the amount of the solubility product or supersaturation of the salt solution may lead to crystallization of its ingredients. The velocity of this process is directly dependent on the disposal number of molecules or ions in the saline. Therefore, urinary stasis due to renal obstruction contributes to stone formation. However, an alteration in the urine pH could also induce crystallization of stone-forming substances.

Furthermore, a deficiency of inhibitors of growth and aggregation of crystals in the urine is also due to calculus formation. Such inhibitors are natural complexes: citrate, pyrophosphates, glycosaminoglycans and nephrocalcin, for example. A decrease in the concentration of these substances in the urine could be consistent with stone formation.

Thus, stone formation seems to be a multifactorial process that is mainly dependent on (1) the urinary concentration of stone-forming substances, (2) activity of natural inhibitors of crystallization, (3) urinary pH, and (4) a disorder of the hydrodynamic system of the urinary tract. However, the central problem in the genesis of urinary calculi is supersaturation with possibly stone-forming substances. Aftercare of patients treated for urinary stones, therefore, should include prevention of supersaturation of the urine with stone-forming substances or conversion of such supersaturation to saturation or undersaturation.

1.6.2
Specific Pathophysiology of Stone Formation

1.6.2.1
Infectious Stones

Infectious stones account for nearly half of all paediatric patients with urolithiasis. The frequency of infectious stones decreases with age, whereas in contrast stone formation resulting from metabolic disorders increases successively. Infectious stones result from a colonization of the urinary tract with urease-producing bacteria. Urease splits urea into ammonium and carbonic dioxide. Ammonium connecting to magnesium and phosphate form a crystal called struvite, which is the most frequent component of infectious stones. Another common component of these stones is apatite (calcium phosphate). The crystallization of struvite or apatite depends on an increase in urinary pH, which has to be at least 7.2. This is usually brought about by the production not only of ammonium but also of ammoniac and hydroxide ions by the bacteria. Urease-producing bacteria are, in declining order of their frequency and clinical relevance, *Proteus mirabilis*, *Klebsiella pneumoniae*, *Pseudomonas aeruginosa* and *Staphylococcus aureus*.

Nevertheless, besides the crystallization of struvite, another important process contributes to infectious stone formation. Infection of the urinary tract and irritation of the urothelium by the small crystals both lead to an increased production of mucoproteins excreted into the urine. This results in early fixation of the crystals, which are usually passed spontaneously, to the wall of the collecting system, contributing to rapid growth of the calculus [51], which could also explain the higher frequency of staghorn calculi in patients with infectious stones.

1.6.2.2
Hypercalciuria

A daily urinary excretion of > 4 mg/kg body weight of calcium is defined as hypercalciuria. The pathogenesis includes resorptive, intrarenal and absorptive disorders. In children, the resorptive form of hypercalciuria is usually due to a long period of immobilization, especially after bone fractures [54], while primary hyperparathyroidism, in contrast to the situation in adults, is rare. Immobilization results in resorption of calcium from the bones. This increases the serum concentration of calcium, with a higher excretion to the urine. Furthermore, the increased serum calcium concentration suppresses the normal production of parathyroid hormone, with a consequent decrease in urinary reabsorption of calcium from the urine. All this combines to cause a rise in the urinary concentration of calcium, which could bind to phosphate or oxalate and crystallize out from the urine.

The renal form of hypercalciuria is the most common in childhood. It reflects a disorder of the reabsorption of calcium in the distal tubules. This is probably due to a defect of the intratubular adenylate cyclase, which normally transforms actions of the parathyroid hormone to the distal tubular epithelium. The renal leak of calcium results in secondary activation of the production of parathyroid hormone by the parathyroid glands, which additionally increases reabsorption of calcium from the bones, with consequent demineralization of the skeletal system.

The absorptive form of hypercalciuria reflects hyperabsorption of calcium from the intestine. The consequent increase in serum calcium concentration initiates a suppression of parathyroid hormone. This elevates the calcium concentration in the urine by way of increased calcium renal excretion and a decrease in calcium reabsorption in the distal tubules (Chap. 4, Case 35).

The intestinal hyperabsorption of calcium in absorptive hypercalciuria is due to a primary increase in activity of 1,25-(OH)-vitamin D [63]. This could be secondary to a renal loss of phosphate, which again initiates an increase in the 1,25-(OH)-vitamin D levels [147].

1.6.2.3
Hyperoxaluria

Oxalate is a end-product of the normal vitamin C metabolism. Hyperoxaluria can arise as a primary condition caused by a genetic alteration or a secondary one, when it is usually due to an intestinal disorder. Both forms usually lead to an increase in the urinary excretion of oxalate to more than 100 mg/day (normal 20–30 mg/day).

Primary hyperoxaluria can be caused by either of two different genetic defects. Type 1 is the result of lacking activity of the enzyme alanine-glycoxylate aminotransferase. Besides oxalate, increased excretion of glyoxylate and glycolic acid can also be observed in these patients. Type 2 results from a deficiency of the enzyme glycerinate-dehydrogenase and is characterized by increased excretion of glycerinate and oxalate. Both types lead to calcification of the renal parenchyma with consequent progressive end-stage renal insufficiency.

Disorders of the gastrointestinal tract can cause increased resorption of oxalate from the intestine, causing endogenous secondary hyperoxaluria. Normally, only 2–10 % of ionic oxalate from the food is resorbed by the intestinal tract. The rest is evacuated, mainly as calcium oxalate. In situations where the concentration of ionic calcium in the food is decreased the concentration of ionic oxalate increases, leading to increased intestinal resorption of it. This is present in patients with an increased excretion of fatty acids because of excretory pancreatic insufficiency (cystic fibrosis) or decreased reabsorption of fatty acids in patients with Crohn's disease, or after surgical resection of the terminal ileum.

Another form of secondary hyperoxaluria may be caused by exogenic factors mainly contributing to increased intake of oxalate from the food or excessive intake of vitamin C (> 4 g/day).

1.6.2.4
Cystinuria

About 6% of paediatric patients with urolithiasis present with cystine stones [107], and 20% of these patients become symptomatic before the age of 15 years. Cystinuria represents a congenital defect of the transport of the amino acids cystine, ornithine, lysine and arginine, which has an autosomal recessive pattern of inheritance. The defect affects the normal reabsorption of these amino acids by the distal renal tubules and the intestinal tract. Whereas the increased excretion of cystine by the intestine remains asymptomatic, an increased concentration of cystine in the urine causes urolithiasis.

Cystine is a substance that is only poorly water soluble. In addition, the solubility is dependent on the pH of the fluid. An acid environment leads to almost complete insolubility of cystine. The maximal solubility limit of cystine is about 25 mg/dl. Higher concentrations inevitably lead to crystallization of cystine, contributing to stone formation (Chap. 4, Case 34).

1.6.2.5
Disorder of the Purine Metabolism

Impairment of different stages in the normal metabolism of purine derivatives may result in the development of different forms of rare, usually congenital, urolithiasis with radiolucent forms of stones. A congenital deficiency of the activity of the enzyme adenine-phosphoribosyl transferase results in an increased concentration of 2,8-dihydroxy-adenine in the urine, which is a poorly water-soluble substance whose solubility, furthermore, is nearly independent of alterations in the urine pH. The disease is rare and affects children at a very young age. A defect of the enzyme xanthine-oxidase with an autosomal recessive mode of inheritance results in formation of xanthine stones in about 40% of the affected children [24]. Another rare cause of renal stone formation is a deficiency of the enzyme hypoxanthine-guanine-phosphoribosyl transferase (Lesch-Nyhan syndrome), which causes an enormously increased concentration

of urate to levels more than 10-fold normal, with subsequent stone formation. However, dietetic causes of urate stone formation are much rarer in children than in adults.

1.6.3
Clinical Presentation and Evaluation

The presence of urinary calculi in young children has to alert the physician to recurrent UTI, functional or morphological disorders and anomalies of the urinary tract, especially neurogenic bladder dysfunction with urinary retention. Older children more frequently present with metabolic disorders.

Whereas in adulthood renal colic is the most frequent acute symptom of urolithiasis, children show more unspecific symptoms, such as poor feeding, nausea, vomiting, constipation and diffuse abdominal pain. Recurrent UTI is frequently the first symptom of urolithiasis. Nevertheless, gross haematuria, dysuria or voiding disorder are not uncommon. Fever, shivering and oligouria should already be regarded as complications. The frequency of spontaneous stone passage is lower than in adults. The cutoff for the probability of spontaneous passage is size under 5 mm. Larger calculi usually need therapeutic intervention. Stones in the lower urinary tract are now rare in central Europe. The most usual symptoms are recurrent UTI, urgency, frequency and gross haematuria.

Clinical evaluation uses the various imaging methods in addition to specific laboratory investigations of urine and blood. Ultrasonography of the urinary tract is currently the most important tool in detecting stones in nearly all parts of the urinary tract. Ultrasound allows sensitive imaging of calculi in the kidney, the proximal and distal ureter and the bladder. The middle part of the ureter is usually accessible only to an unsatisfactory degree by ultrasound. Indirect signs of renal obstruction, such as dilatation of the upper parts of the collecting system, may lead to the diagnosis. Nevertheless, the impossibility of detecting a suspected stone by sonography has resulted in the initiation of IV pyelography, which provides direct visualization especially of calcium-containing urinary calculi. Other stones may be detected as a filling defect in the contrasted collecting system, ureter or bladder. Even though the importance of IV pyelography in the diagnosis of urolithiasis has decreased markedly, it is still strongly recommended before any form of therapeutic intervention, because of its better visualization of the morphology of the urinary tract. VCUG or radionuclear static or diuretic renography may help to detect simultaneous anomalies of the urinary tract contributing to stone formation, such as ureteral obstruction or VUR. Retrograde pyelography and cystoscopy are indicated only in selected cases and can usually be regarded as part of the therapy.

Whereas the imaging methods allow the detection of a urinary calculus, its exact make-up usually remains uncertain. Therefore, several laboratory investigations have been established to detect the possible causes and components of the calculus. Nevertheless, the exact make-up of a urinary stone can only be suspected on the basis of blood and urine analyses and direct physical analysis of the stone itself is necessary to confirm or amend the suspected constituents.

Urinalysis could disclose microhaematuria, leucocyturia, urine pH and crystals. Urine culture may disclose colonization with urease-positive bacteria. Quantitative analysis of the different ingredients of the urine may help to reveal the cause of urolithiasis. The investigations most frequently done are the daily urinary excretion of calcium, phosphate, oxalate, urate and cystine. Special tests, as suspected by Pak and co-workers, for example, can differentiate between the different forms of hypercalciuria [104]. A positive cyanide nitroprussic reaction of the urine indicates the presence of cystinuria. Nevertheless, cystinuria alone is not an inevitable indicator of cystine stone formation.

Blood investigations in paediatric patients with urolithiasis should include the serum concentrations of bicarbonate, calcium, phosphate, urate and parathyroid hormone. Special analyses, e. g. the activity of adenine-phosphoribosyl transferase in lytic erythrocytes, indicate the presence of 2,8-dihydroxyadenine stones.

1.6.4
Therapy

Adequate treatment of urinary calculi in children includes three major principles. There are conservative medical and dietetic approaches, minimal and more invasive approaches, and aftertreatment aimed at the prevention of recurrence. One approach alone is usually not enough to treat and prevent urolithiasis adequately and over a long duration, and a well-considered combination of all provides the best results. The choice of the method to be used as the primary one should take account mainly of the possibility of simultaneously treating the stone and the specific factors in its causation. However, in many cases this is impossible. Therefore, the stone has to be treated first, to prevent secondary damage to the urinary tract. The reason for the stone formation must be analysed and treated later on.

1.6.4.1
Conservative Treatment and Stone Prevention

As in adults, the therapy of the acute symptoms of urolithiasis in children includes adequate analgesia, spasmolysis, treatment of UTI with antibiotics and a increased fluid turnover. Under these conditions about 75% of the calculi that enter the proximal ureter may be passed spontaneously. The others need additional treatment.

The majority of stones that have already become clinically relevant cannot be treated adequately by a conservative approach alone. A combination with invasive measures is commonly needed. The only exception is the case of stones consisting exclusively of urate. As urate crystallizes only in acid environments (pH <6), alkalization of the urine contributes to litholysis and to a decreased size of calculi. Nevertheless, as urate stones are rare in childhood, the clinical relevance of urine alkalization in direct stone therapy can be virtually disregarded. It does, however, have an important place in prevention of stone recurrence (see below). However, medical and dietetic treatments also have important roles in the therapy of the different specific conditions that foster stone formation.

INFECTIOUS STONES ▶ In the case of infectious stones adequate and long-lasting antibiotic treatment adapted to the bacterial susceptibility is necessary. However, as a major part of the bacterial colonization is restricted to the calculus itself, and the local effect of the antibiotics is insufficient, complete stone removal is mandatory to avoid recurrence. Acidulation of the urine worsens the conditions for bacterial growth and impairs phosphate precipitation due to the development of struvite or apatite. The most frequently used medications are substances containing hydrochloric acid or ammonium chloride. Furthermore, restriction of the urinary phosphate concentration also impairs infectious stone formation. This can be done in two ways: reduction of the phosphate food intake and restriction of the intestinal phosphate resorption by aluminium-containing substances.

HYPERCALCIURIA AND HYPEROXALURIA ▶ Thiazide diuretics in a daily dosage of 2 mg/kg body weight increase the tubular re-uptake of calcium, contributing to a lower urine calcium concentration and decreased 1,25-(OH) vitamin D activity in patients with the renal form of hypercalciuria. Additional restriction of the sodium intake and a potassium supplement support the thiazide treatment. Besides dietetic restriction of the intestinal calcium supply, the treatment of absorptive forms of hypercalciuria could be sufficiently supported with sodium cellulose phosphate, which binds intestinal calcium and reduces the intestinal calcium resorption. As the resorption of magnesium is also impaired by sodium cellulose phosphate, a magnesium supplement should be given. The treatment of absorptive hypercalciuria due to renal phosphate loss could be treated by substitution of sodium or potassium phosphate. It is, however, necessary to be aware that the simultaneous presence of UTI and urease-positive bacteria means a markedly increased risk of struvite or apatite stone formation.

The treatment of primary hyperoxaluria should be supported by substitution of vitamin B6 to reduce the oxalate concentration of the urine. Furthermore, medical or dietetic enhancement of the urinary concentration of inhibitors of crystallization, such as citrate, magnesium, and pyrophosphate, improves the solubility of oxalate and may prevent new stone formation. The absorptive form of hyperoxaluria can be treated, paradoxically, with calcium substitution, which impairs intestinal resorption of oxalate by forming insoluble calcium oxalate. Furthermore, increased concentrations of urate in the urine contribute to the precipitation of oxalate. Allopurinol impairs urate formation and should be used to reinforce the treatment of hyperoxaluria.

CYSTINURIA ▶ The urinary excretion of cystine is dependent on the sodium concentration in the urine. Restriction of sodium intake, therefore, contributes to a decreased urinary cystine concentration. Alkalization of the urine promotes better solubility of cystine. Adequate substitution with sodium citrate, sodium bicarbonate or acetazolamide increases the urine pH, which should ideally be around 8.0.

Complexors could create compounds with poorly soluble or insoluble substances that improve the solubility dramatically. The D-penicillamine-cysteine complex is about 50-fold as soluble as cystine. The substance can be given by mouth. The main side effects are exanthema, rheumatic symptoms, pancytopenia, proteinuria and vitamin B6 antagonism. Alpha mercapto-propionylglycine shows the same characteristics as D-penicillamine but a higher efficacy with fewer side effects. The main problem is a possible loss of function during long-term application. Another potent inductor of the formation of the better soluble cysteine from cystine is the presence of vitamin C. Substitution of high doses of vitamin C, therefore, is a common measure in the treatment of cystinuria. The risk of inducing oxalate stones is very low.

METAPHYLAXIS ▶ The majority of conservative medical or dietetic measures have no direct effect on existing urinary calculi, but can influence the conditions promoting stone formation and assist in this way in prevention of stone recurrence. A restricted fluid intake contributes to stone formation, because the concentration of the substances contained in the urine is increased by renal water re-uptake. An adequate fluid intake, therefore, is the first measure in prevention of stone recurrence, regardless of the specific reasons for stone formation.

Besides the formation of the infectious struvite or calcium-apatite stones, a basic environment of acidic urine supports crystallization of nearly all other stone-forming urinary ingredients. Alkalization of the urine, therefore, is a major component of adequate preventive treatment against stone recurrence. Furthermore, long-term treatment with inhibitors of crystal aggregation or complexors may prevent new stone formation, especially in patients with calculi due to congenital metabolic disorders.

1.6.4.2
Invasive Treatment

Especially in paediatric patients, the benefit it is thought would accrue from invasive instrumental or operative therapy of urinary calculi has to be weighed precisely against other options. If necessary, in principle the same methods of stone treatment are available for children as for adults. Besides extracorporeal shock-wave lithotripsy (ESWL), all transurethral or percutaneous methods of modern urological endoscopy and open surgical procedures are established treatments for urinary calculi. The method selected depends mainly on the stone's location and size and the age of the patients.

EXTRACORPOREAL SHOCK-WAVE LITHOTRIPSY ▶ If possible, preference in any treatment of urolithiasis in children should be given to ESWL, because of its minimally invasive nature and high efficacy. Except in the mid-part of the ureter, the method allows efficient treatment of stones at nearly all locations in the urinary tract. Shock waves generated piezo-electronically or physically outside the body are focused and applied to the stone to initiate its disintegration. The stone is located by fluoroscopy or ultrasound, which should be used in children whenever this is feasible. As one session of ESWL needs about 2500–3000 impulses and the patient has to keep still throughout the 30–40 minutes needed for the session, general anaesthesia is indispensable for this procedure in paediatric patients. The treatment is usually well tolerated even by very young children and can be repeated after a short interval (not less than 3 days) if the stone disintegration is unsatisfactory or incomplete.

Nevertheless, in spite of its minimally invasive character, ESWL could also inflict major damage on the kidney, as not every shock wave applied hits the stone directly and some can instead hit the surrounding renal parenchymatous and vascular structures. Valid data on long-term effects of ESWL given for kidney function are still lacking.

The most common complications of ESWL are haematuria, pyelonephritis and intrarenal or subcapsular haematoma, which rarely has to be treated by open surgical revision. Such secondary effects as ureteral obstruction caused by passage of stone fragments must be expected, depending on the primary stone size, and these require auxiliary interventions, e.g. ureteral stenting or percutaneous nephrostomy, especially if the case is complicated by pyelonephritis.

The success rate of ESWL is absolutely satisfactory. The rate of complete freedom from stones is about 80%, although a substantial proportion of the patients need at least two or more sessions of treatment [124]. Thus, especially in patients with huge stones, the risk of renal damage, radiation exposure and general anaesthesia from multiple ESWL sessions has to be weighed against the risks of other, more invasive, procedures that may provide higher efficacy.

ENDOSCOPIC TREATMENT ▶ Depending on a stone's location, there are two possible endoscopic approaches to the upper urinary tract. Renal stones can be instrumented by percutaneous nephroscopy, whereas ureteral stones are better reached by transurethral ureteroscopy. Both methods have gained increasing popularity for use in paediatric patients as modern fibreoptic techniques have allowed the development of smaller endoscopes with similar optic and functional qualities.

The indications for percutaneous nephrolitholapaxy are huge calyceal, pelvic or uncomplicated staghorn stones [74]. The procedure needs general anaesthesia. Unproblematic access to the kidney and wide connections between the calyces and the renal pelvis detectable by preoperative IV pyelography are the major conditions for the success of this treatment. The puncture of the kidney under ultrasonographic control should pass the renal parenchyma only for a short distance. After endoscopic visualization, the stone can be disintegrated by sonic or laser litholapaxy. The stone fragments can be evacuated from the collecting system directly under visual control. A percutaneous nephrostomy allows the postoperative passage of residual fragments, and bleeding from the puncture channel can also be staunched.

The main side effects of this method are bleeding complications and usually temporary impairment of renal function. The efficacy of the procedure is high, even though in the case of huge stones more than one session may be necessary. Alternatively, a second approach to residual fragments can be made by ESWL. Nevertheless, in selected cases, percutaneous nephrostolithotomy is an efficient alternative to ESWL and to open surgical procedures.

Especially in the case of distal and mid-ureteral stones when spontaneous passage has failed to occur, a direct transurethral endoscopic approach to the ureter via ureteroscopy is indicated to harvest the stone at once or after laser lithotripsy. Paediatric endoscopes down to a diameter of 9.5 F allow this approach at least in children younger than 12 months, especially if the ureter has been stented for at least 2 days. However, the most frequent indication of transurethral instrumentation in paediatric patients with urolithiasis is auxiliary ureteral DJ-stenting before or after ESWL. Furthermore, spontaneous stone passage can be eased by ureteral stenting and the stone can be resited in a location where it is more easily accessible to ESWL. Therefore, a combination of both methods has a high efficacy and minimizes the risk to the young patients.

OPEN SURGERY ▶ In spite of the high efficacy of ESWL and the increasing popularity of endoscopic methods of lithotripsy, there are still indications for an open surgical approach in paediatric urolithiasis. Complicated staghorn stones and stones secondary to anomalies of the upper urinary tract are common reasons for nephropyelolithotomy or ureterolithotomy. Stones due to ureteropelvic junction obstruction, for example, are harvested during pyeloplasty. Other anomalies, such as horseshoe kidney or renal dystopia, decrease the efficacy of ESWL or endoscopic methods because of the specific anatomical features. Nevertheless, open stone surgery is only necessary with adequate renal function. A precise preoperative evaluation of the renal function by radionuclear renal scintigraphy is therefore mandatory. In cases with severe restricted renal function a simple nephrectomy involves less perioperative risk than an attempt to harvest the stone.

1.7
Vesico-ureteral Reflux

The incidence of reflux in children is about 1%, even though some authors have found this anomaly in up to 18.5% of their own cases [70]. Reflux is a common finding in children with antenatally diagnosed dilatation of the upper urinary tract [159]. Reflux is seen in 70% of children younger than 1 year with UTI. The frequency decreases continuously with age, declining to 5.2% in adults [9]. Even though 85% of reflux cases are in female subjects, among boys presenting with UTI the incidence of reflux is double that in girls. There is a genetic component in the origin of reflux, although the mode of inheritance is not clear. Most authors suggest a polygenic mode of transmission. However, Noe et al. propose a dominant inheritance with variable penetrance [101].

1.7.1
Aetiology and Pathogenesis

1.7.1.1
Primary Reflux

Primary reflux is caused by a congenital anomaly of the ureterovesical junction. As in normal children, on its way to the orifice the ureter tunnels through the bladder mucosa for a distance that is equivalent to about double its own diameter. In primary reflux this distance is significantly shorter [105]. This means a ureter with both a large calibre and a short intravesical length may cause reflux. The short length of the submucosal section of the ureter in primary reflux is mainly caused by an abnormal position of the ureteral orifice in the vesical trigone. The most common finding is lateralization of the orifice. This is probably caused by a lower evagination of the ureteric bud from the mesonephric duct early in fetal development. Another explanation is impaired anchoring of the ureteral orifice in the bladder trigone owing to muscular insufficiency. This would result in lateralization of the orifice during bladder filling.

1.7.1.2
Secondary Reflux

Secondary reflux is caused by subvesical obstruction with consequent elevation of the intravesical pressure. The obstruction may be anatomical or functional. Posterior urethral valves is the most common anatomical diagnosis in secondary reflux in children. The more frequent functional causes of secondary reflux are neurogenic or nonneurogenic voiding disorders with a significant decrease in bladder compliance or increase in intravesical pressure. Although the normal ureterovesical junction resists acute elevations of intravesical pressure to over 100 cmH$_2$O, chronic stress damages its antireflux mechanism [69]. Children with involvement of the spinal cord in particular have an elevated risk of developing reflux.

Secondary reflux can also occur during lower UTI. The inflammation causes a decrease in bladder compliance and also an increase in intravesical pressure by way of inhibition of bladder contractions. Furthermore, endotoxins of gram-negative bacteria may cause atonia of the ureteric muscles, thereby affecting the antireflux mechanism of the ureterovesical junction. This is why VCUG for diagnosis of VUR should not be planned during episodes of acute UTI.

1.7.2
Clinical Presentation

The initial symptom in the majority of children with reflux is UTI with episodes of high fever. In addition, the patients have dysuria, pyuria or urinary frequency. In contrast to adults, in children pyelonephritis causes more gastrointestinal symptoms than flank pain. Some patients with reflux report flank pain even without evidence of UTI, especially during voiding or when the bladder is full.

Only in newborn babies are the symptoms unspecific. Whereas high fever is very uncommon in these children, lethargy or just not doing well leads to the diagnosis.

Untreated chronic reflux in children causes renal scarring. This leads to a continuous loss of renal parenchyma with consequent insufficiency of renal function, which is known as reflux nephropathy (Chap. 4, Case 25). The majority of renal scarring in reflux is associated with recurrent UTI. Nevertheless, antenatal primary high-grade reflux is frequently associated with morphological renal damage in the absence of infectious disease (primary dysplasia). It has been suggested that this phenomenon is caused by obstruction during the early fetal development of the upper urinary tract. Usually, these patients show a primary impairment of renal function in the affected kidney (Chap. 4, Case 23) Chronic reflux nephropathy may also be associated with arterial hypertension.

1.7.3
Clinical Evaluation

The clinical evaluation of VUR is divided into two different subgroups. One subgroup is subsumed under documentation of the presence of reflux, and the other under symptoms caused by VUR, especially UTI.

1.7.3.1
Documentation of UTI

UTI is the most common clinical symptom of VUR. Timely evaluation of UTI is highly recommended as it makes an early start of specific treatment possible, which may prevent major damage to the renal functional tissue. The urine samples of the patients should be investigated microscopically. But even more important is the establishment of a urine culture to test for bacterial colonization and determine what antibiotic therapy should be given. Urine collection should be oriented to the age of the patients and the probability of external contamination. The most reliable way of avoiding contamination is to collect urine by suprapubic needle aspiration, if possible under ultrasonic guidance. Simultaneous bladder voiding may complicate the procedure and increase the risk of a false puncture. Furthermore, the needle trauma may cause iatrogenic microhaematuria, leading to misinterpretation. Nevertheless, any growth of bacteria after needle aspiration must be followed by further evaluation.

Another very reliable way of avoiding external contamination is to collect urine by bladder catheterization after sufficient disinfection around the urethral orifice. Growth of more than 10^3 colonies per millilitre of urine should prompt further evaluation. In older children with sufficient voiding control, urine evaluation by midstream urine analysis may lead to representative results. More than 10^5 colonies are considered to be significant. Often used, but not reliable, is urine collection via bags that are attached to the genitalia of the little patients to collect spontaneously voided portions. The risk of contamination is very high. The method is therefore not advisable and should be avoided whenever possible. Nevertheless, growth of more than 10^5 colonies should still be regarded as significant, but identification of the bacteria is important to allow differentiation between real UTI and contamination.

1.7.3.2
Voiding Cysto-urethrography

The most important and sensitive tool that can be used to detect VUR is VCUG, whether fluoroscopic or radionuclear techniques are used. The cystography should be performed without anaesthesia and muscle relaxants if possible. Furthermore, as acute bladder infection can affect intravesical pressure or the ureterovesical junction, VCUG should be performed some weeks after adequate therapy of an episode of acute UTI.

Both forms of cystography need bladder catheterization to administer the contrast medium. Reflux may be expected during the filling phase and the voiding phase. Thus, to exclude reflux, both phases need to be observed by the investigator. Furthermore, the sensitivity of detecting reflux by cystography increases if more than one cycle of filling and voiding per investigation is observed.

The decision between radionuclear or conventional (fluoroscopic) cystography is dependent on the extent of anatomical damage of the bladder and kidney expected, as radionuclear cystography is not capable of showing any anatomical detail of the bladder or upper urinary tract. However, without suspected functional impairment of the bladder, nuclear cystography is more sensitive in detecting reflux than the conventional method but involves significantly less radiation exposure. Therefore, the method is particularly suitable for following reflux in patients already diagnosed with the disease.

1.7.3.3
Ultrasonography

Nowadays, the majority of children with higher grades of reflux are diagnosed during the peripartal period. The dilatation of the upper urinary tract in these patients is normally found by fetal ultrasound evaluation during routine antenatal controls. Within days after birth a control ultrasonography is performed. In the case of persisting dilatation of the ureter, renal pelvis and/or calices, VCUG is indicated. Especially when dilatation is bilateral the suspected diagnosis of VUR must be confirmed as a matter of urgency in the newborn period.

In cases of low-grade reflux without dilatation of the upper urinary tract, routine B-mode ultrasonography cannot detect reflux but does serve as a sensitive tool for the evaluation of renal damage, so that it has almost replaced IV pyelography in this context. Volumetry of the kidneys by ultrasound may detect impaired renal growth of the affected side and compensatory growth of the contralateral side as a sign of chronic renal damage by persisting reflux. Additionally, renal scarring may be suspected, but not definitively proven, on the basis of ultrasound investigation.

Ultrasound cysto-urethrography using sonicated human albumin as contrast medium has been shown to detect VUR very sensitively in clinical studies [8], but the procedure is not yet adequately established.

1.7.3.4
^{99m}Tc-DMSA Uptake

Intravenous administration of ^{99}technetium-labelled DMSA is used to investigate renal perfusion and thereby represent the amount of the regularly functioning proximal tubuli. The uptake of the contrast medium correlates with the glomerular filtration rate [143]. Infectious disease, such as pyelonephritis, impairs the regular uptake of ^{99m}Tc-DMSA, thus showing damaged renal tissue very specifically and sensitively as scars caused by loss of perfusion of the renal cortex. DMSA uptake therefore plays a major part in evaluation of the effects of VUR on renal tissue. Its results strongly influence decisions about what further treatment will be adequate.

1.7.3.5
IV Pyelography

IV Pyelography gives information on the renal function, damaged renal tissue and anatomy of the upper and lower urinary tract. However, it now plays only a minor role in the evaluation of VUR. Most of the information can be much more easily and more sensitively obtained by ultrasonography or renal scintigraphy with minimal radiation exposure or none at all. Nonetheless, IV pyelography is more sensitive in the evaluation of additional anatomical alteration of the urinary tract, as reflux is often combined with other genitourinary anomalies, such as ureteral duplication or bladder diverticula.

1.7.3.6
Urethrocystoscopy

Endoscopy of the lower urinary tract has only a minor role in detecting VUR, but provides sensitive information on anatomical details causing or caused by the disease. It may detect subvesical obstruction. In particular, the evaluation of the proximal urethra in boys in whom posterior urethral valves are suspected provides the possibility of diagnosis and therapy by the same procedure. Furthermore, endoscopy of the bladder detects abnormal positioning and configuration of the ureteral orifice (Fig. 12). Even though the value in terms of predicting the degree of reflux by these findings is uncertain, they may help the urological surgeon to plan the extent and method of the operative treatment and should therefore be performed preoperatively in any patient with VUR.

1.7.3.7
Urodynamics

Every patient in whom secondary reflux is suspected should be evaluated by urodynamic studies to check for any intravesical pressure increase, instability of the detrusor muscle, voiding disorder or infravesical obstruction. The complete urodynamic evaluation includes cystomanometry, uroflowmetry and electromyography of the pelvic floor. It should be combined with a fluoroscopic voiding cystography, because massive VUR may impair interpretation of the results by increasing bladder capacity, thereby mimicking increased bladder compliance.

1.7.4
Grading

In the early 1960s preliminary attempts were made to find a specific grading system for VUR. Based on the findings of VCUG, different systems were proposed, focusing on different morphological alterations such as widening of the ureter or calices during voiding or the filling phase of the bladder. The currently used international classification is a fusion of the two most frequently used grading systems of Heikel and Parkkulainen and Dwoskin and Perlmutter [76] (Fig. 13).

1.7.5
Therapy

The main goal of any therapy for VUR is to avoid damage to the renal parenchyma by recurrent upper UTI. Most cases of reflux in children resolve spontaneously. Especially in low-grade reflux (grade I–II), in which the ureter still has a normal calibre, the rates of spontaneous resolution are between 62 % and 85 % [36, 66]. It is rarer for higher grades of reflux to resolve spontaneously. Studies of patients with grade

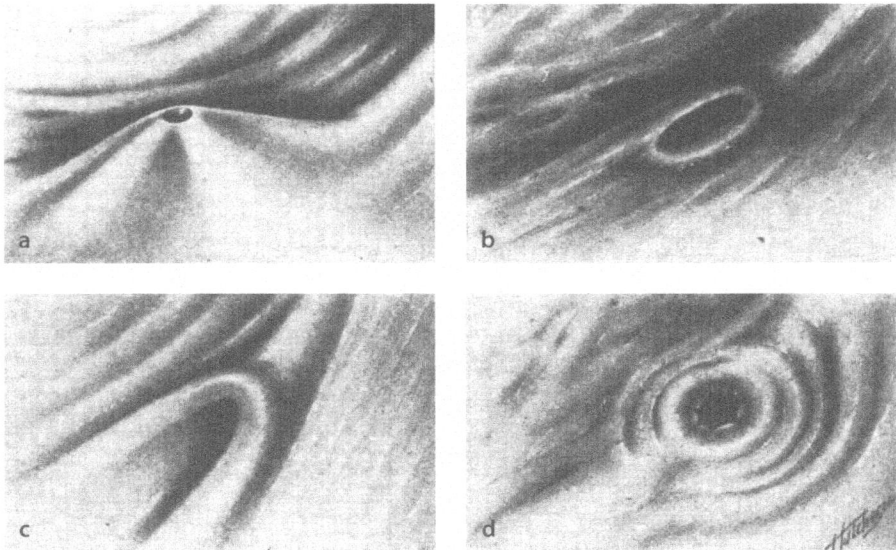

Fig. 12a–d. Typical variants of the configuration of the ureteral orifice in vesicoureteral reflux (VUR). **a** Normal; **b** stadium; **c** horseshoe; **d** golf hole

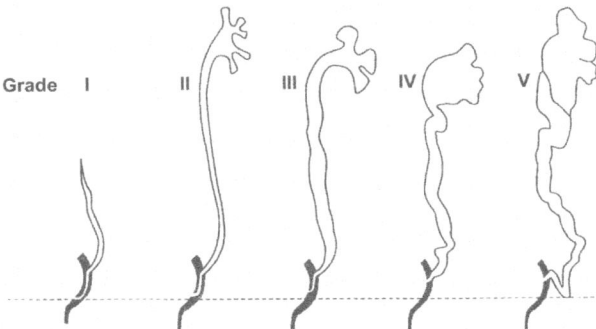

Fig. 13. International classification of the different grades of VUR. Notice the shortened intramural distance of the distal ureter with increasing grade of reflux

IV–V reflux showed a spontaneous resolution rate of only 9–30% [94, 131]. The resolution of reflux is also dependent on the age of the patients at diagnosis. The younger the patient the greater the likelihood of complete spontaneous resolution of the disease. In addition, the grade of reflux may decline during age.

Spontaneous resolution of reflux may be due to a changing or decreasing ratio between the ureteral diameter and its submucosal distance during ageing. Furthermore, maturation of the bladder during its growth causes an increase in bladder capacity, a decrease in intravesical pressure, especially during voiding, and a consequent increase in bladder compliance that may contribute to resolution of the reflux. Spontaneous resolution of reflux can be expected throughout the whole of the longitudinal growth period of childhood, but its probability decreases with age.

However, primary symptomatic VUR, if maturation does not take place during further development of the bladder, requires operative correction. In the case of secondary reflux, the timely treatment of the secondary causes, such as voiding disorders, promises complete resolution of reflux and avoids alterations in the anatomy of the ureterovesical junction, which could result in irreparable injury. The management of normal bladder filling and emptying, therefore, is one of the most important goals of this treatment. It involves reducing the bladder outlet resistance and normalizing the intravesical pressure by surgical or medical means.

However, after exclusion or sufficient treatment of secondary causes, the decision on whether to treat reflux conservatively or surgically has to be made individually, with due consideration for reflux grade, grade of renal damage, age and sex of the patient and parental compliance, even though a conservative approach may be justified in almost every case. Nevertheless, the question of whether conservative or surgical treatment can prevent progressive reflux nephropathy is still under discussion [134].

1.7.5.1
Medical Treatment

Most lower grade refluxes resolve spontaneously. Therefore, medical treatment mostly includes the avoidance of reflux nephropathy caused by recurrent UTI. One of the most important parts of the management of reflux is the diagnosis followed by rapid and adequate treatment of the first symptomatic urinary infection. After the evaluation of reflux, any patient without suggestive serious nephropathy should be treated by a conservative approach to allow possible resolution or down-grading of reflux. Therefore, antibiotic prophylaxis should be continued for at least 1 year. The dosage is at most half, but more frequently a fifth, of the therapeutic dosage of the drug selected for use. Especially in toilet-trained children, it should be given once daily at night, because the night is the longest period of urine storage in the bladder, with the highest risk of the development of UTI. The medication used depends on the age of the patients. Children younger than 3 months should be treated with amino-penicillin derivatives. Older children, in whom the biliary function has matured, should be treated with trimethoprim alone, a combination of trimethoprim and sulfamethoxazole, or nitrofurantoin. The last involves the lowest risk of intestinal complications, as the substance is maximally concentrated in the urine. Additionally, oral cephalosporins can be used for long-term antibiotic prophylaxis.

Intermittent treatment of recurrent UTI without prophylaxis during the free intervals more frequently leads to renal scarring and is therefore highly ineffective and should not be performed.

The main problem of long-term antibiotic treatment is parental compliance. To avoid misunderstandings, it is important to give the parents brief information, before any decision is made on therapy, about the risks of reflux nephropathy and complications of the medical management as they compare with the chance of a spontaneous resolution of the disease as the patients get older. Whenever problems are expected with the parental compliance over a sufficiently long period, a surgical approach should be favoured even in cases of symptomatic lower grade reflux, to avoid any renal damage.

The follow-up of reflux patients managed medically includes a urine culture every 3 months to detect breakthrough infections. In addition, ultrasonic investigations of the kidneys and bladder and a VCUG should be performed once yearly. If beginning reflux nephropathy is suspected, a ^{99m}Tc-DMSA uptake is helpful to detect renal scarring and decreasing renal function. Breakthrough infections, increases in renal scarring and a decrease in renal function are unambiguous signs of failing conservative treatment and require surgical correction of the reflux.

1.7.5.2
Operative Treatment

The goal of any operative treatment of VUR is to establish an antirefluxive mechanism of the ureterovesical junction. This can be obtained by increasing compression of the transvesical part of the ureter during bladder filling and increasing intravesical pressure. In addition, the normal bladder function should not be impaired by the result of the operation. Most of the operative approaches that can be adopted in reflux therefore use a ureterocystoneostomy with submucosal tunnelling of the distal ureter. The length of the submucosal distance should be at least 5 times the ureteral diameter [105]. Success rates of up to 99% are not uncommon in centres where a lot of experience has accumulated [37]. Meanwhile, there are many different techniques of antireflux surgery. They can be divided into endoscopic techniques, open surgical extravehicular techniques, and open surgical intra- or transvesical techniques. The latter again are subdivided into suprahiatal and infrahiatal techniques, which are defined by the original position relative to the position of the neo-orifice after ureteral reimplantation. A selection of the different operative approaches currently most often used are detailed below.

ENDOSCOPIC TREATMENT ▶ Endoscopic approaches in VUR provides lesser operative trauma and a short stay in hospital, and therefore maximal parental compliance. The major problem of these techniques lies in the lower success rates, especially in higher grades of reflux related to the open surgical techniques. In general, endoscopic treatment of reflux can be managed as an outpatient procedure. The minimally invasive character of the operation offers the possibility of using the method as an alternative to long-term antibiotic prophylaxis, especially when parental compliance is low.

The procedure is simple. During cystoscopy a tissue-augmenting substance is injected into the lamina propria behind the submucosal distal part of the refluxive ureter. The position of the ureteral orifice is raised. The depot serves as an abutment, against which the orifice is fixed to provide a better seal during bladder filling or voiding.

The substances most frequently used are Teflon (polytetrafluoroethylene), bovine collagen and dextranomers. There is most experience with Teflon. The use of Teflon in endoscopic management yields excellent results, especially in low-grade refluxes. Success rates up to 92% are reported, but are dependent on the grade of reflux and the number of repeated

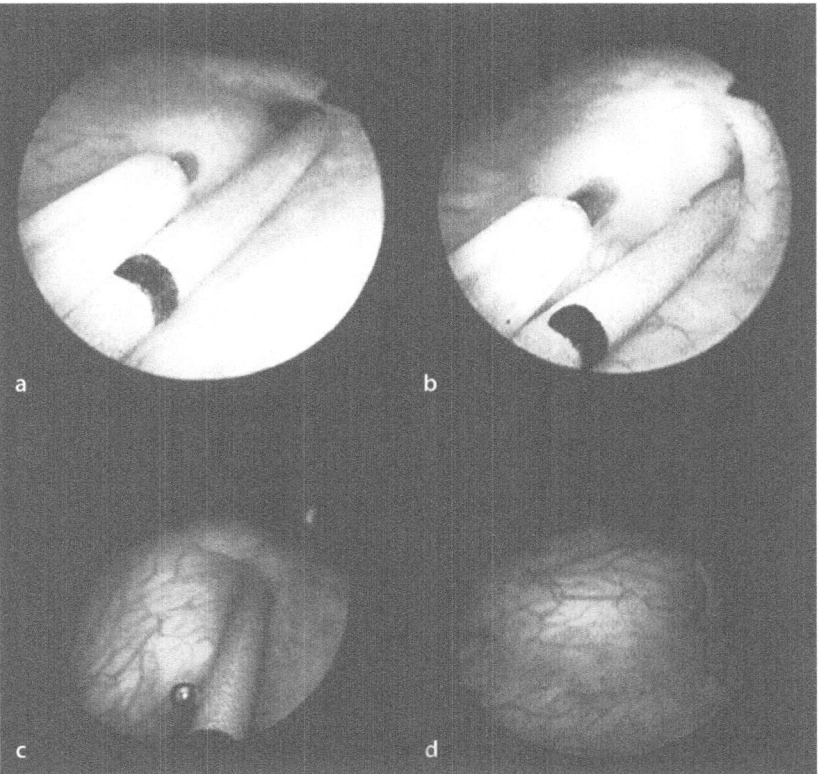

Fig. 14a–d. Endoscopic treatment of vesicoureteral reflux. **a** Positioning of the injection needle caudally of the ureteral orifice (stented with a ureter catheter). **b** Injection of the bulk-ing agent with consecutive augmentation of the dorsal wall of the orifice. **c, d** Completed injection **a** before and **d** after removal of the ureter catheter

treatments. The major disadvantage of Teflon is its tendency to migrate not only locally but also over distances, which may lead to granuloma in the lung, brain and the lymphatic system.

Therefore, alternative substances have been tested. Bovine collagen cross-linked with glutaraldehyde has also been used to correct reflux. The initial results of various authors were promising, but long-term results showed very high rates of recurrences, which were attributed to the tendency of collagen to disappear with time.

Dextranomers mixed with sodium hyaluronate solution (Deflux) can also be used as a tissue-augmenting substance in endoscopic correction of reflux. The results are promising. Nevertheless, long-term results are not yet available. However, it seems that Deflux combines the advantages and efficacy of Teflon with a lack of its negative side effects and is currently, therefore, the most promising material for use in endoscopic reflux surgery (Chap. 4, Case 26) [115] (Fig. 14).

EXTRAVESICAL APPROACH ▶ Open surgical techniques in VUR have a very high success rate. As they are invasive procedures the patients should be hospi-talized for some days. The extravesical techniques reduce the length of stay in hospital and the periop-erative complication rate, because the bladder stays closed without urinary contamination of the structures surrounding the bladder.

One of the most popular extravesical approaches in reflux is the technique developed and described almost simultaneously by Lich [79] in the US and Gregoir [49] in Europe.

The strategy is to embed the ureter in a submucosal tunnel without opening the bladder. The distal ureter is prepared for its insertion into the bladder. The muscular layer of the detrusor muscle is incised along a length of 4–5 cm down to the mucosa without injuring it. The incision runs from the uretero-vesical junction in a cranial, slightly lateral, line. The ureter is then laid on the mucosa, and the detrusor muscle is closed over it, creating the antirefluxive mechanism (Fig. 15).

The Lich-Gregoir technique is easy and successful in up to 98% [6]. It does have some disadvantages. The ureteral orifice has to be positioned orthotopically. Para-ureteral diverticula may cause problems. Furthermore, the mobilization of the bladder may damage nerves to the bladder, resulting in impaired

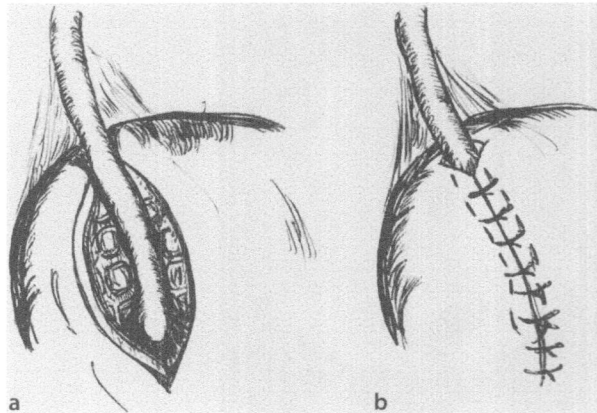

Fig. 15a, b. Principle of ureterocystoneostomy by Lich-Gregoir technique. **a** Incision of the external bladder wall down to the mucosa. **b** Closure of the bladder wall over the embedded distal part of the ureter

bladder drainage and urinary retention. Therefore, the technique should not be used for a bilateral approach to VUR.

INTRA- OR TRANSVESICAL APPROACH ▶ The intra- or transvesical techniques in antireflux surgery can allow correction of any grade and form of VUR. The perioperative trauma is greater than with an extravesical approach. The stay in hospital is therefore slightly longer. The complication rate is slightly higher. Nevertheless, because of their exceptionally high success rates – up to 99% [17] – intravesical approaches are used very frequently. Although many different techniques of extra- or transvesical ureteral reimplantation have been described, only a few of them are discussed below.

The technique described in 1958 by Politano and Leadbetter [111] is still especially popular. The strat-

egy is to create a new and adequate submucosal course of the ureter after complete reimplantation of the refluxive ureter (Fig. 16). The major disadvantage of the original procedure is the transvesical "blind" separation of the bladder wall from the peritoneum. This manipulation contains a risk of injuring intraperitoneal structures, especially bowel perforation, with possible lethal consequences.

Another very efficient technique of ureteral reimplantation was presented by Cohen [31]. The strategy is to elongate the submucosal course of the ureter via a reimplantation from the original insertion place across the trigonum (Fig. 17). Especially in bilateral reflux, the technique avoids extended bladder mobilization with the risk of neurogenic disorder. Furthermore, the risk of damaging peritoneal structures is minimized by the exclusively transvesical approach. The success rates, at up to 99% [20], are equal to those obtained with the Politano-Leadbetter technique. The major disadvantages of the Cohen cross-trigonal technique are the problems that must be expected with later retrograde endoscopic manipulation at the ureter (Chap. 4, Case 25).

As an alternative, ureteral reimplantation by the psoas hitch technique is very efficient. The strategy is to mobilize the lateral part of the bladder from the pelvis and fix it to the psoas muscle proximal to the iliac vessels (Fig. 18). This means that the technique offers the possibility of bridging an insufficient ureteral length caused by injury of the distal ureter. Furthermore, the manoeuvre allows the formation of extra long submucosal tunnels, which offers the option of reimplanting ureters with badly distended distal diameter without further modelling. The psoas hitch technique is generally used in cases

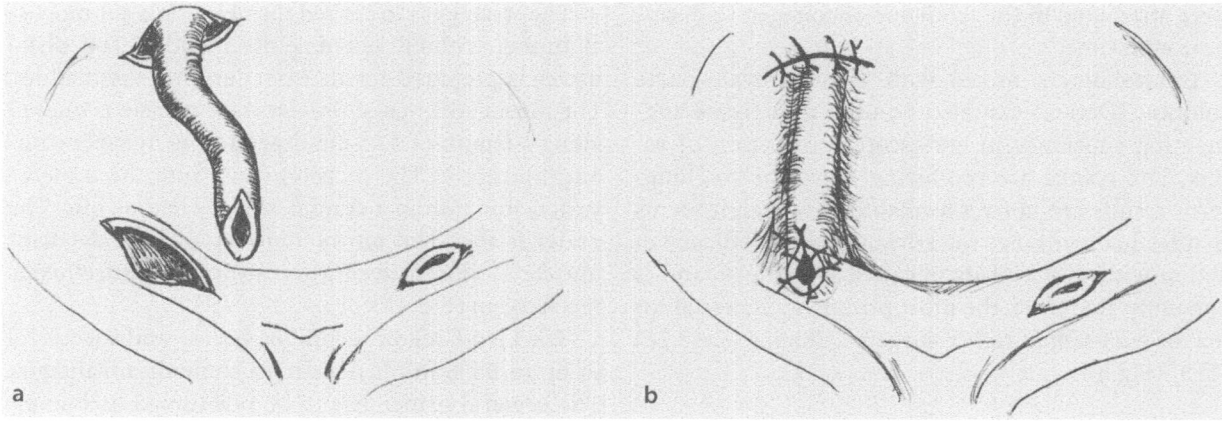

Fig. 16a, b. Principle of ureterocystoneostomy by Politano-Leadbetter technique. **a** Situs after mobilization of the refluxive ureter and reinsertion via the newly created hiatus after retrovesical cranial preparation. **b** Ureteral reimplantation after submucosal tunnelling

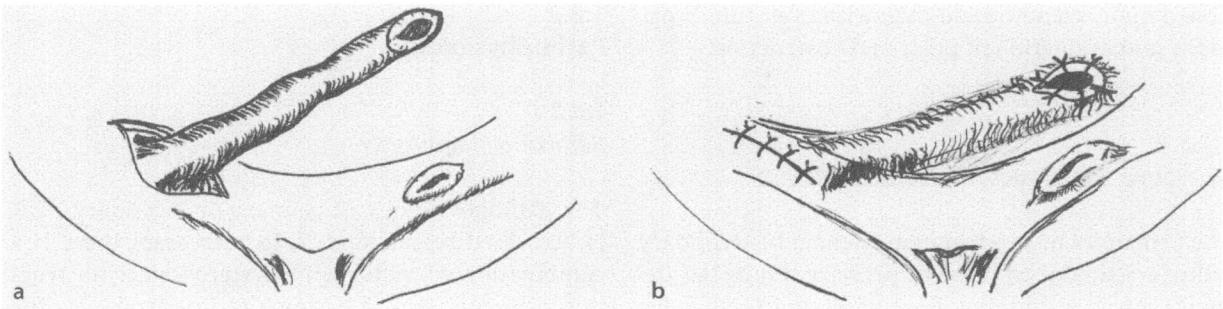

Fig. 17 a, b. Principle of ureterocystoneostomy in cross-trigonal technique (Cohen). **a** Transvesical mobilization of the distal refluxive ureter. **b** Ureteral reimplantation after submucosal tunnelling cross over the trigone

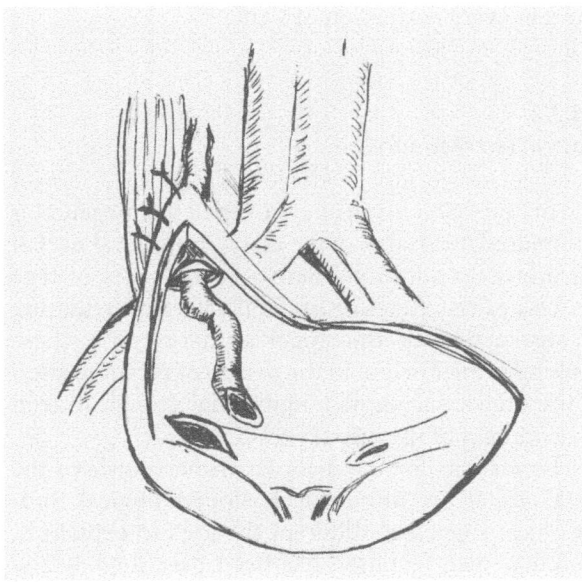

Fig. 18. Modification of ureterocystoneostomy in psoas-hitch technique. Following explantation of the refluxive ureter the bladder is mobilized on the same side and hitched to the psoas muscle cranial to the pelvic vessels. The new hiatus of the ureter is created at the hitched part, and the ureter is reimplanted after submucosal tunnelling in a manner analogous to the Politano-Leadbetter technique

of recurrent reflux or obstruction after failed prior reimplantation. But the technique is also frequently used as a first choice in antireflux surgery. The success rates are similar to those of other trans- or intravesical techniques.

1.7.5.3
Postoperative Outcome and Follow-up

COMPLICATIONS ▶ While the open surgical techniques, especially, yield very high success rates, there are typical complications of ureteral reimplantation. Insufficient length of the submucosal tunnel causes persistent reflux, which results in re-operation. However, there may also be transient reflux of the contralateral, unaffected, ureter, which is secondary to trigonal oedema with dislocation of the contralateral orifice and consequent shortening of the submucosal course of the distal ureter. Persistence of postoperative contralateral reflux is extremely rare, and the management, therefore, is conservative.

Ureteral obstruction after reimplantation is also a common complication. Ischaemia of the distal part of the ureter with consequent development of scar tissue with a tendency to shrink leads to obstruction. In these cases, reoperation is unavoidable. Another explanation for obstruction is angulation of the ureteral insertion, which causes increasing obstruction with increasing bladder volume. In most cases the neo-implantation of the ureter was too far lateral. Persistent obstruction by angulation needs reoperation.

Postoperative transient obstruction is observed more frequently and is caused by trigonal oedema or submucosal bleeding in the region of the neo-implantation. In general, reoperation is not necessary, even if transient percutaneous nephrostomy is needed.

FOLLOW-UP ▶ After surgical correction of VUR the patients have to be followed up carefully. Long-term antibiotic prophylaxis should be performed for at least 6 weeks postoperatively, but if possible up to the first radiological assessment 3 months after the operation. At this time a radionuclear or fluoroscopic VCUG should be performed to re-evaluate the postoperative outcome. After documentation of the operative success the antibiotic prophylaxis can be stopped. Further controls should include urinalysis, blood pressure evaluation and ultrasound investigations of the kidneys. Renal scars, hydronephrosis, impaired renal growth or recurrent urinary infections requires a new evaluation with cysto-urethrography and evaluation of postrenal obstruction.

1.7.5.4
Operative Techniques in Secondary Reflux

The principles of surgical management of secondary reflux are similar to those of primary reflux, but the indications are different. First of all, the reasons for secondary reflux must have been treated. The main goal is to reduce intravesical pressure, which is frequently caused by subvesical obstruction and/or neurogenic dysfunction of the bladder. After successful treatment of the subvesical obstruction, conservative strategies using anticholinergic agents are indicated. Patients without adequate response to conservative management should undergo augmentation of the bladder, using different segments of the bowel, for example. This procedure can be combined with ureteral reimplantation in the augmented part of the bladder. Only persistent secondary reflux in patients with normal intravesical pressure should be planned for isolated antireflux surgery using the same techniques as for primary reflux.

1.8
Megaureter

1.8.1
Definition

The term 'megaureter' means an inhomogeneous group of anomalies of the ureter without a specific entity. The anomalies have only dilatation of the ureter in common, which is caused by different pathologies of the urinary tract. Depending on these differences, the spectrum of megaureter is divided into subgroups. The management of each particular subgroup varies considerably depending on the specific reason for it. The conditions referred to as megaureter are classified into four major subgroups by cause of dilatation. There are (1) refluxing, (2) obstructed, (3) nonrefluxing and nonobstructed, and (4) refluxing and obstructed megaureters. Each subgroup is divided further into primary or secondary causes (Table 1).

1.8.2
Pathophysiology

1.8.2.1
Refluxing Megaureter

The pathophysiology of primary or secondary VUR is described in section 1.7. In rare cases there is a combination of reflux and ureterovesical obstruction, which is caused by impaired peristalsis in the distal intramural part of the affected ureter. As in these cases conservative management of reflux involves a risk of losing kidney function, recognition of this phenomenon is mandatory and has to be kept in mind in every evaluation of VUR.

1.8.2.2
Obstructed Megaureter

The main reason for primary obstructed megaureter is impaired peristalsis of the distal intramural part of the ureter. In addition, there are rare cases of true stenosis of the ureter or ureteral valves contributing to obstruction of the upper urinary tract. These cases have their origin in the period of recanalization of the ureter during its longitudinal growth in fetal development of the urinary tract.

The reasons for the disorder in peristalsis of the distal ureter are unknown. Histopathological findings have suggested different theories to explain it. Muscular disorientation has been described, which would alter the normal cooperation of muscular fibres that is needed for normal peristaltic movement of a tubular system [92]. Other authors have suggested both muscular hypoplasia and muscular hypertrophy, interstitial fibrosis of the ureteral wall and increased collagen deposition in the intracellular space as contributory factors in impaired peristalsis [93, 102]. The question of why only the distal part of the ureter is affected remains unanswered, but it is suggested that the ureterovesical junction and the ureteropelvic junction are the last areas to be recanalized during normal fetal development of the ureter. Recent studies suggest a genetics-based defect of the subtype-2 angiotensin II receptor, which may lead to impaired muscular development of the ureter [52].

Table 1. Megaureter

Reflux		Obstruction		Nonrefluxing + nonobstructed		Refluxing + obstructed	
Primary	Secondary	Primary	Secondary	Primary	Secondary	Primary	Secondary

A secondary obstructed megaureter is caused by external impairment of the ureterovesical junction. This form of megaureter is commonly associated with decompensated voiding disorders caused by neurogenic or nonneurogenic bladder dysfunction or infravesical obstruction. All lead to intravesical pressure elevation, causing larger discrepancies between intraureteral and intravesical pressure. This causes impaired transportation of urine by normal ureteral peristalsis, with consequent hyperplasia of muscle fibres of the distal ureteral wall.

Another possible cause of secondary megaureter is fibrosis of the bladder wall around the transmural part of the ureter, caused by chronic infection of the bladder wall. This would also impair the peristalsis of the distal ureter.

Other causes of secondary obstructed megaureter resulting from ureterovesical junction obstruction, such as bladder diverticula or ureteroceles, are described elsewhere.

1.8.2.3
Nonrefluxing, Nonobstructed Megaureter

The diagnosis of nonrefluxing, nonobstructed megaureter is made after exclusion of any other reason. In these patients the dilatation of the upper urinary tract has no influence on kidney function or renal urinary output. The pathophysiology remains completely unknown. So-called secondary nonrefluxing nonobstructed megaureter may be caused by excessive urine production as a result of diabetes mellitus or insipidus or other polyuric nephropathies. Primary causes of nonrefluxing, nonobstructed megaureter may be alterations of ureteral compliance during development of the upper urinary tract. There may also be problems with the normal configuration of the ureteral wall. There is evidence of an altered deposition of interstitial matrix proteins such as collagen or elastin in these megaureters [41]. Another probable cause of nonrefluxing, nonobstructed megaureter is a transient functional ureterovesical obstruction that does not disturb kidney function and therefore does not lead to further evaluation. In spite the presence of an obstruction, increased compliance of the ureter may explain the unaltered kidney function.

The tendency to more restrained management of the dilated upper urinary tract in children has shown that most megaureters formerly classified and treated as primary obstructed megaureter would now be classified in the nonrefluxing, nonobstructed subgroup without the need for specific therapy (Chap. 4, Case 26).

1.8.3
Clinical Presentation and Evaluation

Most cases of megaureter are detected before birth by antenatal routine ultrasound screening investigations and therefore present without clinical symptoms. Others frequently present with upper UTI. In newborns lethargy or failure to thrive are frequent symptoms. In older children episodes of flank pain or stone transit may lead to the diagnosis.

The most important diagnostic tool for the evaluation of megaureter is ultrasonography. It allows classification by the grade of dilatation of the upper urinary tract. Furthermore, it allows an assessment of the status of the renal parenchyma and of the bladder configuration and therefore presents information on the severity of the disease and, to a certain degree, its underlying cause. Ultrasonography is the investigation of choice for serial follow-up of conservatively managed megaureter. The most common findings in patients with megaureter of any origin are a dilatation of the intra- and extrarenal collecting system and concomitant dilated distal ureter, which can be easily identified as a retrovesical tubular liquid formation.

Once the presence of megaureter is suspected, reflux must be excluded or confirmed by VCUG. Furthermore, the investigation yields information about bladder configuration and the quality of the urethra, which may indicate a neurogenic disorder of the bladder or subvesical obstruction.

In some cases, especially if an operative therapy is planned, IV pyelography (IVP) may be useful to obtain additional information about the morphology of the upper urinary tract and the distinct location of the ureteral obstruction. Nevertheless, IVP also provides some information about renal function and urinary excretion, but has lost its importance in the diagnosis of megaureter, as radionuclear imaging is more sensitive for differentiation of renal obstruction from renal dilatation.

Diuretic renography allows the evaluation of significant obstruction of the upper urinary tract and a differential quantification of the function of both kidneys in one investigative unit. The most frequently used radiolabelled tracer is Tc^{99}-mercapto-acetyl-3-glycine (^{99m}Tc-MAG_3), which is filtered and cleared by the kidney.

Any interpretation of ^{99m}Tc-MAG_3 clearance has to consider the volume of the affected system and the renal filtration rate to avoid false-positive evidence of obstruction, because the washout of the tracer depends on its distribution inside the collecting system. A delayed washout from a heavily dilated system, therefore, is not a significant sign of obstruction. The result of ^{99m}Tc-MAG_3 clearance that has the strongest validity is the exclusion of obstruction. Any suspicion of obstruction should be related to the differential kidney function. Unaffected kidney function does not exclude functional obstruction, but allows follow-up without the need for immediate therapy.

1.8.4
Therapy

The decision on therapy is dependent on the type of megaureter to be treated. There is general consent about the therapeutic strategies of refluxing and obstructed megaureters. But the problem is to achieve reliable classification of the subgroup of nonobstructive megaureter, with a consequent lack of a uniform concept of treatment for these patients. Nevertheless, even in cases of sufficient treatment of a megaureter, hydro-ureteronephrosis may persist. This causes difficulties with interpretation of the results of follow-up investigations. In these cases, regular evaluation of kidney function is needed to differentiate insufficiently treated patients from those with simple dilatation of the upper urinary tract.

1.8.4.1
Refluxing Megaureter

Primary refluxing megaureter without loss of renal function can be followed up with long-term antibiotic prophylaxis. Only in cases with no tendency to improvement, decreasing renal function, or breakthrough infections is an operative correction indicated. The techniques are described in section 1.7.5.2. Secondary refluxing megaureter requires treatment of its primary causes (Chap. 4, Case 23).

1.8.4.2
Obstructive Megaureter

Primary obstructive megaureter derives from obstruction at the ureterovesical junction. Therefore, the goal of any form of treatment is to widen this stenosis. Endoscopic techniques are ineffective and involve a high risk of postoperative reflux because of the stenosis in the intramural part of the ureter. Thus, open operative strategies are required, with the goal of resection of the distal (stenotic) part of the ureter and subsequent ureteral reimplantation.

Now that hydro-ureteronephrosis can already be diagnosed antenatally on routine ultrasonographic evaluation of the fetus, the timing of an operative correction of obstructive megaureter has to be rethought. There is evidence that surgical correction in children under the age of 8 months has a higher complication rate, even in experienced hands [109]. Nevertheless, if surgical correction is required at an earlier age, e.g. in cases with massive dilated ureters and poor kidney function, a temporary urinary diversion by pyelocutaneostomy or distal ureterocutaneostomy may be indicated until the child is old enough for a definitive correction (Chap. 4, Case 15). Any other patients should be admitted for surgical correction during their 2nd year of life. Even if they have already been diagnosed before birth, the definitive correction can be delayed with careful supervision of the renal function of the affected kidney and prevention of upper UTI.

The treatment of a secondary obstructed megaureter requires specific therapy for its primary causes.

1.8.4.3
Nonobstructed Nonrefluxing Megaureter

With the more frequent use of "wait-and-see" strategies, the management of prenatally diagnosed megaureter has changed within the last few years. Several studies had shown that the majority of megaureters formerly classified as obstructed are the nonobstructed variants that do not need surgical correction [65, 82]. As there is no reliable test of obstruction, in the past many patients with nonobstructed megaureters were operated on at very young ages. The physiological improvement of the maturing kidney was misinterpreted as a benefit of the operation. Therefore, several patients had been operated on unnecessarily.

Thus, every child with prenatally diagnosed hydro-ureteronephrosis with unaltered renal function and without UTI should be followed up conservatively. In cases of UTI and normal kidney function long-term antibiotic prophylaxis is indicated. Under these conditions, the rate of spontaneous improvement of hydro-ureteronephrosis of nonobstructed megaureters is over 50% [58] (Chap. 4, Case 16). A decrease in kidney function or breakthrough infections indicates operative correction.

1.8.5
Operative Techniques

The goal of any operation on obstructed megaureters is to resect the stenotic part of the distal ureter followed by a reimplantation in an antireflux manner. The techniques used are similar to those of reflux (see section 1.7.5.2). Some authors prefer transvesical mobilization of the distal ureter analogous to the Cohen or Politano-Leadbetter procedure even in obstructed megaureters. In general this is only possible with slightly dilated ureters. On the basis of our experience, we prepare the distal ureter outside the bladder in any case and then dissect it from the bladder and go into the bladder to create the neo-hiatus and the submucosal tunnel for the reimplantation. Others use the psoas hitch technique as their first choice.

The actual difference between the surgical correction of reflux and of obstructed megaureter lies in the management of the sometimes massive dilatation of the distal ureter. As the length of the submucosal tunnel has to be at least 4–5 times the ureteral diameter, massive dilatation would need a very long tunnel. In normal bladders there is not enough space for such tunnels. One strategy is to elongate the distance by the psoas hitch technique (Fig. 18). The other possibility is to reduce the ureteral diameter, as is described in several different techniques and known as "modelling" the ureter.

The diameter can be reduced by folding the distal part of the ureter after creating two lumens by means of a suture. The other possibility is to resect a part of the distal ureteral wall and adapt the edges by a suture to create a smaller lumen. This procedure is called 'ureteral tapering' (Fig. 19). The most frequent problems are reflux caused by a too short submucos-

al tunnel, scarry reobstruction most probably caused by ischaemia of the distal ureter, or too drastically enforced modelling of the distal ureter.

1.9
Obstructive Uropathy

Renal obstruction is caused by several different urological disorders. Although the causes of these diseases are different, their effects on renal function and morphology are at least equivalent and they can, therefore, be subsumed under the term 'obstructive uropathy'.

Obstruction of the kidney can occur in all parts of the urinary tract, but besides the variants of obstruction of the lower (subvesical) parts, which are described in section 1.3, there are two areas along the ureter that are particularly susceptible to obstruction. These are the ureteropelvic junction (UPJ) and the ureterovesical junction (UVJ). Both these areas can be affected by different alterations, which in turn will lead to renal obstruction. The pathophysiology, clinical presentation and clinical evaluation of both forms of obstruction of the upper urinary tract are similar, and they are discussed together below.

1.9.1
Pathophysiology

Renal obstruction is defined as an impediment to urinary drainage from the upper collecting system, which leads to progressive dilatation of the upper urinary tract. But dilatation alone does not prove that an obstruction is present. Unambiguous obstruction will lead to a lasting increase in intrarenal pressure,

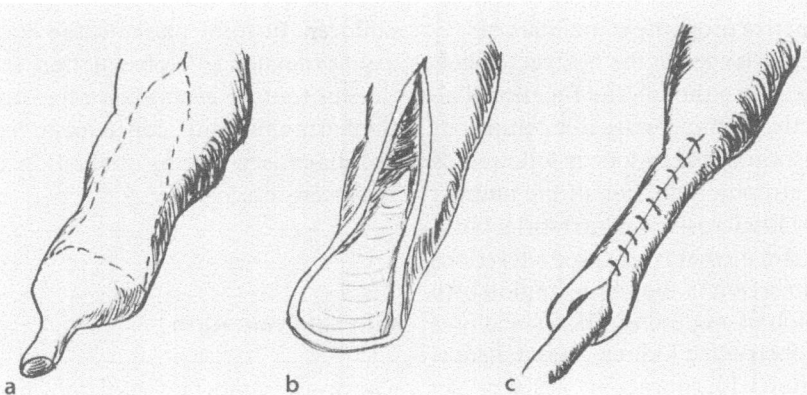

Fig. 19a–c. Principle of ureter "modelling". **a** Incision line for the resection of the stenosis and the surplus ureteral wall (*dotted line*). **b** Status after explantation of the distal ureter out of the bladder wall. **c** Closure of the distal ureter over a ureteric stent in preparation of the ureteral reimplantation into the bladder

which in turn influences the efficacy of glomerular filtration and tubular function. The kidney can withstand this situation for a while. After this period, progressive structural changes of the renal parenchyma will be followed by impairment of renal function.

The typical morphological and functional changes made to the kidney by renal obstruction, regardless of the specific reasons for it, are summarized in the term 'obstructive uropathy'.

Congenital obstructive uropathy remains one of the most frequent reasons for children's end-stage renal insufficiency. The morphological alterations of the kidney tissue caused by renal obstruction are described in many studies, but up to now the exact mechanisms leading to these alterations are only partly understood. However, in the last 10–15 years a great deal of effort, especially in animal models, has been invested into attempts to shed some light on the phenomenon of obstructive uropathy.

First of all, differentiations between acute and chronic and between complete or partial obstruction are needed. Cases of acute and/or complete obstruction in children are very rare. In most cases acute obstruction is caused by ureteral obliteration resulting from urolithiasis.

Congenital obstructive uropathy is caused by chronic partial renal obstruction that begins even in the fetal period. Complete or early subtotal renal obstruction in the fetus leads to renal dysplasia, or even renal agenesis. In contrast to renal obstruction of the mature kidney, obstruction of the developing kidney impairs normal organogenesis. The exact mechanisms are not clear. The majority of cases of congenital renal obstruction seen by the paediatric urologist are milder variants of the disease. Nevertheless, even mild obstruction can harm renal development and function. The challenge is to differentiate this from simple dilatation of the upper urinary tract. Therefore, complete understanding of the pathophysiology of obstructive uropathy is mandatory.

The morphological changes in the obstructed kidney are well documented, although the functional alterations leading to these changes are not completely understood. Obstruction of the kidney is followed by progressive tubular atrophy, reduction of the number of glomeruli, glomerulosclerosis, and interstitial fibrosis [25]. One of the main mediators of these alterations caused by renal obstruction is the renin–angiotensin system. The expression of angiotensin II, especially, is up-regulated in the obstructed kidney. Angiotensin II causes vasoconstriction with consequent ischaemia of the renal tissue, which leads to renal scarring. Furthermore, angiotensin II stimulates the expression of several growth factors, such as epidermal growth factor or transforming growth factor-β1 (TGF-β1), which in turn is one of the main mediators of the development of interstitial fibrosis. Additionally, angiotensin II controls the apoptotic activity of tubular cells in particular, and therefore modulates cellular growth [67]. Studies with animal models have shown that apoptosis is the main factor responsible for the induction of tubular atrophy and consequent loss of renal tissue in chronic obstructive uropathy [146].

Although the morphological and molecular alterations of obstructed kidneys are largely similar in both acute obstruction and chronic obstruction in the adult, the main difference in congenitally obstructed kidneys is the additional impairment of normal organogenesis and organ growth by the disease. This requires early identification and therapy of renal obstruction to protect normal organ development and thereby preserve normal kidney function. Therefore, a reliable marker of early obstruction, which unfortunately is still lacking, would improve the prognosis of congenital renal obstruction.

1.9.2
Clinical Presentation

In this era of antenatal ultrasound as a routine tool in normal monitoring of pregnancies, the diagnosis of hydronephrosis has already been made by the time of birth in the majority of patients. But some patients miss out on this and may present in early childhood with recurrent UTI, stone disease, haematuria or more unspecific symptoms, such as failure to thrive or symptoms of malnutrition. In some patients hydronephrosis is not discovered until a mostly asymptomatic abdominal mass is palpated.

Older children frequently report flank pain or upper abdominal pain, especially during micturition. Recurrent UTI are more frequent than in younger children. In some patients, the diagnosis of hitherto asymptomatic UPJ obstruction is made by chance during routine evaluation after blunt abdominal or flank trauma with consequent haematuria. Others are diagnosed during evaluation of arteriovascular hypertension.

1.9.3
Clinical Evaluation

The most important tool for the detection of hydronephrosis is ultrasonography. In cases known since the antenatal period, further screening investigation should be performed at short intervals in the newborn period. Once persistent or progressive hydronephrosis is diagnosed, the underlying reasons for it must be evaluated. The kidney function should be monitored. The presence of VUR has to be excluded or confirmed by a voiding cystography. The most important tool for discrimination of renal obstruction from simple dilatation is nuclear diuretic renography. This allows observation of renal function and drainage of the collecting system in a single investigation. The criteria of obstruction are impaired kidney function and/or a delay in renal washout of nuclear contrast medium. The method is highly sensitive, but its specificity remains unsatisfactory. However, there is a lack of alternative methods.

Evidence of UTI, stone disease or flank pain confirms the presence of renal obstruction even in cases in which diuretic renography gives normal results.

The importance of IV pyelography in the evaluation of renal obstruction has decreased, but especially when morphological details are required it has major advantages over diuretic renography. Therefore, in cases with duplicated collecting systems or ureteral valves IV pyelography still has a place. Other tools, such as duplex colour sonography or magnetic resonance urography, may be used in addition in special cases but are not currently used routinely in evaluation of children with obstructive uropathy.

1.9.4
Clinical Management

The main goal of the management of renal obstruction is to protect kidney function by avoiding renal damage from recurrent infections or progressive increase of the intrarenal pressure. Even today, there are no tools that allow the unambiguous diagnosis of renal obstruction. Nonetheless, the sonographic, radiographic and radionuclear methods available permit a valid assessment of the underlying disorder, which becomes more precise with increasingly standardized methods and the more clearly defined criteria of assessment.

Several patterns of clinical management of obstructive uropathy have been proposed. The following suggested pattern is a consensus work of the German Arbeitsgemeinschaft Pädiatrische Nephrologie and the Paediatric Urology Committee of the Deutsche Gesellschaft für Urologie. It offers a possible strategy for the management of antenatally diagnosed dilatation of the upper urinary tract (Fig. 20).

When a renal dilatation is diagnosed later, after birth, the principles of management are still similar. Ultrasonographically discovered dilatation of the kidney requires radionuclear diuretic renography. Renal obstruction combined with significant (>7%)

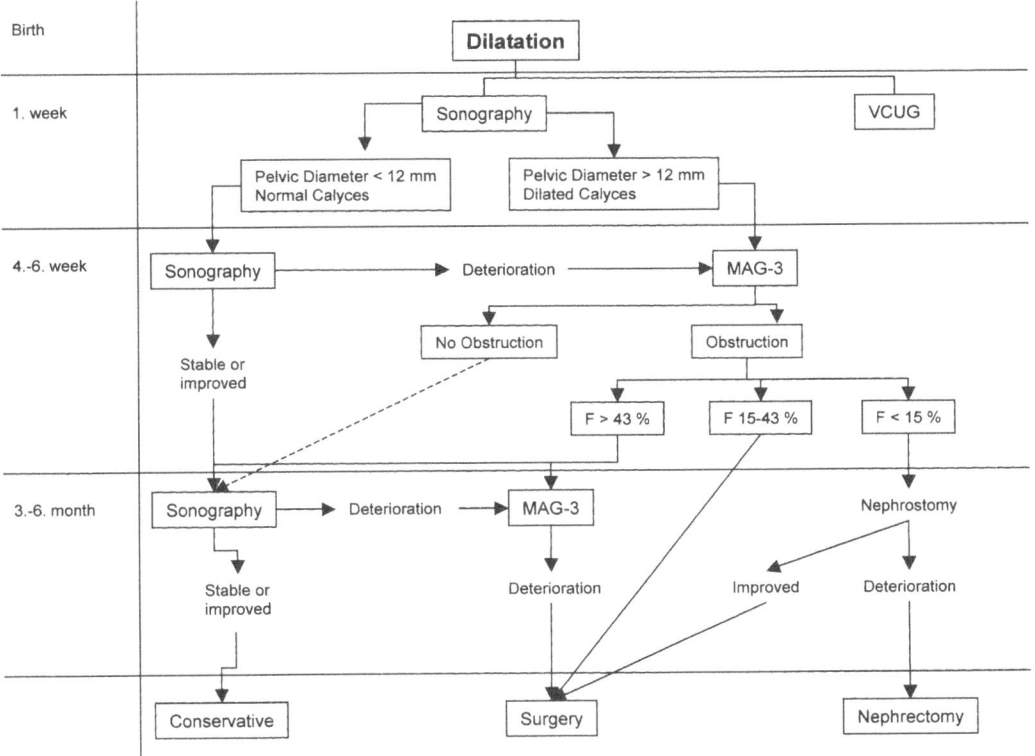

Fig. 20. Management of connatal dilatation of the upper urinary tract

loss of kidney function is an indication for immediate operative correction. Evidence of impaired renal drainage with no effect on kidney function should be followed up according to a short-term schedule (Chap. 4, Cases 11 and 12). Recurrent upper UTI, stone disease or pain is an indication for operative correction, even if kidney function is normal or normal renal drainage is assumed.

The value of antibiotic prophylaxis in the conservative management of the dilated upper urinary tract is controversial. There is still a lack of results from prospective randomized studies dealing with this subject. Thus, any decision has to be made individually for each patient. Frequent reasons are status post pyelonephritis in a dilated system, bilateral dilatation and megaureter. Especially in cases with unilateral dilatation of the renal pelvis, there is no need for routine long-term antibiotic prophylaxis.

1.9.5
Ureteropelvic Junction Obstruction

Ureteropelvic junction (UPJ) obstruction is the most common cause of antenatal dilatation of the urinary tract. About 80% of all dilated renal units are due to UPJ obstruction [18]. Since ultrasound has become a routine tool in prenatal fetal observation, the majority of cases with UPJ obstruction are known before birth. Boys are twice as often affected as girls. The left kidney is predominant. Bilateral involvement occurs in 10–40% of cases [59]. As there is a familial accumulation of UPJ obstruction over more than one generation, an autosomal dominant pattern of inheritance has been suggested [29].

There is a high incidence of other urological anomalies associated with UPJ obstruction. Some authors report that up to 50% of their patients with UPJ obstruction show other analogous urological disorders [77]. Besides the involvement of the contralateral kidney in up to 40% there is higher frequency of contralateral dysplastic kidney disease (Chap. 4, Case 4). Contralateral renal agenesis occurs in at least 5% [59]. Furthermore, UPJ obstruction is frequently associated with VUR, which may aggravate obstructive uropathy but may also result in increased narrowing of the UPJ. However, the majority of cases of UPJ obstruction combined with VUR show minor grades of reflux, mainly caused by bladder infections with no influence of the degree and prognosis of obstruction.

1.9.5.1
Aetiology

The aetiology of UPJ obstruction remains incompletely understood. UPJ obstruction is divided into three major subgroups by cause: (1) intrinsic (idiopathic), (2) extrinsic (aberrant vessel) or (3) secondary.

INTRINSIC UPJ OBSTRUCTION ▶ For intrinsic UPJ obstruction Whitacker firstly hypothesized impaired drainage of urine to the proximal ureter by the inability of the renal pelvis to initiate normal transport of urine boluses by peristaltic movements. This occurs in cases of only little funnel-shaped configuration of the pyeloureteral junction [152]. This theory of a discontinuity of normal muscular contractions over the distance of the pyeloureteral junction is supported by anatomical studies showing attenuated connections between the muscle fibres because of an abnormal interposition of extracellular matrix [50]. Other authors have implicated muscular hyperplasia of muscle fibres in the pyeloureteral area in the causation of UPJ. However, it is not clear whether the hyperplasia is due to obstruction or whether the obstruction itself is due to the muscular hyperplasia [139]. Another more embryological approach to explain UPJ obstruction cites incomplete recanalization of the physiologically solid phase during normal ureteral development in the fetus [120].

There are other rare alterations of the UPJ that may lead to intrinsic obstruction. In general these are disorders resulting from persistent embryological structures such as ureteral valves or polyps.

EXTRINSIC UPJ OBSTRUCTION ▶ In children extrinsic UPJ obstruction is most frequently due to an aberrant or early-branching central renal vessel that passes ventrally from the UPJ or proximal ureter. The vessel leads to the lower kidney pole and compresses the proximal ureter, which results in obstruction (Chap. 4, Cases 10 and 13). Stephens suggested the development of a secondary intrinsic stenosis of the UPJ by chronic extrinsic obstruction. The lasting compression of the ureteral tissue may result in ischaemia of this area and also leads to progressive fibrosis [140]. Other authors reject the presence of solitary extrinsic UPJ obstruction in children. They suggest a simultaneous intrinsic involvement of the UPJ that is due to incomplete relief of obstruction after elimination of the aberrant vessel. However, there is a consensus that vascular compression of the proximal ureter is the main reason for UPJ obstruction in adults.

SECONDARY UPJ OBSTRUCTION ▶ Secondary UPJ obstruction may occur in cases with widely dilated ureters because of high-grade primary or secondary VUR. This is due to progressive elongation of the ureter with consequent kinking near the more firmly fixed UPJ, which leads to obstruction.

1.9.5.2
Therapy

The main principle in the therapy of UPJ obstruction is to protect kidney function. Otherwise, there has to be a clear differentiation between asymptomatic dilatation of the upper urinary tract and significant obstruction. Surgical intervention can also cause kidney damage. The pros and cons of any operative treatment therefore have to be weighed conscientiously. A possible strategy for the clinical management of congenitally dilated upper urinary tract is shown in Fig. 20.

If a conservative strategy is decided on, antibiotic prophylaxis is not routinely necessary. The indications for ureteral stenting or percutaneous nephrostomy are limited to patients with septic complications due to a urinary obstruction that is resistant to conservative treatment. If possible, intermittent drainage of the dilated collecting system should be avoided before any final operative therapy, to preserve optimal conditions for the surgery (Chap. 4, Case 9).

The basic aim of any operative correction of UPJ obstruction is to attain normal urinary drainage from the renal pelvis to the upper ureter, which can be managed in different ways. Several methods have been proposed.

The open surgical procedures can be subdivided into dismembered techniques with complete disconnection of the renal pelvis and the proximal ureter or flap techniques using flaps from the dilated renal pelvic wall to widen the pyeloureteral junction. The operative goal of all of these techniques is a widely patent and watertight pyeloureteral anastomosis that is tension free. Only dismembered pyeloplasty allows full resection of the abnormal obstructive ureteral segment.

One of the most popular methods was first described in 1949 by Anderson and Hynes [4]. They performed a dismembered pyeloplasty, creating an elliptical anastomosis of the spatulate proximal ureter with the lower portion of the partially resected renal pelvis (Fig. 21a–c). The operation is usually performed via a flank incision directly ventral to the tip of the 12th rib. The exposure of the renal pelvis and the proximal ureter is excellent. The technique allows correction of nearly any form of UPJ anomaly

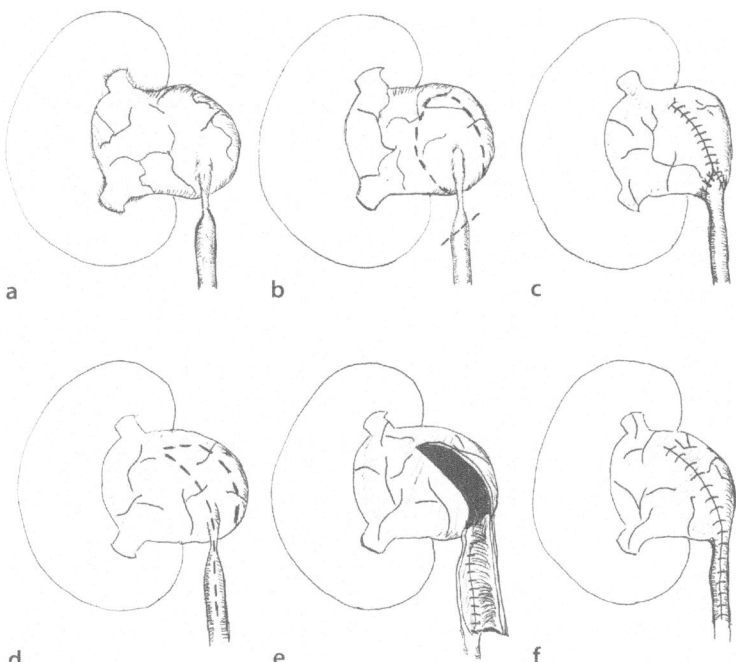

Fig. 21a–f. Principles of pyeloplasty for ureteropelvic junction obstruction (*dotted lines* incision lines). **a–c** Anderson-Hynes technique [4] with resection of the stenotic segment of the proximal ureter and a part of the dilated renal pelvis. **d–f** Flap technique (Culp-DeWeerd [33]) bridging the narrow segment of the proximal ureter

except long strictures of the proximal ureter. It also allows uncomplicated correction of the extrinsic form of UPJ obstruction by an aberrant lower pole vessel.

The flap techniques were originally designed to reconstruct the pyeloureteral junction after high insertion of the proximal ureter. Nowadays, for routine pyeloplasty they have been almost completely replaced by the dismembered techniques. Nevertheless, there are still indications for the flap techniques, especially in cases with long strictures of the proximal ureter segment. The technique first described in 1951 by Culp and DeWeerd [33] is a typical example of a flap-using pyeloplasty. A spiral flap to be raised from the lateral part of the renal pelvic wall must be outlined. Then the incision of the medial margin of the flap is elongated via the narrow segment of the pyeloureteral junction. The length of the flap is dependent on the length of the proximal ureter that has to be bridged. The apex of the flap is then rotated down to the most inferior end of the ureteral incision and anastomosed to the margins of the ureterotomy. Finally, the renal pelvis is closed cranial to the ureteropelvic junction (Fig. 21 d – f).

Although both endoscopic and laparoscopic techniques are used as alternatives for the treatment of UPJ obstruction in adults, sometimes with excellent results, their use is not recommended in paediatric patients.

1.9.6
Ureterovesical Junction Obstruction

The area that is the second most frequent site of obstruction of the upper urinary tract in childhood is the ureterovesical junction (UVJ). The consequence of UVJ obstruction is dilatation of the whole of the upper urinary tract from the intrarenal part down to the distal ureter. Although there are different reasons for UVJ obstruction the clinical presentation is subsumed under the term 'obstructive megaureter'. The different reasons for obstructive megaureter are presented below. By analogy with the reasons for UPJ obstruction these can be subdivided into intrinsic (ureteral) and extrinsic (extraureteral).

1.9.6.1
Primary Obstructive Megaureter

The most frequent intrinsic cause of UVJ obstruction is congenitally impaired drainage of urine from the distal ureter into the bladder. This problem is gener-

ally known as primary obstructive megaureter (POM). The aetiology is described in section 1.8.2.2. Much more rarely, POM is caused by a real narrowness of the intramural transvesical part of the distal ureter which originates from incomplete recanalization of the ureter during fetal development (see also section 1.1.2). The clinical presentation and diagnosis are described above (section 1.8.3), although interpretation of the diuretic renography is more complicated than in cases with UPJ obstruction.

The clinical management of POM is similar to that of UPJ obstruction (Fig. 20), except that antibiotic prophylaxis is recommended in asymptomatic cases with no influence on the kidney function. Interestingly, the frequency of significant primary congenital obstruction is much lower at the UVJ than at the UPJ. Therefore, the probability of spontaneous improvement is higher, and in most cases conservative management should be the strategy of choice. In other cases, in which kidney function is affected or there is progressive dilatation of the upper urinary tract, surgical correction is recommended. Some of the different operative techniques are presented in section 1.8.5.

1.9.6.2
Secondary Obstructive Megaureter

Restriction of the normal urinary drainage from the distal ureter into the bladder from an extraureteral origin leads to secondary obstructive megaureter (SOM). The impairment may result from a hypertrophied ureteral wall, which is generally caused by recurrent cystitis or neurogenic or subvesical obstructive voiding disorders. The hypertrophied ureteral wall impairs the peristaltic movement of the ureter for a normal forward movement of the urine.

The clinical presentation of SOM is characterized mainly by the primary disorder leading to obstruction. This emphasizes the importance of a careful evaluation of the upper urinary tract even in patients with suspected disorder of the lower parts of the tract. The evaluation is similar to that in POM. The therapy of SOM usually requires treatment of the primary causes. During this period, antibiotic prophylaxis should be administered to protect the kidney from further infections. In cases with a marked loss of kidney function intermittent supravesical urinary diversion may be indicated. Only in cases with persistent UVJ obstruction after successful treatment of these causes is specific treatment of the obstruction necessary. The operative strategies are similar to those applied in POM.

1.10
Paediatric Oncology

Neoplastic disease is the second most frequent reason for death in childhood following accidents. The general incidence of malignant neoplasm in children under 15 years of age is about 15/100000. After cancers of the haematopoietic system, urogenital neoplasm, with nearly 20%, represents the most important malignant diseases in childhood. Cancers that affect the urogenitalia are nephroblastoma, germ cell tumours, pelvic rhabdomyosarcoma and, to some extent, neuroblastoma.

The embryological characteristics of most neoplasms occurring in childhood contribute to an excellent response to multimodal forms of therapy. Combinations of surgical treatment, radiotherapy and polychemotherapy provide a cure even in metastatic disease in nearly 70% of the patients. However, to obtain such success rates, treatment of the children in specially trained, equipped and experienced paediatric oncology centres is strongly recommended. Most treatments of paediatric neoplasms are performed according to standardized therapeutic regimens and are controlled by international multicentre studies. The main goal of these studies is to optimize the therapeutic efficacy, decrease toxicity and prevent long-term side effects.

1.10.1
Wilms' Tumour

Max Wilms was the first to described a characteristic blastemal renal tumour in paediatric patients in 1899, which he called a nephroblastoma. Its incidence is about 1/100000. About 90% of the children are affected before the 7th year of life. The majority of them are diagnosed between 2 and 4 years of age. While the disease becomes more and more infrequent after the age of 10 years, nephroblastoma has also been observed in adults in rare cases. There is no sex or side predominance. Up to 7% of nephroblastomas are bilateral. Furthermore, a familiar predisposition is observed in about 1% of cases.

Wilms' tumour is frequently associated with other congenital anomalies. Children with sporadic aniridia or asymmetrical body development (hemihypertrophy) frequently develop nephroblastoma. Furthermore, distinct combinations of congenital anomalies, such as Beckwith-Wiedemann syndrome (hemihypertrophy, microcephaly, macroglossia, visceromegaly and mental retardation) or WAGR syndrome (Wilms' tumour, aniridia, genitourinary anomalies, mental retardation) are associated with Wilms' tumour (Chap. 4, Case 37).

These associations of nephroblastoma with other congenital anomalies suggests a genetically determined neoplastic predisposition. Koufos et al. observed a loss of allelic heterozygosity of chromosome 11p in patients with WAGR syndrome , leading to the discovery of the Wilms' tumour gene (*WT1*) [72]. Region p13 is next to the aniridia gene, which explains the association of Wilms' tumour and aniridia.

The *WT1* gene is characterized as a recessive tumour suppressor gene that loses its regulatory function by way of two consecutive mutations (two-hit hypothesis). Whether the first mutation occurs in the metanephric blastema or not until later in the developing kidney determines the extent of associated genitourinary anomalies and possibly whether both kidneys are affected or only one.

In the case of sporadic affliction of one kidney the second mutation always occurs in the mature kidney and initiates tumour development [68].

The presence of a second Wilms' tumour gene (*WT2*) was postulated, again by Koufos and co-workers, when they observed a cytogenic alteration of chromosome 11 region p15 associated with the Beckwith-Wiedemann syndrome [73]. Whether other genetic factors – and if so which – play a part in the pathogenesis of nephroblastoma is not known.

1.10.1.1
Classification of Nephroblastoma

Nephroblastoma derive from persisting primitive fetal metanephrogenic structures. The tumour is characterized as an embryonic tumour with undifferentiated blastemic portions and epithelial and mesenchymal differentiated portions combining to give an extremely heterogeneous and multifarious histological appearance. Depending on the expression of these possible different components, the nephroblastoma can be subdivided into triphasic biphasic and monophasic tumours. The prognosis of the different subtypes of nephroblastoma correlates with the expression of the different cell differentiation types, leading to a basic classification into tumours with favourable, intermediate and unfavourable prognoses. With more sarcomatous or anaplastic portions found in the tumour the prognosis becomes less favourable [11]. Although the classification of 'unfavourable prognosis' applies to only 10% of patients, it accounts for nearly 60% of deaths from the disease. The therapeutic strategy, therefore, is oriented to this classification.

1.10.1.2
Clinical Presentation and Evaluation

Wilms' tumour can still be asymptomatic even in its metastatic stages. Therefore, the first symptom is frequently a palpable or visible abdominal mass. Occasionally, the diagnosis of a renal tumour is an incidental diagnosis on abdominal sonography. About 30% of the children present with abdominal symptoms, to the point of acute abdomen after intraperitoneal rupture of the tumour. Acute flank pain can be caused by haemorrhage into the tumour, which is frequently followed by fever and anaemia. Gross haematuria is rare, whereas up to 25% of the children show microhaematuria. The differential diagnosis includes neuroblastoma, retroperitoneal malignant lymphoma, rhabdoid tumour and benign tumours such as cystic nephroma (benign multilocular cyst).

The leading investigations in the diagnosis of Wilms' tumour are abdominal ultrasonography and computed or MR tomography. Because of their multifarious tissue differentiation and frequent spontaneous intratumoral bleeding, the appearance of nephroblastoma is highly heterogeneous on ultrasound. The investigation allows distinct assignment of the tumour to the kidney in the majority of cases. Furthermore, the presence of a tumour thrombus that has passed via the renal vein into the vena cava, something that occurs in about 20% of nephroblastomas, can be reliably detected by the method.

Table 2. Clinical staging of nephroblastoma

Stage	Description
I	Tumour limited to the kidney and completely excised. No rupture of tumour
II	Tumour extends beyond the kidney but is completely excised - Penetration into perirenal tissue - Regional lymph node metastasis - Penetration into extrarenal vessels or tumour thrombus - Penetration into the ureter - Infiltration of the peritoneum
III	Residual tumour, no distant metastases - Tumour biopsy before surgical removal - Peritoneal metastases - Lymph node metastases beyond the regional drainage - Macroscopic residual tumour - Microscopically positive margins
IV	Distant metastases
V	Bilateral synchronous or metachronous nephroblastoma

Nevertheless, the standard investigation for the diagnosis of Wilms' tumour is CT or MRI scan of the abdomen. These allow precise imaging of the tumour and of surrounding structures for reliable evaluation of the primary distribution of the tumour, bilateral renal involvement and possible local or distant tumour progression. As in the ultrasound findings, Wilms' tumour also presents as a highly heterogeneous mass on the tomographic investigations. As the majority of the nephroblastomas metastasize primarily to the liver and lung, CT of the thorax should be included in the normal routine clinical staging of the disease. Bone scans and evaluation of the brain are recommended in cases of suspected rhabdoid tumour or clear cell sarcoma. However, besides the histopathological differentiation of Wilms' tumours, the clinical dissemination of the tumour led to an internationally accepted classification system (Table 2).

1.10.1.3
Therapy

The necessity of a stage- and histology-adapted therapy of Wilms' tumour was proven by prospective multicentre nephroblastoma-studies in the US [National Wilms' Tumour Study (NWTS)], in Germany (Gesellschaft für Pädiatrische Oncology und Haematology [GPOH]) and Europe (Society International d' Oncologie Pédiatrique [SIOP]). Currently the therapy of nephroblastoma is based on the fifth protocol of the NWTS ($NWTS_{-5}$) or the corporate protocol of the SIOP/GPOH ($SIOP_{93-01}$/GPOH).

The two protocols differ fundamentally in their primary therapeutic approaches. Whereas the $NWTS_{-5}$ protocol recommends primary surgical removal of the tumour followed by adjuvant or radiochemotherapy, the $SIOP_{93-01}$/GPOH protocol requires primary chemotherapy followed by surgical removal of the remaining tumour in children older than 6 months. The aim of this approach is to reduce the tumour size and its local dissemination (downstaging) to facilitate the surgical operation and reduce the risk of intraoperative tumour burst, which results in more intense postoperative therapy including additional radiotherapy and yields a higher rate of completely removed tumours [85]. Only in children younger than 6 months does primary operative tumour resection promise better results, because in the majority of these patients the presence of a stage-I nephroblastoma of low-grade malignancy is probable, which could be treated sufficiently by isolated surgical removal.

The chemotherapy of nephroblastoma basically contains dactinomycin and vincristine, combined with Adriamycin for disease in stage III or higher. Residual tumours or tumours of primary high-grade malignancy are primarily treated according to a high-risk protocol containing a combination of carboplatin, ifosfamide, Adriamycin and etoposide. Radiotherapy is recommended only for patients with locally advanced (stages III-IV, N+) or residual tumour. This is due to a high rate of secondary long-term side effects, especially the development of secondary cancers, which may occur in about 17% of irradiated patients.

The operative therapy of Wilms' tumour should achieve not only removal of the tumour, if possible complete, but also local intraabdominal staging, including evaluation of the local lymph nodes. The primary tumour should be removed by radical nephrectomy. Only in bilateral involvement is an organ-sparing strategy indicated, if possible bilaterally but at least on the kidney that is less severely affected. Open surgical biopsy should be avoided to minimize the risk of local tumour cell dissemination. The radical retroperitoneal lymphadenectomy itself does not influence the prognosis of the disease but allows better adaptation of the postoperative therapy. If possible, a complete removal of residual metastatic tumour masses after chemotherapy is additionally recommended. Mutilating surgery should be avoided whenever possible.

Bilateral nephroblastoma should be regarded as an isolated entity as far as prognosis and therapeutic approaches are concerned. The coincidence of associated congenital urogenital anomalies is 4-fold that in unilateral involvement. The patients are usually younger at the time of diagnosis.

Whereas the prognosis of synchronous involvement (7% of all nephroblastomas) correlates with the histological and clinical stage on the side where disease is more advanced and is therefore comparable to that with unilateral involvement, metachronous occurrence, which is rarer (1.7%), is associated with a distinctly poorer prognosis [136]. Especially in these patients local downstaging by preoperative chemotherapy is essential to optimize the conditions for organ-sparing surgery.

The prognosis of Wilms' tumour of low and intermediate malignancy, with an overall survival rate of at least 80%, is excellent. Just the patients with unfavourable histology still have an unsatisfactory prognosis.

1.10.2
Neuroblastoma

Neuroblastoma is the most frequent malignant solid neoplasm in children. The incidence is 1.1/100000 children younger than 15 years per year. Most (90%) of these tumours occur during the patients' first 5 years of life. The median age at diagnosis is 21 months [60]. Compared with Wilms' tumour, they are less frequently associated with other congenital anomalies.

1.10.2.1
Aetiology and Pathogenesis

The nephroblastoma derives from cells of the embryological neural crest forming the sympathetic ganglia and the medullary part of the adrenal gland. The tumour can, therefore, arise from any point on the neural crest. The most frequent points of origin, in declining order, are the adrenal gland (50%), retroperitoneum (28%), thorax (12%), neck (5%) and multiple foci (1%) [100]. The histological appearance of neuroblastoma may be very heterogeneous. Hughes, therefore, postulated a histological grading system. He correlated the grade of malignancy of the tumour with its content of ganglion differentiated cells, from the highly differentiated ganglioneuroblastoma to the undifferentiated small round cell tumours [53]. Nevertheless, tumour grading has only a minor role in neuroblastoma. Neither histological nor biochemical evaluation can reflect the malignant potential of the tumour. However, molecular biological characteristics, such as the amplification of the *N-myc* oncogene of the tumour, allow clear differentiation of a group of patients with an extremely unfavourable prognosis [26]. It is still not clear whether a potentially less malignant tumour changed into a more aggressive variant by re-amplifying the oncogene or the amplification defines a basically different new tumour entity. However, the evaluation of the *N-myc* amplification has become an essential part of the diagnosis of neuroblastoma.

A special feature of the tumour biology of neuroblastoma is its capability of spontaneous regression. Neuroblastoma screening investigations of children younger than 1 year reflect a distinctly higher incidence of the disease than could statistically be expected [32]. This may be explained by a high spontaneous regression rate even in metastatic stages. This is supported by a nearly complete lack of *N-myc* amplification in neuroblastoma of children younger than 12 months, compared with about 30% in older children or children with advanced tumour stages.

1.10.2.2
Clinical Presentation and Evaluation

Neuroblastoma is nearly asymptomatic in its early stages. Common unspecific symptoms such as weight loss, fever, and local bone pain indicate that the disease is already in an advanced stage. Rare but characteristic symptoms are nasal obstruction and epistaxis in aesthesioneuroblastoma, protrusio bulbi with orbital involvement (Chap. 4, Case 38), and Horner's syndrome with involvement of the cervical sympathetic nerves. There is a tendency for paravertebral, and especially abdominal, tumours to extend through the intervertebral foramen. The resulting so-called dumbbell-shaped tumour may compress the spinal cord. As this is frequently asymptomatic in the early stages, paravertebral tumour manifestation calls for additional evaluation of the spinal area to avoid neurological damage.

The majority of neuroblastomas attract attention in routine screening programmes. These screening investigations detect the urinary excretion of the products of catecholamine metabolism, vanillylmandelic acid and homovanillic acid, produced by the tumour. The increased catecholamine metabolism is also reflected in increased serum concentrations of catecholamines.

Once a neuroblastoma is suspected, the primary tumour should be evaluated by ultrasound investigation, computed tomography or MR tomography. A very sensitive method of detecting regions with increased catecholamine metabolism is scintigraphy using ^{131}I-meta-iodobenzylguanidine (^{131}mIBG). The radioisotope is taken up by the adrenergic secretory vesicles into the tumour. The method is suitable for the detection and location of the primary tumour as well as detection of metastases.

Because of its tendency to metastasize to the bones and bone marrow, diagnostic bone marrow aspiration is a mandatory diagnostic tool in the evaluation of neuroblastoma. Metastatic spread to the liver, lung, skin or brain is less common. Nevertheless, evaluation of these organs is recommended.

However, the diagnosis of neuroblastoma is confirmed by surgical exploration and resection of the primary tumour and its local lymph node stations followed by histological evaluation. Combined with the imaging and laboratory investigations, the results of the operation allow clinical classification of neuroblastoma. The actual classification is based on the international criteria for neuroblastoma diagnosis, staging and response (INSS) (Table 3).

1.10.2.3
Therapy

Neuroblastoma represents a heterogeneous group of tumours with different tumour biological characteristics contributing to different therapeutic approaches. The most important prognostic factors are the clinical tumour stage and the age of the patient at the time of diagnosis. Other significant factors are amplification of the N-myc oncogene, increased serum concentration of lactate dehydrogenase, and a decreased number of thrombocytes.

The intensity of the therapy must be stratified depending on the different biological features of neuroblastoma in very young patients and on whether the tumour is locally limited or widespread. The ongoing neuroblastoma study NB97 therefore established three groups requiring different intensities of treatment [100].

Table 3. International classification of the clinical stages of neuroblastoma (INSS). Survival rates from Neuroblastoma Study NB$_{79}$-NB$_{90}$ of the German Society of Paediatric Oncology and Haematology

Stage	Description	5-year-survival
I	Tumour confined to the organ or structure of origin	85%
IIa	Tumour extending beyond the organ or structure of origin but not crossing the midline. Incomplete surgical resection. No regional lymph node involvement	
IIb	Tumour extending beyond the organ or structure of origin but not crossing the midline. Complete or incomplete surgical resection. Ipsilateral regional lymph node involvement	85%
III	Tumour extending beyond the organ or structure of origin and crossing the midline. Ipsilateral or contralateral regional lymph node involvement	
IV	Distant metastases to distant lymph nodes, bone, bone marrow, liver or other organs	23%
IV-S	Tumour localization analogue to stage I or II with dissemination to one or more of the following sites: liver, skin or bone marrow. Only children younger than 12 months	79%
	Overall 5-year-survival	80%

1. Observation group
   - Infants with stage I–III or IV-S without *N-myc* amplification
   - Children with stage I or stage II, with near-complete surgical resection without *N-myc* amplification
2. Standard risk
   - Infants with stage II–III with pulmonary or renal insufficiency or neurological symptoms without *N-myc* amplification
   - Children with unresectable stage II–III tumours without *N-myc* amplification
   - Patients in group 1 with progressive disease under observation
3. High-risk patients
   - All patients with *N-myc* amplification
   - Patients with stage IV neuroblastoma

The first step in the treatment of neuroblastoma is surgical exploration of the tumour. The aim is complete resection of the tumour and regional lymph node staging. The harvesting of tumour tissue is essential, with immediate evaluation of the *N-myc* amplification for indications as to the further therapeutic strategy that should be adopted.

Depending on the postoperative classification, patients in the observation group are merely followed up for 6–12 months without further therapy. If necessary, residual tumour can be resected in a second operation. Patients showing progression of disease are crossed over to the therapeutic regimen for the standard-risk group.

In the standard-risk group the surgical exploration of the primary tumour is followed by chemotherapy. The therapy consists of two different medical blocks in each cycle. Block 1 consists in the administration of cisplatin, etoposide and vindesine, while block 2 consists in administration of a combination of vincristine, dicarbazine, ifosfamide and Adriamycin. Infants are treated with a less toxic protocol consisting of Adriamycin, vincristine and carboplatin. Residual tumour should be resected in a second operation.

Improving the prognosis of high-risk patients is the most important challenge in the therapy of neuroblastoma. In spite of intensive high-dose chemotherapy with autologous stem cell suspension and a subsequent distinct elevation of the therapeutic morbidity, earlier studies showed a hardly changed survival rate of only about 25% in this group. This led to a reduction of the doses given in chemotherapy and the establishment of alternative experimental therapeutic approaches for advanced neuroblastoma, such as targeted radiation therapy with radiolabelled mIBG and monoclonal antibodies against human neuroblastoma cells. Nevertheless, the success rates in patients with high-risk tumour are still unsatisfactory.

1.10.3
Testicular Tumours in Children

Testicular tumours in childhood account for 1–2% of all solid tumours. In contrast to adults, in whom about 95% of testicular tumours are germ cell tumours, the corresponding rate in children is only 60–75%. Benign testicular tumours in childhood account for 25–33% of the patients, and most of these are Sertoli-cell tumours (15%) and Leydig cell tumours (20%) [136].

Maldescensus testis is associated with testicular neoplasm. The anomaly is one of the most direct causes of the development of testicular cancer. About 10% of all testicular tumours arise from maldescended testes. The risk of tumour development in undescended testes is 35-fold that in normally descended testes. The risk further correlates with the degree of testicular dislocation: 5% of abdominal testes develop a tumour, as opposed to 1% of testes in the groin area.

A histological classification of testicular tumours in childhood is given in Table 4 [62].

Table 4. Histological classification of testicular tumours in childhood

Histological class	Tumours
I	Germ cell tumours – Yolk-sac tumour – Teratoma – Teratocarcinoma – Seminoma
II	Gonadal stoma tumour – Leydig cell tumour – Sertoli-cell tumour – Intermediates
III	Gonadoblastoma
IV	Tumours of supporting tissue – Fibroma – Leiomyoma – Haemangioma
V	Lymphoma and leukaemia
VI	Tumour-like lesions – Epidermoid cyst – Hyperplastic nodule due to congenital adrenal hyperplasia
VII	Secondary tumours
VIII	Tumours of adnexa

Histological differentiation of the different tumour types is essential. It leads to stratification of the therapeutic strategies. Furthermore, the histological subtypes of testicular tumours show an age-specific distribution of occurrence. About 70% of patients with yolk-sac tumour are younger than 2 years, and 80% of patients with teratoma are younger than 4 months. Paediatric seminoma is rare.

1.10.3.1
Clinical Presentation, Evaluation and Therapy

A testicular tumour in childhood becomes obvious as a hard, indolent swelling of the testicle. The finding has to be differentiated from testicular torsion, epididymitis, groin hernia and hydroceles (Chap. 4, Case 27). It must be emphasized that in children about 25% of testicular tumours are clinically associated with hydroceles. Nevertheless, a normal clinical examination of the testis does not exclude a testicular tumour. Advanced tumour with lymphatic or haematogenous metastases could become apparent as a palpable abdominal mass or other symptoms arising from the metastases, e.g. dyspnoea or anaemia. Important tumour markers of testicular tumours are the serum concentration of alpha fetoprotein (aFP) and β-human-chorionic gonadotropin (βHCG). Especially yolk sac tumours express aFP, whereas teratocarcinomas predominantly express βHCG. Seminomas only express βHCG in about 20% of cases.

The diagnosis of the primary tumour is made in an intraoperative frozen section of a specimen taken from the affected testis via a groin incision. In the case of a malignant tumour, the testis must be removed completely at the internal inguinal annulus. Benign lesions should be resected completely from the testis, protecting as much testicular tissue as possible.

Once the diagnosis has been confirmed by histopathological examination, examination for lymph node involvement and haematogenous metastases is recommended. As the first lymphatic stations of testicular tumour are the retroperitoneal lymph nodes near the renal vessels, a CT scan of the abdomen provides the most reliable information on this area. Furthermore, possible mediastinal or pulmonary metastases should be evaluated by conventional X-ray or CT scan of the thorax. A bone scan or brain scan is only recommended in patients with symptoms suggesting possible metastasis to these regions. Together with the histological evaluation of the primary tumour, the results of the clinical evaluation contributes to a clinical classification system (Table 5),

which in turn is used to stratify the therapeutic approaches.

The principles of the treatment of testicular malignant tumours in children in current use are:
1. Refrain from radiotherapy.
2. Refrain from primary retroperitoneal lymphadenectomy.
3. Do not give adjuvant therapy in stage I A yolk-sac tumour or teratoma.

This contributes to a preference for chemotherapy over primary surgery or radiotherapy, which is a basic difference from the therapy strategies used in adults, where primary chemotherapy and primary retroperitoneal lymphadenectomy are alternatives and radiotherapy is still standard in stage I–II B seminoma.

Malignant testicular tumours should be treated after inguinal orchidectomy with two cycles of chemotherapy containing cisplatin, vinblastine and bleomycin (stage I A–II B). More advanced stages are treated with a combination of cisplatin, etoposide and bleomycin. Except in stage I A, all other patients who show no evidence of residual tumour and negative tumour markers are treated with an-

Table 5. Clinical staging of testicular tumours in children

Clinical stage	Characteristics
I	No metastases detectable
IA	– Tumour confined to the testis and epididymitis
IB	– Infiltration of the spermatic or tumour in undescended testis
IC	– Infiltration of the scrotal skin or transscrotal operation
II	Lymph node metastases beneath the diaphragm
IIA	– Lymph nodes <2 cm diameter
IIB	– Lymph nodes 2–5 cm in diameter
IIC	– Lymph nodes >5 cm in diameter
IID	– Palpable abdominal mass or fixed inguinal tumour
III	Mediastinal and/or supraclavicular lymph node metastases
IIIA	– Mediastinal and/or supraclavicular lymph node metastases
IIIB	– Minimal pulmonary metastatic disease: <5 metastases <2 cm in diameter
IIIC	– Advanced pulmonary metastatic disease: >5 metastases or >5 cm in diameter
IV	Generalized advanced disease – Haematogenous metastases in liver, bones, CNS – Persisting tumour marker without evidence of metastases

other cycle of their particular chemotherapy. When there is evidence of residual tumour masses and/or persisting tumour markers, complete resection of all affected sites is recommended if possible. In patients with elevated markers in isolation, without evidence of organ involvement, a modified retroperitoneal lymphadenectomy is recommended. This is followed by three cycles of a combination of cisplatin, etoposide and ifosfamide when the histology has shown vital tumour cells. This stratification of a combination of surgical and chemotherapeutic strategies for the treatment of testicular tumour in children contributes to the excellent prognosis of the disease. The survival rates are better than 90%.

1.10.4
Rhabdomyosarcoma of the Pelvis

Sarcoma deriving from soft tissue is a common solid tumour of the urogenital tract. Rhabdomyosarcoma is the most common soft tissue sarcoma in childhood. It arises from mesenchymal cells normally forming striated muscle cells. This tumour could, therefore, develop from almost any place where striated muscle cells are located. About 20% of rhabdomyosarcomas affect structures of the urogenital tract [71]. The median age at diagnosis is 6 years. There is no gender predominance.

Rhabdomyosarcomas are aggressive tumour entities with a pronounced tendency to infiltrate the surrounding structures and lymphogenous or haematogenous metastasis. About 20% of the patients have evidence of widespread disease by the time of diagnosis [75].

Typical locations of rhabdomyosarcoma of the urogenital tract are:
1. Bladder or prostate
2. Spermatic cord
3. Uterus and vagina

The principles of the treatment of rhabdomyosarcoma include complete surgical resection of the tumour, unless this would make a mutilating operation unavoidable. In these cases harvesting of a representative specimen for a precise histological classification is recommended. As the tumour is usually chemosensitive, tumours preoperatively assessed as inoperable should first be treated with chemotherapy using agents selected from vincristine, dactinomycin, Adriamycin, ifosfamide, etoposide, cyclophosphamide and carboplatin. The therapy may induce downstaging of the tumour with consequent improvement of the operative outcome.

Table 6. Clinical staging of rhabdomyosarcoma in children

Stage	Definition
I	Localized disease, completely removed, no lymph node involvement
IA	– Tumour confined to organ of origin
IB	– Tumour infiltrating beyond the organ of origin
II	Microscopic residual disease or regional lymph node involvement
IIA	– Microscopic residual disease, no lymph nodes
IIB	– Lymph node involved, completely resected, no residuals
IIC	– Lymph node involved, microscopic residual disease
III	Incomplete removal or biopsy with gross residual disease
IV	Distant metastases or lymph node involvement beyond the regional stations

Depending on the postoperative status or the clinical presentation at the time of diagnosis, for inoperable patients the clinical staging system presented in Table 6 was postulated as a result of the American Intergroup Rhabdomyosarcoma Study (IRS).

1.10.4.1
Rhabdomyosarcoma of the Bladder or Prostate

Patients with rhabdomyosarcoma of the bladder frequently present with haematuria or transurethral prolapse of parts of the tumour. Involvement of the prostate causes subvesical obstruction with strangury, frequency, urgency, and urinary retention. Regional lymph node involvement is frequently found.

Complete tumour resection is usually impossible unless radical cystectomy or prostatectomy is needed. Only cases with rhabdomyosarcoma of the bladder roof allow organ-sparing complete resection of the tumour. However, in the majority of cases a representative biopsy taken for diagnosis is followed by a primary chemotherapy. If there is a complete remission of the tumour after chemotherapy, no further surgical intervention is necessary. In cases with residual tumour after chemotherapy radiotherapy is recommended. Only in patients with residual tumour after chemo- and radiotherapy is operative resection of the tumour indicated, if necessary by cystoprostatectomy or exenteration.

1.10.4.2
Paratesticular Rhabdomyosarcoma

Paratesticular rhabdomyosarcoma arises from mesenchymal structures of the spermatic cord. It may be associated with a hydrocele or present as a relatively tender scrotal mass. The tendency to lymphogenic spread is higher than in other testicular tumours. A careful evaluation of the retroperitoneal lymph nodes is therefore recommended. The treatment of choice is inguinal semicastration followed by chemotherapy and, in cases with residual tumour after chemotherapy, retroperitoneal lymphadenectomy. Patients older than 10 years have a worse prognosis [153]. In these patients a primary retroperitoneal lymphadenectomy is recommended even when there is no clinical evidence of lymph node involvement.

1.10.4.3
Rhabdomyosarcoma of Vagina or Uterus

Rhabdomyosarcoma of the vagina usually presents as the so-called sarcoma botryoides prolapse of the introitus. This tumour does not infiltrate the pelvic structures and has an excellent prognosis [153]. Primary radical resection of the tumour is mostly impossible without removal of the complete vagina. But as the tumour shows good chemosensitivity and radiosensitivity, the resection of residual tumour is commonly possible without severe damage to the vagina.

Rhabdomyosarcoma of the uterus is a very rare disease affecting older girls during puberty. Chemosensitivity of this tumour is poor. Primary radical hysterectomy is therefore the therapy of choice.

References

1. Abeshouse BS, Bhisitkul I (1959) Crossed renal ectopia with and without fusion. Urol Int 9:63
2. Allen TD (1970) Congenital ureteral strictures. J Urol 104:196
3. Amar A (1975) The clinical significance of renal caliceal diverticulum in children: Relation to vesicoureteral reflux. J Urol 113:255
4. Anderson JC, Hynes W (1949) Retrocaval ureter: a case diagnosed preoperatively and treated successfully by a plastic operation. Br J Urol 21:209
5. Ansell JE (1983) Exstrophy and epispadias. In: Glenn JF (ed) Urologic surgery. Lippincott, Philadelphia
6. Arap S, Abrao EG, Menezes de Goes G (1981) Treatment and prevention of complications after extravesical antireflux technique. Eur Urol 7:263
7. Argueso RL, Ritchey ML, Boyle ET et al (1992) Prognosis of patients with unilateral renal agenesis. Nephrol 6:412
8. Atala A, Share JC, Paltiel HJ et al (1994) Sonicated albumin in the detection of vesicoureteral reflux in humans. Soc Pediatr Urol Newslett 8:6
9. Baker R, Maxted W, Maylath J et al. (1966) Relation of age, sex, and infection to reflux: data indicating high spontaneous cure rate in pediatric patients. J Urol 95:27
10. Beck AD (1971) The effect of intrauterine urinary obstruction upon the development of the fetal kidney. J Urol 105:784
11. Beckwith JB, Palmer NF (1978) Histopathology and prognosis of Wilms' tumor. Result from the first national Wilms' tumor study. Cancer 41:1937
12. Ben-Chaim J, Jeffs RD, Reiner WG et al (1996) The outcome of patients with real bladder exstrophy in adult life. J Urol 155:1251
13. Bernstein J, Slovis TL (1992) Polycystic diseases of the kidney. In: Edlman CM (ed) Kidney. Little Brown, Boston
14. Bichler KH, Strohmeyer WL, Kom S (1985) Urolithiasis im Kindesalter. Monatsschr Kinderheilkd 133:256
15. Blythe B, Passerini GG, Camuffo C et al (1993) Endoscopic incision of ureteroceles. Intravesical versus ectopic. J Urol 149:556
16. Boyden EA (1931) Description of a horseshoe kidney associated with left inferior vena cava and disc shaped suprarenal glands, together with a note on the occurrence of horseshoe kidneys in human embryos. Anat Rec 51:187
17. Brannon W, Oschner MG, Rosencrantz DR et al (1973) Experiences with vesicoureteral reflux. J Urol 109:46
18. Brown T, Mandell J, Lebowitz RL (1987) Neonatal hydronephrosis in the era of ultrasonography. AJR Am J Roentgenol 148:959
19. Bukowski TP, Perlmutter AD (1994) Reduction cystoplasty in the prune belly syndrome: a long-term follow-up. J Urol 152:2113
20. Burbige K (1991) Ureteral reimplantation: a comparison of results with the cross-trigonal and Politabno-Leadbetter techniques in 120 patients. J Urol 146:1352
21. Busch R, Huland H (1984) Correlation of symptoms and results of direct bacterial localization in patients with urinary tract infections. J Urol 132:282
22. Campbell MF (1930) Renal ectopy. J Urol 24:187
23. Campbell MF (1970) Anomalies of the ureter. In: Campbell MF, Harrison JH (eds) Urology. Saunders, Philadelphia
24. Carpenter TO, Lebowitz RL, Nelson D et al (1986) Hereditary xanthinuria presenting in infancy with nephrolithiasis. J Pediatr 109:307
25. Chevalier RL (1999) Molecular and cellular pathophysiology of obstructive uropathy. Pediatr Nephrol 13: 612
26. Christiansen H, Sahin K, Berthold F et al (1995) Comparison of DNA-aneuploidy, chromosome 1 abnormalities, myc-n amplification and CD 44 expression as prognostic factors in neuroblastoma. Eur J Cancer 31:541
27. Churchill BM, McLorie GA, Khoury AE et al (1990) Emergency treatment and follow-up of posterior urethral valves. Urol Clin North Am 17:343
28. Coffey RC (1921) Transplantation of the ureter into the large intestine in the absence of a functioning bladder. Surg Gynecol Obstet 32:383
29. Cohen B, Goldman SM, Kopilnick M et al (1978) Ureteropelvic junction obstruction: its occurrence in 3 members of a single family. J Urol 120:361

30. Cohen N, Berant M (1976) Duplications of the renal collecting system in the hereditary osteo-onychdysplasia syndrome. J Pediatr 89:261

31. Cohen SH (1975) Ureterozystoneostomie: eine neue Antirefluxtechnik. Aktuel Urol 6:1

32. Craft AW, Parker L (1996) Screening for neuroblastoma: 20 years and still no answer. Eur J Cancer 32A:1540

33. Culp OS, DeWeerd JH (1951) A pelvic flap operation for certain types of ureteropelvic obstruction. Preliminary report. Mayo Clin Proc 26:483

34. Cussen LJ (1977) Valves of the ureter. In: Bergman D, Docket JW Jr (eds) Urinary system malformations in children. Birth defects: original article series vol 13. Liss, New York

35. Domenech-Mateu JM, Gonzales-Compta X (1988) Horseshoe kidney: a new theory on its embryogenesis based on a study of a 16-mm human embryo. Anat Rec 222:408

36. Duckett JW (1983) A "conservative" analysis. Am J Kidney 3:139

37. Duckett JW, Walker RD, Weiss R (1992) Surgical results: international reflux study in children-United States branch. J Urol 148:1674

38. Ellerker AG (1958) The extravesical ectopic ureter. Br J Surg 45:344

39. Engel RM, Wilkenson HA (1970) Bladder exstrophy. J Urol 104:699

40. Ericson NO, Ivemark BI (1958) Renal dysplasia and pyelonephritis in infants and children: primitive ductules and abnormal glomeruli. Arch Pathol 66:264

41. Escala JM, Keating MA, Boyd G et al (1989) Development of elastic fibers in the upper urinary tract. J Urol 141:969

42. Felson B, Cussen LJ (1975) The hydronephrotic type of congenital multicystic disease of the kidney. Semin Roentgenol 10:113

43. Field PL, Stephens FD (1974) Congenital urethral membranes causing urethral obstruction. J Urol 111:250

44. Fontaine E (1997) Long-term results of renal transplantation in children with prune-belly syndrome. J Urol 158:892

45. Fowler RJ, Stephens FD (1963) The role of testicular vascular anatomy in the salvage of high undescended testes. In: Stephens FD (ed) Congenital malformations of the rectum, anus, and genitourinary tract. Williams and Wilkins, Baltimore

46. Gearhart JP, Leonard MP, Bingers JK et al (1992) The Cantwell-Ransley technique for repair of epispadias. J Urol 148:851

47. Gittes RF (1984) Congenital megacalyces. Monogr Urol 5:1

48. Gleason PE, Kelalis PP, Husmann DA et al (1994) Hydronephrosis in renal ectopia: Incidence, etiology and significance. J Urol 151:1660

49. Gregoir W, Van Regermorter GV (1964) Le reflux vesicoureteral congenital. Urol Int 24:119

50. Hanna MK, Jeffs RD, Sturgess JM et al (1976) Ureteral structure and ultrastructure, part II. Congenital ureteropelvic junction obstruction and primary obstructive megaureter. J Urol 116:725

51. Hinman F (1979) Directional growth of renal calculi. J Urol 121:700

52. Hohenfellner K, Hunley TE, Schloemer C et al (1999) Angiotensin type 2 receptor is important in the normal development of the ureter. Pediatr Nephrol 13:187

53. Hughes M, Marsden HB, Palmer MK (1974) Histological patterns of neuroblastoma related to prognosis and clinical staging. Cancer 34:1706

54. Hwang TIS, Hill K, Snell P (1988) Effect of prolonged bedrest on the propensity of renal stone formation. J Clin Endocrinol Metab 66:109

55. Ives E, Coffey R, Carter CO (1980) A family study of bladder exstrophy. J Med Genet 17:139

56. Jacobson SH, Eklöf O, Erikson CG et al (1989) Development of hypertension and uremia after pyelonephritis in childhood: 27-year follow-up. BMJ 299:703

57. Jodal U (1987) The natural history of bacteriuria in childhood. Infect Dis Clin North Am 1:713

58. Johnson HW, Gleave M, Coleman GU et al (1987) Neonatal renomegaly. J Urol 138:1023

59. Johnston JH, Evans JP, Glassberg KI et al (1977) Pelvic hydronephrosis in children: A review of 219 personal cases. J Urol 117:97

60. Kaatsch P, Haaf G, Michaelis J (1995) Childhood malignancies in Germany – methods and results of a nationwide registry. Eur J Cancer 31A:993

61. Kaplan BS, Kaplan P, Rosenberg HK (1989) Polycystic kidney disease in childhood. J Pediatr 115:867

62. Kaplan GW (1983) Testicular tumors in children. AUA Update series 2: lesson 12

63. Kaplan RA, Haussler MR, Deftos U (1977) The role of 1,25-dihydroxyvitamin D in the mediation of intestinal hyperabsorption of calcium in primary hyperparathyroidism and absorptive hypercalciuria. J Clin Invest 59:756

64. Kapoor R, Saha MM (1987) Complete duplication of the bladder, common urethra and external genitalia in the neonate. A case report. J Urol 137:1243

65. Keating MA, Retik AB (1989) Management of failure of ureterocystoneostomy. In: McDougal WS (ed) Difficult problems in urologic surgery. Year Book Medical Publishers, Chicago

66. King LR, Kazmi SO, Belman AB (1974) Natural history of vesicoureteral reflux: outcome of a trial of nonoperative therapy. Urol Clin North Am 1:144

67. Klahr S (2001) Urinary tract obstruction. Semin Nephrol 21:133

68. Knudson AG, Strong LC (1972) Mutation and cancer: a model for Wilms' tumor of the kidney. JNCI 83:313

69. Koff SA (1992) Relationship between dysfunctional voiding and reflux. J Urol 148:1703

70. Kollermann VMW (1974) Überbewertung der pathogenetischen Bedeutung des vesiko-ureteralen Refluxes im Kindesalter. Z Urol 67:573

71. Koscielniak E, Jürgens H, Winkler K (1992) Treatment of soft tissue sarcoma in childhood and adolescence. Cancer 70:2557

72. Koufos A, Hansen MF, Lampkin BC et al (1984) Loss of alleles at loci on human chromosome 11 during genesis of Wilms' tumor. Nature 309:170

73. Koufos JJ, Grundy P, Morgan K et al (1989) Familial Wiedemann-Beckwith syndrome and a second Wilms' tumor locus map 11p15. Am J Hum Genet 44:711

74. Kurzrock EA, Huffmann JL, Hardy BE et al (1996) Endoscopic treatment of pediatric urolithiasis. J Pediatr Surg 31:1413

75. Lawrence W, Hays DM, Heyn R et al (1987) Lymphatic metastases with childhood rhabdomyosarcoma. A report from the Intergroup Rhabdomyosarcoma Study. Cancer 60:910

76. Lebowitz RL (1992) The detection and characterization of vesicoureteral reflux in the child. J Urol 148: 1640

77. Lebowitz RL, Griscom NT (1977) Neonatal hydronephrosis: 146 cases. Radiol Clin North Am 15:49

78. Leiter E (1972) Horseshoe kidney: Discordance in monozygotic twins. J Urol 108:683

79. Lich R, Howerton LW, Davis LA (1961) Recurrent urosepsis in children. J Urol 86:554

80. Liddle RM, Rosenbaum DM, Blumhagen JD (1989) Delayed radiologic appearance of bilateral thoracic ectopic kidneys. AJR Am J Roentgenol 152:120

81. Lister J, Singh H (1973) Pelvicalyceal cysts in children. J Pediatr Surg 8:901

82. Liu HYA, Dhillon HK, Yeung CK et al (1994) Clinical outcome and management of prenatally diagnosed primary megaureters. J Urol 152:614

83. Livingston WD, Collins TL, Novick DE (1981) Incidental renal masses. Urology 17:257

84. Loder RT, Guilboux J, Bloom DA (1992) Musculoskeletal aspects of prune-belly syndrome. Am J Dis Child 146: 1224

85. Ludwig R, Weirich A, Pötter R et al (1992) Präoperative Chemotherapie des Nephroblastoms. Vorläufige Ergebnisse der Therapiestudie SIOP-9/GPO. Klin Padiatr 204:204

86. Mackie GG, Stephens FD (1975) A correlation of renal dysplasia with position of the ureteral orifice. J Urol 114:274

87. Maizels M, Stephens FD (1980) Valves of the ureter as a cause of primary obstruction of the ureter: anatomic, embryologic and clinical aspects. J Urol 123:742

88. Maizels M, Stephens FD (1979) Renal ectopia and congenital scoliosis. Invest Urol 17:209

89. Malek RS, Kelalis PP, Burke EC (1971) Ectopic kidney in children and frequency of association of other malformations. Mayo Clin Proc 46:461

90. Mannhardt W, Schofer O, Schulte-Wissermann K (1986) Pathogenic factors in recurrent urinary tract infections and renal scar formation in children. Eur J Pediatr 145:330

91. McHugh K, Stringer DA, Hebert D et al (1991) Simple renal cysts in children: diagnosis and follow up with US. Radiology 178:383

92. McKinnon KC (1977) Primary megaureter. Birth Defects 13:15

93. McLaughlin AP, Pfister RC, Leadbetter WF et al (1973) The pathophysiology of primary megaloureter. J Urol 109:805

94. McLorie GA, McKenna PH, Jumper BM et al (1990) High grade vesicoureteral reflux: Analysis of observational therapy. J Urol 144:537

95. Mesrobian HGJ, Kelalis PP, Hrabovsky E et al (1985) Wilms' tumor in horseshoe kidneys: a report from the national Wilms' tumor study. J Urol 133:1002

96. Monfort G, Guys JM, Bocciardi A et al (1991) A novel technique for reconstruction of the abdominal wall in the prune belly syndrome. J Urol 146:639

97. Moore KL (1996) Embryologie: Lehrbuch und Atlas der Entwicklungsgeschichte des Menschen. Übersetzt und bearbeitet von E. Lütjen-Decroll, 4th edn. Schattauer, Stuttgart

98. Muecke EC (1964) The role of the cloacal membrane in exstrophy: the first successful experimental study. J Urol 92:659

99. Nakayama DK, Harrison MR, de Lorimier AA (1986) Prognosis of posterior urethral valves presenting at birth. J Pediatr Surg 21:43

100. NB90 Gesellschaft für Pädiatrische Onkologie und Hämatologie (1990) Multizentrische therapiebegleitende Studie zur Behandlung von Kindern und Jugendlichen mit Neuroblastom. Study protocol of 30 December 1990

101. Noe HN, Wyatt RJ, Peeden JN et al (1992) The transmission of vesicoureteral reflux from parent to child. J Urol 148:1869

102. Pagano P, Passerini G (1977) Primary obstructed megaureter. Br J Urol 49:469

103. Pagon RA, Smith DW, Shepard TH (1979) Urethral obstruction malformation complex: a cause of abdominal muscle deficiency and the "prune-belly". J Pediatr 94:900

104. Pak CYC, Britton F, Peterson R (1980) Ambulatory evaluation of nephrolithiasis: classification, clinical presentation and diagnostic criteria. Am J Med 62:19

105. Paquin AJ (1959) Ureterovesical anastomosis: the description and evaluation of a technique. J Urol 82:573

106. Patton BM, Barry A (1952) The genesis of exstrophy of the bladder and epispadias. Am J Anat 90:35

107. Pavanello L, Rizzoni B, Dussini N et al (1981) Cystinuria in children. Eur Urol 7:139

108. Perlmutter AD (1976) Reduction cystoplasty in prune-belly syndrome. J Urol 116:356

109. Peters CA, Mandell J, Lebowitz RL et al (1989) Congenital obstructed megaureters in early infancy: Diagnosis and treatment. J Urol 142:641

110. Peters DJM, Spruit L, Saris JJ et al (1993) Chromosome 4 localization of a second gene for autosomal dominant polycystic kidney disease. Nat Genet 5:359

111. Politano VA, Leadbetter WF (1958) An operative technique for the correction of vesicoureteral reflux. J Urol 79:932

112. Potter EL (1952) Pathophysiology of the fetus and newborn. Year Book Medical Publishers, Chicago

113. Potter EL (1965) Bilateral absence of ureters and kidneys: a report of 50 cases. Obstet Gynecol 25:3

114. Potter EL (1972) Normal and abnormal development of the kidney. Year Book Medical Publishers, Chicago

115. Puri P (2000) Endoscopic correction of vesicoureteral reflux. Curr Opin Urol 10:593

116. Reeders ST, Bruenning MH, Comey G et al (1986) Two genetic markers closely linked to adult polycystic kidney disease on chromosome 16. Br Med J 292:851

117. Reinberg Y, deCastano I, Gonzalez R (1992) Influence of initial therapy on progression of renal failure and body growth in children with posterior urethral valves. J Urol 148:532

118. Rittenberg MH, Hulbert WC, Snyder HM et al (1988) Protective factors in posterior urethral valves. J Urol 140:993

119. Royer P, Habib R, Mathieu H et al (1962) L'hypoplasie renale bilaterale congenitale avec reduction du nombre et hypertrophie des nephrons chez l'enfant. Ann Pediatr 38:133

120. Ruano-Gill D, Coca-Payeras A, Tejedo-Maten A (1975) Obstruction and normal re-canalization of the ureter in the human embryo: its relation to congenital ureteric obstruction. Eur Urol 1:287

121. Scherz HC, Kaplan GW, Packer MG et al (1989) Ectopic ureteroceles: surgical management with preservation of continence-review of 60 cases. J Urol 142:538

122. Schrott KM, Sigel A, Schott G (1983) Frühzeitige Total-rekonstruktion der Blasenexstrophie. In: Rodeck R (ed) Verhandlungsbericht der Deutschen Gesellschaft für Urologie, 35. Meeting, 21–24 September. Springer, Berlin Heidelberg New York

123. Schulman CC (1976) The single ectopic ureter. Eur Urol 2:64

124. Schulz-Lampel D, Lampel A, Lazica M et al (1997) Extracorporeal shockwave lithotripsy in childhood. Urologe A 36:200

125. Sen S, Beasley SW, Ahmed S et al (1992) Renal function and vesicoureteral reflux in children with ureteroceles. J Pediatr Surg 7:192

126. Shapiro ELH, Jeffs RD (1984) The inheritance of classical bladder exstrophy. J Urol 132:308

127. Share JC, Lebowitz RL (1989) Ectopic ureterocele without ureteral and calyceal dilatation (ureterocele disproportion): findings on urography and sonography. AJR Am J Roentgenol 152:567

128. Sharma SK, Bapna BC (1986) Surgery of the horseshoe kidney- an experience of 24 patients. Aust NZ J Surg 56:175

129. Shindo S, Bernstein J, Arant BSJ (1983) Evolution of renal segmental atrophy (Ask-Upmark kidney) in children with vesicoureteral reflux: Radiographic and morphologic studies. J Pediatr 102:847

130. Sigel A (2000) Anomalien bzw. Fehlbildungen der Harnorgane. In: Sigel A, Ringert RH (eds) Kinderurologie. Springer, Berlin, Heidelberg, New York

131. Sigel A (2000) Neurogene Harnblase – urologische Relevanz spinaler Dysraphie. In: Sigel A, Ringert RH (eds) Kinderurologie. Springer, Berlin, Heidelberg, New York

132. Silvermann FM, Huang N (1950) Congenital absence of the abdominal muscles associated with malformations of the genitourinary and alimentary tracts. Report of cases and review of the literature. Am J Dis Child 80:9

133. Skoog SJ, Belman AB, Majd M (1987) A nonsurgical approach to the management of primary vesicoureteral reflux. J Urol 138:941

134. Smellie JM, Barratt TM, Chantler C et al (2001) Medical versus surgical treatment in children with severe bilateral vesicoureteric reflux and bilateral nephropathy: a randomized trial. Lancet 357:1329

135. Smith DW (1970) Recognizable patterns of human malformation. Saunders, Philadelphia

136. Snyder HM, DFÁngio G, Evans AE et al (1998) Pediatric oncology. In: Walsh PC, Retik AB, Vaughn ED Jr, Wein AJ (eds) Campbell's urology. Saunders, Philadelphia

137. Spencer JR, Maizels M (1987) Inhibition of protein glycolization causes renal dysplasia in the chick embryo. J Urol 138:94

138. Stamey TA (1975) A clinical classification of urinary tract infections based upon origin. South Med J 68:934

139. Starr NT, Maizels M, Chou P et al (1992) Microanatomy of and morphometry of the hydronephrotic "obstructed" renal pelvis in asymptomatic infants. J Urol 148:519

140. Stephens FD (1982) Ureterovascular hydronephrosis and the "aberrant" renal vessel. J Urol 128:984

141. Stephens FD (1983) Congenital malformation of the urinary tract. Praeger, New York

142. Tank ES (1986) Experiences with endoscopic incision and open unroofing of ureteroceles. J Urol 136:241

143. Taylor A (1982) Quantification of renal function with static imaging agents. Semin Nucl Med 12:330

144. Thompson GJ, Pace JM (1937) Ectopic kidney: a review of 97 cases. Surg Gynecol Obstet 64:935

145. Timmons JWJ, Malek RS, Hattery RR et al (1975) Calyceal diverticulum. J Urol 114:6

146. Truong L, Petrusevska G, Yang G et al (1996) Cell apoptosis and proliferation in experimental chronic obstructive uropathy. Kidney Int 50:200

147. Tschöpe W, Ritz E, Schmidt-Gayk H (1980) Is there a renal phosphorous leak in recurrent renal stone formers with absorptive hypercalciuria? Eur J Clin Invest 10:381

148. Wall B, Wachter HE (1952) Congenital ureteral valve: its role as a primary obstructive lesion: classification of the literature and report of an authentic case. J Urol 68:684

149. Ward JN, Nathanson B, Draper JW (1965) The pelvic kidney. J Urol 129:677

150. Weiner ES, Lawrence S, Hays D et al (1994) Retroperitoneal node biopsy in childhood paratesticular rhabdomyosarcoma. J Pediatr Surg 29:171

151. Weyrauch HM (1939) Anomalies of the renal rotation. Surg Gynecol Obstet 69:183

152. Whitacker RH (1975) Some observations and theories on the wide ureter and hydronephrosis. Br J Urol 47:377

153. Wierrani F, Zoubek A, Grin W et al (1996) Das Sarcoma botryoides der kindlichen Vagina – ein Weichteilsarkom mit guten Heilungschancen. Geburtshilfe Frauenheilkd 56:441

154. Winberg J, Anderson HJ, Bergström T et al (1974) Epidemiology of symptomatic urinary tract infections in childhood. Acta Pediatr Scand S252:1

155. Woodard JR, Parrot TS (1978) Orchiopexy in the prune belly syndrome. Br J Urol 50:348

156. Woodard JR, Zucker J (1990) Current management of the dilated urinary tract in prune belly syndrome. Urol Clin North Am 17:407

157. Young HH, Frontz WA, Baldwin JC (1919) Congenital obstruction of the posterior urethra. J Urol 3:289

158. Zarbo A, Kay R (1986) Ureterosigmoidostomy in bladder exstrophy: a long-term follow-up. J Urol 136:396

159. Zerin JM, Ritchey ML, Chang AC et al (1993) Incidental vesicoureteral reflux in neonates with antenatally detected hydronephrosis and other renal abnormalities. Radiology 187:157

Diagnostic Procedures in Paediatric Uroradiology

A. Leenen

2.1
Introduction

The paediatric genitourinary tract can be affected by congenital and acquired disorders. Although some entities can be diagnosed clinically, radiological imaging and diagnostic work-up are often necessary. Therefore, the primary goal of paediatric renal imaging is to provide information about the nature and extent of disease. Knowledge of clinical and laboratory data and of therapeutic regimens influences the choice of modality and is a first-step in reducing overall exposure to medical radiation. Radiologists and referring physicians must be familiar with technique, limitations and interpretation of the numerous imaging modalities available for evaluating the urinary tract and with the indications for them. This chapter presents a brief survey of the current role of high-resolution ultrasonography (US), X-ray procedures, computed tomography (CT) and magnetic resonance imaging (MRI) in paediatric uroradiology, together with the specific findings that each can yield and any controversies about them.

2.2
Ultrasonography

Ultrasonography is the most important part of the initial work-up of children with known or suspected renal disease. Except for the renal function, this imaging modality in combination with colour or power Doppler mode has been shown to be capable of demonstrating almost every aspect of urinary tract pathology. It gives a rapid anatomical overview, especially with regard to shape and size of the kidneys and dilatation of the collecting system. Advantages of this modality are low costs, lack of radiation, widespread availability, absence of side effects and excellent anatomical resolution. A point of difference from other imaging techniques is that the diagnostic value of real-time US is strongly correlated with the examiner's skill and the degree of patient cooperation. These hazards interfere with the evaluation of the efficacy of this modality in clinical tests.

2.2.1
Grey-scale US

2.2.1.1
Technique

The cornerstone of sonographic pre- and postnatal evaluation of the urinary tract is conventional grey-scale US. Depending on the size of the child, postnatal examinations can be performed with 3.5- to 7.5-MHz phased-array sector or linear-array transducers. The use of a high-frequency linear transducer with graded compression of the abdomen is frequently beneficial in imaging of the ureter and can rule out renal fusion anomalies or calculi (Fig. 1).

Sonograms of bladder, retrovesical space, and kidneys have to be obtained with the patients in the supine and/or prone position in multiple planes with the highest possible frequency that still allows adequate tissue penetration. Images of the kidneys ac-

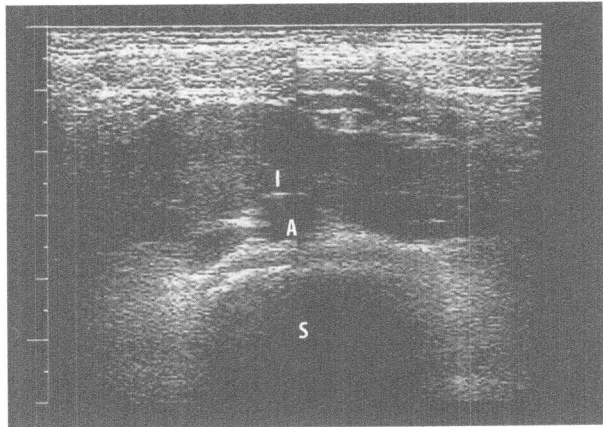

Fig. 1. Horseshoe kidney. Transverse sonogram in an 8-year-old boy demonstrates an isthmus of renal parenchyma (*I*) anterior to the spine (*S*) and the aorta (*A*) connecting the lower poles of the kidneys. Note the high resolution in the near field using a linear array 7.0 MHz transducer

quired in the supine position allow optimal visualisation of upper renal poles using liver and spleen as acoustic windows, while lower renal poles are better visualised with the child lying prone. In a young child who is not yet toilet trained the bladder has to be examined first, and often during the course of the examination, to evaluate spontaneous voiding. Postvoid examinations of kidneys and bladder are useful in children with hydronephrosis and/or megaureter and suspected bladder dysfunction.

Sedation or patient preparation is rarely required. The infant must be adequately hydrated, as otherwise any dilatation of the collecting system can be missed. Cooperative children are asked not to void for several hours before the examination. Because of physiological dehydration, renal ultrasound in the neonate should not be done until after the 3rd day of life; in fact it is better to delay it until the 2nd or 3rd week after birth unless findings of prenatal US or physical stigmata indicate a possible need for imaging and intervention.

US appears to be an ideal method for evaluating renal dimensions. Measurements of kidney size should be taken in maximum longitudinal and transverse planes in the supine or contralateral decubitus position [24, 40] and the renal volume calculated from outer kidney diameters using the volume formula for an ellipsoid. Correlation of renal length to body height and renal volume to bodyweight in growth charts provide objective information about renal development [41]. However, morphometric data must be carefully interpreted owing to interobserver variability of measurements and atypical variants in kidney outline. Single measurements of parenchymal thickness are of limited value owing to large variations in cortical depth.

In cases of ureteropelvic junction obstruction conventional sonography can be followed by administration of frusemide, parenteral 0.5 mg/kg bodyweight or oral 1 mg/kg bodyweight. In this well-known diuresis sonography [59] repeated measurements of the maximum transverse diameter of the collecting system are obtained after 10–90 min. The normal state is characterised by no increase at all or only a moderate increase in pelvicaliceal diameters, with a return to the basal condition in less than 60 min. In cases of severe obstruction, pyelectasis increases and fails to return to the former condition within 150 min [132].

2.2.1.2
Clinical Applications

PRENATAL US ▶ Owing to the widespread use of obstetric US, most congenital anomalies affecting the fetal genitourinary system are detected prenatally. This screening has resulted in a marked increase in the number of neonates referred for uroradiological evaluation and seems to be responsible for the decline in the diagnosis of obstructive uropathy in children with urinary tract infection (UTI) [4]. The normal fetal kidney is visible at about the 18th to 20th week of gestation, and a strong correlation exists between renal length and gestational age [27]. Antenatal examination includes evaluation of the renal pelvis, the echostructure of the parenchyma, the volume of amniotic fluid and the fetal bladder. Complete urine flow impairment (UFI) in fetal life leads to atrophy of the renal parenchyma, while partial or intermittent obstruction causes dilatation of the excretory system and can be due to a delay in normal ureter maturation [87, 105]. However, in cases of UFI maternal or fetal intervention is virtually never indicated and most newborns are asymptomatic.

The most common pathologic finding in fetal US is hydronephrosis due to ureteropelvic junction obstruction [19, 39, 69]. Several parameters have been described to differentiate normal dilatation from hydronephrosis. These include morphometric measurements such as renal pelvic antero-posterior diameter (APD) and the pelvic-to-renal APD ratio seen on the transverse view. A renal-to-pelvic APD ranging from 3 to 10 mm can occur in normal fetuses, while a diameter of >10 mm or progressive caliectasis indicates severe hydronephrosis [11, 60]. Other pathologic findings are, in declining order of frequency, ureterovesical junction obstruction, duplex anomalies with upper-pole hydronephrosis, posterior urethral valves with oligohydramnion, vesicoureteric reflux (VUR), multicystic dysplastic kidney disease and other rare conditions, such as prune-belly syndrome [19, 31, 43].

POSTNATAL US ▶ Postnatal US examination can confirm or exclude prenatal findings indicating abnormalities of renal number, position, size and fusion. About 20–25% of prenatally discovered renal abnormalities do not persist postnatally, while 20% of cases with hydronephrosis are detected for the first time in postnatal examinations [39].

US is the modality of choice for detecting hydronephrosis or megaureter. The renal pelvis and calices are not visible without excess fluid intake or overdistension of the bladder [44]. However, small pelvic fluid collections with no clinical significance can be found in 41–75% of healthy neonates [47, 163] and in older children after a change of position. Transient visualisation of the distal ureter with a small lumen should be considered a normal finding. After confirmation of hydronephrosis and megaureter postnatally, uroradiological work-up is needed to establish their significance. Dilatation of the collecting system is not synonymous with obstruction, and even marked dilatation may disappear in the first months of life. However, US can identify hydronephrotic renal units that are at risk of deterioration. Homsy et al. [69] concluded that moderately or markedly dilated renal units (renal pelvis more than 1.5 cm) are an indication of hydronephrosis with a poor outcome. The Society for Fetal Urology has developed a grading system to determine the extent of upper urinary tract dilatation, evaluating the appearance of the calices, the renal pelvis and parenchyma and the size of the retrovesical ureter [49]. Correlation of grade 3 or 4 hydronephrosis on US (dilatation of renal pelvis and calices throughout the kidney with/without thinning of the parenchyma) with results of diuresis renography showed high sensitivity and specificity in the detection of obstruction [98]. Diuresis sonography after good hydration seem to be useful to differentiate pelviureteric junction obstruction from dilatation without flow impairment [129, 132] and can be used in follow-up studies during treatment and after surgery. Follow-up US evaluation 4–6 weeks after the birth of all newborns with prenatal hydronephrosis and a normal postnatal sonogram is necessary to rule out significant obstruction missed on the initial examination [39].

US is commonly used in the primary investigation of children with suspected renal parenchymal or cystic disease (Fig. 2). In general, echogenicity of the renal cortex equals that of adjacent liver parenchyma in the first few months of life and shows decreasing echogenicity with weight and age (Fig. 3) [47, 62, 71]. Sonographic findings of renal parenchymal disease include increased cortical echogenicity and absence of corticomedullary differentiation (Fig. 4). However, renal echogenicity fails to be a reliable index of severity of glomerular disease as judged by renal biopsy.

The role of grey-scale US in UTI lies primarily in identification of surgically correctable findings such as renal abscess or congenital anomalies. US is not very effective in differentiating upper from lower urinary tract involvement, and clinical studies suggest a low impact of renal US on patient management in children with UTI [3, 67, 106]. Sonographic findings in severe pyelonephritis are renal enlargement, loss of corticomedullary differentiation and thickening of renal pelvis and/or ureter wall [126]. UTI can lead to permanent renal damage, due to scarring or reflux nephropathy. Because of low sensitivity and specificity, grey-scale US seems to be of limited value in detection of reflux nephropathy and mild degrees of renal scarring [150].

Conventional US is a poor screening method for the detection and grading of VUR [48, 50]. However, VUR can be suggested in the presence of a small kidney, a renal pelvis with changing dimensions during examination, a dilated distal ureter and uroepithelial

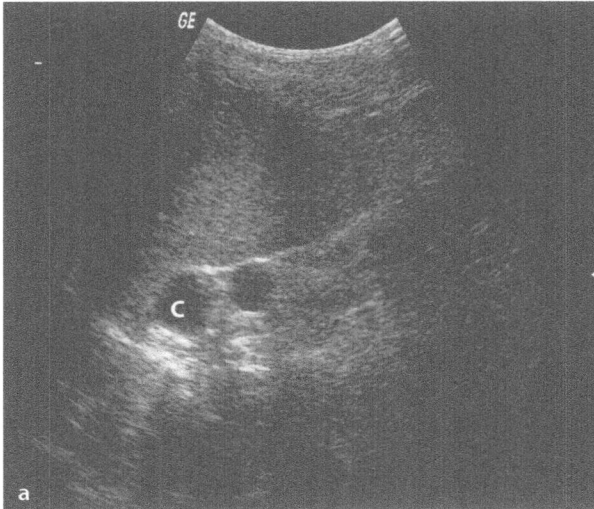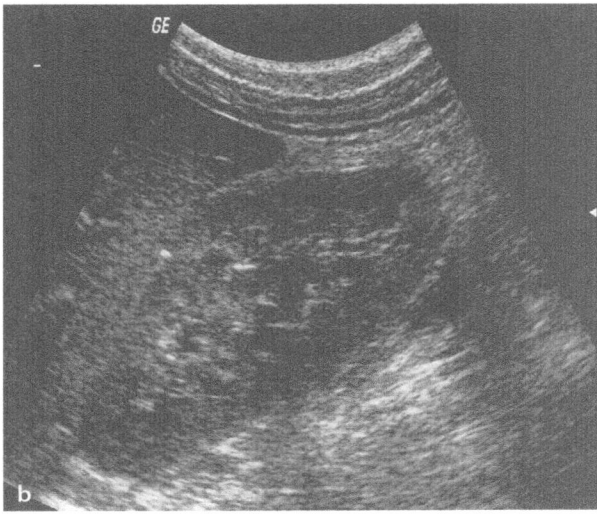

Fig. 2a, b. Multicystic dysplastic kidney. **a** Longitudinal sonogram of the left flank in a 2-year-old girl demonstrates two cysts (*C*) in the area of the left kidney. **b** Longitudinal scan of the normal right kidney in the same child shows compensatory hypertrophy

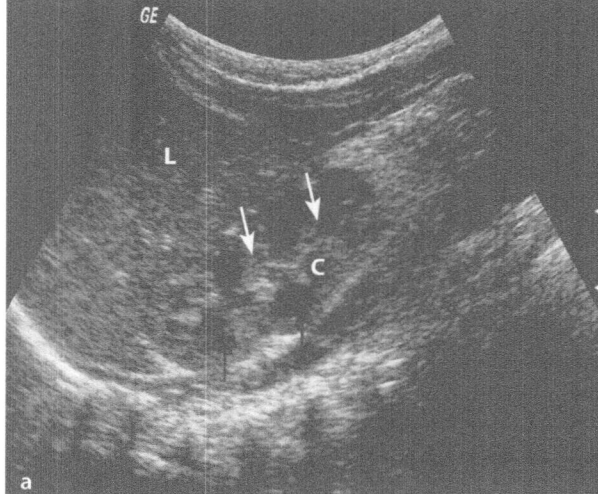
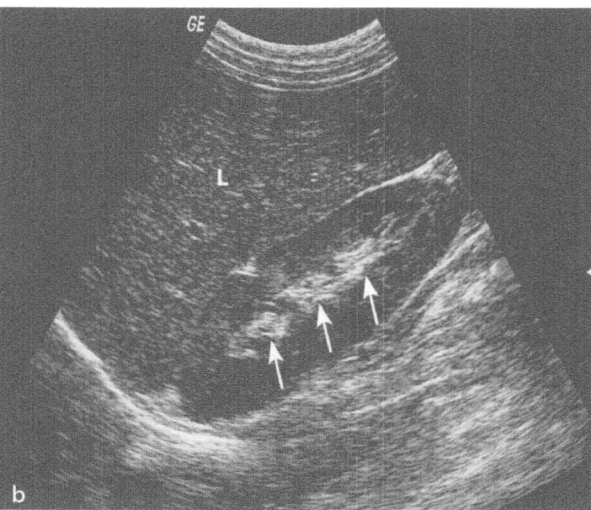

Fig. 3 a, b. Normal renal anatomy. **a** Neonatal kidney. Echogenicity of the cortex (*C*) equals that of the adjacent liver (*L*). Note the prominent, hypoechoic medullary pyramids (*closed arrows*). The central renal sinus (*open arrows*) is only slightly visible. **b** In this 10-year-old child, longitudinal scan of the right kidney reveals an adult pattern. The renal cortex (*C*) is less echogenic than the liver (*L*); the renal pyramids are imperceptible and the renal sinus (*open arrows*) is echogenic. Note the normal junctional parenchymal defect (*closed arrow*) at the upper pole of the kidney

thickening. In high-grade VUR, dilatation of the collecting system has to be differentiated from hydronephrosis or hydroureter due to obstruction.

US is a reliable modality in the evaluation of nephrolithiasis and nephrocalcinosis, with a sensitivity of 96% [30]. In general, stones in the renal pelvis and the calices and at the ureterovesical junction are easily identified sonographically and, depending on their size, may or may not show acoustic shadowing.

Acoustic shadowing is usually detected with calculi greater than 5 mm. Renal stones in the ureter are often associated with obstructive hydronephrosis. US is capable of showing earlier stages of nephrocalcinosis than are plain radiographs.

Because of its multiplanar imaging capability, US remains the modality of choice for initial evaluation of primary or secondary renal tumours (Figs. 5, 6). US can reliably differentiate between intra- and ex-

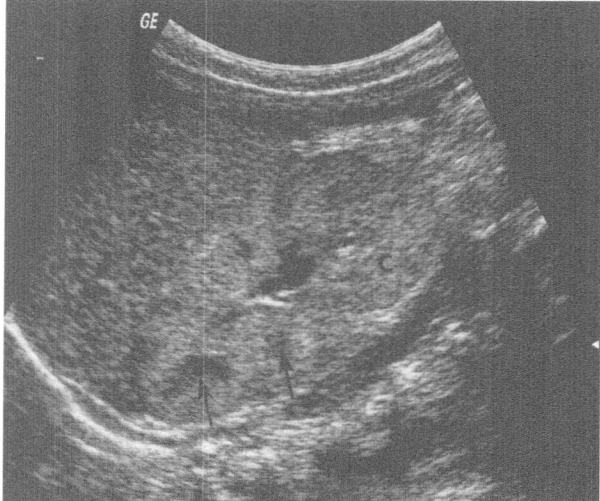

Fig. 4. Congenital nephrotic syndrome. Longitudinal sonogram of an enlarged neonatal kidney demonstrates increased echogenicity of the renal cortex (*C*). The pyramids (*arrows*) are small, and corticomedullary differentiation is reduced

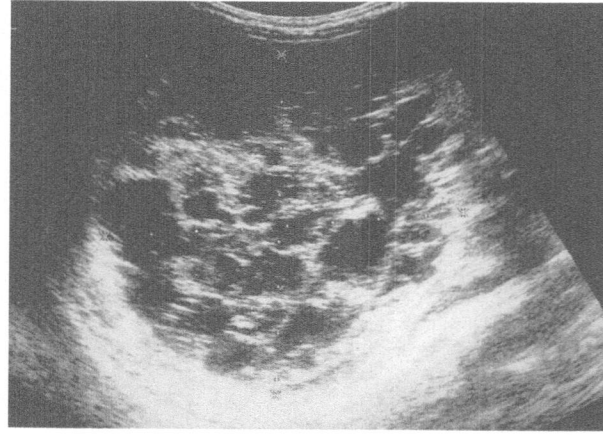

Fig. 5. Multilocular cystic nephroma. Transverse sonogram of the upper pole of the right kidney in a 9-month-old girl shows a predominantly anechoic, septated mass without solid components

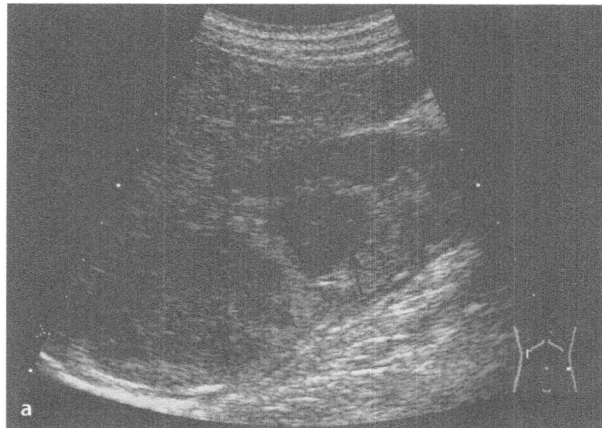

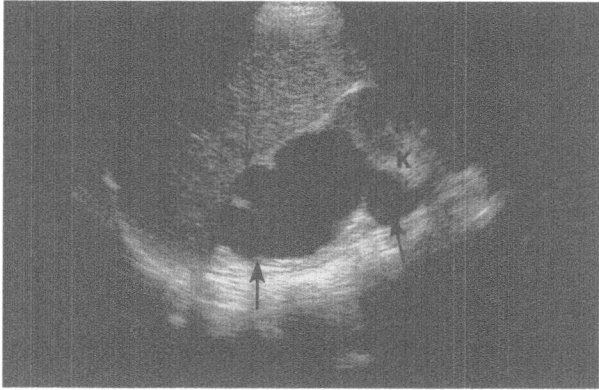

Fig. 7. Urinoma after blunt abdominal trauma. Longitudinal sonogram in a 7-year-old child demonstrates anechoic fluid collection (*arrows*) at the upper pole of the right kidney (*K*)

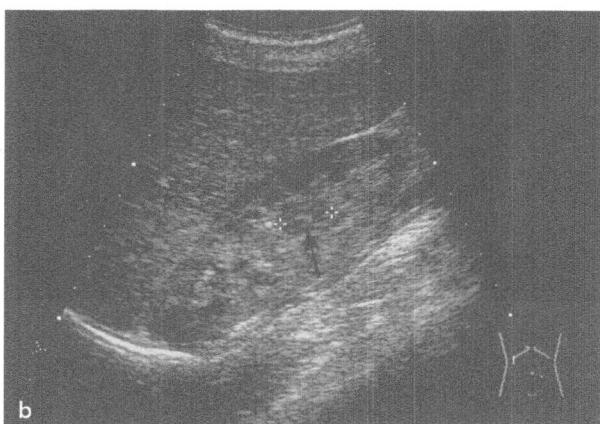

Fig. 6a, b. Renal involvement in non-Hodgkin's lymphoma. **a** Longitudinal sonogram in a 6-year-old boy reveals hypoechoic masses (*arrows*). **b** Control scan 5 days after beginning of therapy demonstrates significant tumour reduction

trarenal tumours such as Wilms' tumour and neuroblastoma and can rule out invasion of such surgically relevant vascular structures as the retrohepatic portion of the IVC and the right atrium. In the cooperative child, US often allows better evaluation of the IVC than contrast-enhanced CT examinations [118]. In the pre- and postoperative periods of therapy, US accurately demonstrates tumour reduction and can rule out local recurrence.

US, even in combination with duplex and colour Doppler, is of limited value in the evaluation of arterial hypertension and renal vascular disease. Possible features in renal artery stenosis are size reduction of the affected kidney and increased cortical echogenicity of the contralateral kidney [46]. US is helpful in the assessment of acute renal cortical or medullary necrosis, but of only limited value in the evaluation of acute tubular necrosis.

Blunt abdominal trauma is a common problem in the paediatric age group. Although computed tomog-

raphy (CT) is the modality of choice in the evaluation of serious abdominal injuries, US is relatively sensitive in identifying lacerations, subcapsular or perirenal haematoma and urinoma (Fig. 7). In combination with duplex and/or colour Doppler it can rule out major vascular injuries.

Conventional US in combination with duplex and colour Doppler remains the primary imaging modality for evaluation of both medical and surgical complications of renal transplantation. Acute rejection can be associated with enlargement of the grafted kidney, decreased sinus fat, abnormal echogenicity of renal cortex and/or pyramids and increased wall thickness of the renal collecting system [145]. US depicts perirenal fluid collections, ureteral obstruction and vascular alterations.

US is the primary imaging modality in evaluation of the lower urinary tract. The thickness of a normal bladder wall varies most with the degree of filling and only minimally with age and gender [76]. US can easily demonstrate the irregularly thickened bladder wall in neurogenic bladder dysfunction. The evaluation of post-voiding bladder volume allows estimation of the extent of emptying without invasive catheterisation and is superior to measurements with MRI [65, 66, 157]. A variety of malformations of the bladder may be encountered, such as duplication, diverticula or urachal remnants. Normal allantoic remnants without symptoms and signs of infection are a common finding in newborns and even older children [23, 167]. US examination is of value in evaluating neoplasms of the lower urinary tract, e.g. rhabdomyosarcoma, and can demonstrate extravesical fluid associated with bladder injury.

2.2.2
Doppler US

The development of Doppler US with its capability to depict renal perfusion added a new dimension to the imaging of the genitourinary tract and provides a useful adjunct to real-time US imaging.

2.2.2.1
Technique

Doppler imaging is based on the Doppler effect, which changes the frequency of the reflected sound wave and is used in duplex Doppler (combination of grey-scale US with pulsed Doppler), colour and power Doppler. The power Doppler mode (colour Doppler energy, amplitude-coded colour Doppler) is independent of Doppler angle and modulated by signal amplitude, but lacks information about direction and flow velocity. Compared with colour Doppler US it gives better visualisation of renal vasculature and perfusion [22, 33, 125]. Unfortunately, power Doppler US is very sensitive to motion and difficult to perform in an uncooperative child.

In Doppler examinations, Doppler settings (transducer frequency, wall filter, pulse repetition frequency and sample volume) are adjusted according to the expected flow rate and the lowest possible beam-to-vessel angle has to be used. The resistance to flow is generally measured by the resistive index (RI). RI is calculated from the formula: RI = peak systolic velocity – end diastolic velocity/peak systolic velocity × 100. The RI decreases with age; the normal RI of the renal vessels in children above 6 years is less than 0.7, most of such children having RIs of approximately 0.6 [91].

2.2.2.2
Clinical Applications

Power Doppler US, with its ability to show hypovascular lesions, seems suitable for use in the diagnosis of acute pyelonephritis with its excellent specificity, but it is less sensitive than CT, renal cortical scintigraphy and MRI (Fig. 8) [9, 33, 99, 162]. A normal colour Doppler US examination can exclude major renal injury [121] and readily identify the formation of arteriovenous fistulas after renal biopsy [102, 124]. In combination with conventional US it provides useful information about allograft dysfunction in renal transplantation [70, 107]. In renal neoplasms, US and duplex and colour Doppler combined allow

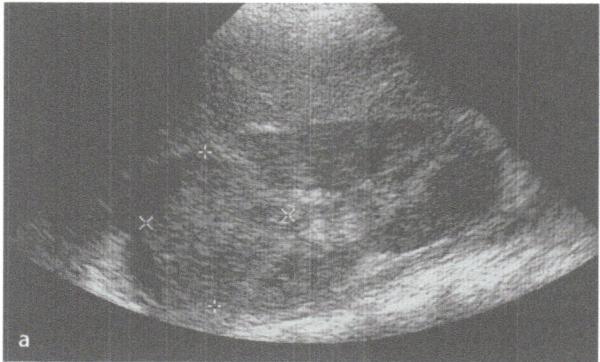

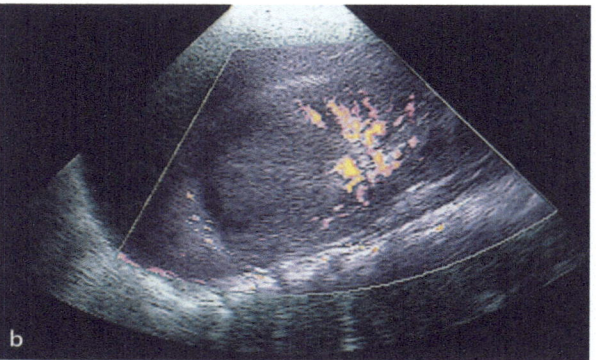

Fig. 8 a, b. Focal bacterial nephritis in process of progressing to abscess formation. **a** Longitudinal sonogram of a 4-year-old child with characteristic clinical findings demonstrates a focal area of increased echogenicity (*crosses*) with a small fluid collection at the upper pole of the right kidney. **b** Power Doppler US allows differentiation between normal renal parenchyma and area of decreased perfusion

direct visualisation of a tumour thrombus in the main renal vein and inferior vena cava and depicts the thrombotic material in renal vein thrombosis. The role of Doppler US in the diagnosis of renal artery stenosis remains controversial. Owing to false-positive and false-negative results, Doppler US seems to be of limited value as a screening modality (Fig. 9) [18, 21, 57].

Colour Doppler US is sensitive in demonstrating ureteric jets and may be an adjunct to conventional US in evaluating patients with VUR [51, 77, 110, 137]. Duplex Doppler US with or without stimulated diuresis seem to be a useful method for differentiating pelviureteric junction obstruction from a dilated collecting system without restriction to urinary outflow [112, 115, 116, 129, 142]. In a study by Kessler et al. [85] using duplex Doppler sonography, patients with unilateral dilatation and obstruction at the pelviureteric junction had significantly higher RIs in cortical renal arteries than patients with unilateral dilatation without obstruction. Intravenous administration of normal saline and frusemide improves the

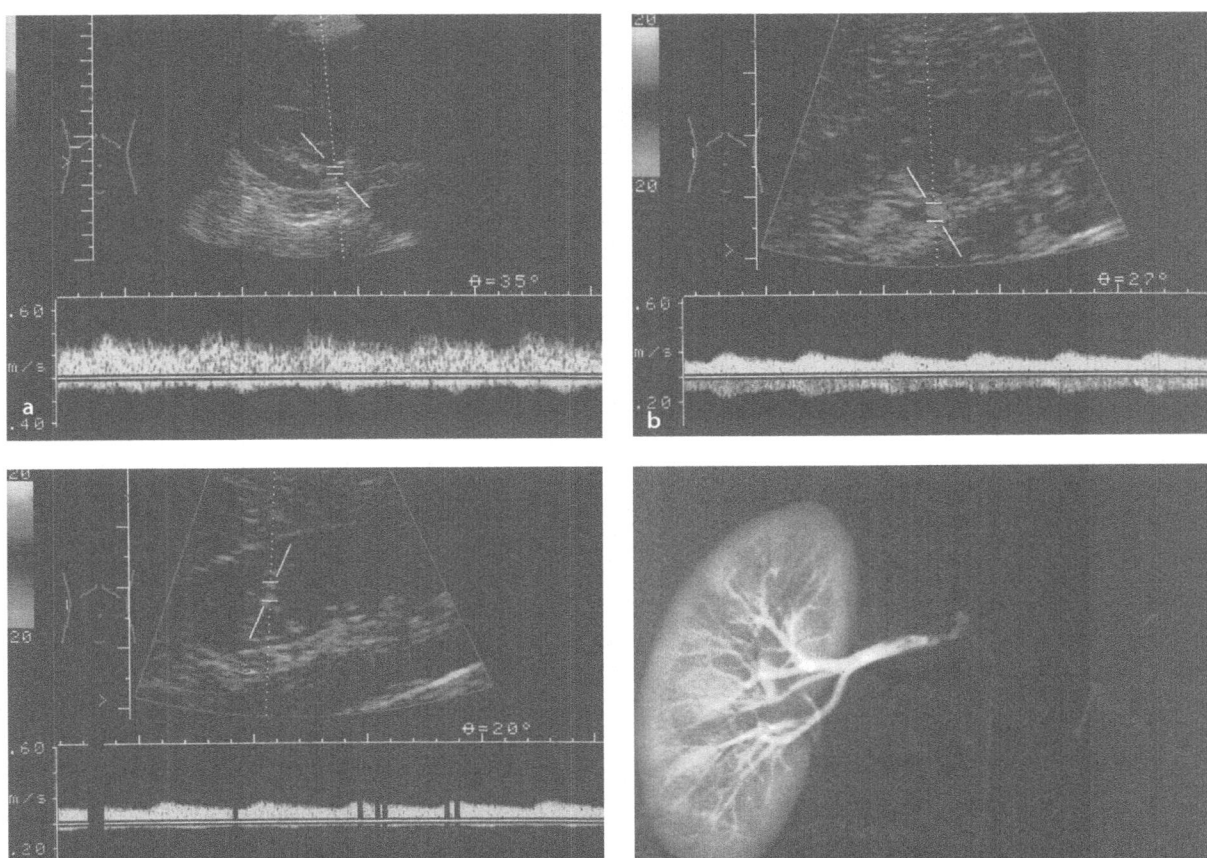

Fig. 9a–d. Renal artery stenosis due to fibromuscular dysplasia in a 12-year-old boy. **a–c** Duplex Doppler US of **a** main renal artery, **b** a segmental renal artery and **c** an interlobar renal artery depicts characteristic dampening of the arterial waveforms. **d** Evaluation of the proximal right renal artery with digital subtraction angiography prior to percutaneous transluminal angioplasty confirms significant stenosis (*arrow*)

sensitivity and specificity of duplex Doppler US in detection of relevant obstruction [141].

2.2.3
Contrast-enhanced Voiding US

VUR is the most common abnormality of the genitourinary tract in the paediatric age group, with a high incidence in children with recurrent UTI. VUR is almost always due to incompetence of the ureterovesical junction and not secondary to infection or obstruction. The primary imaging modalities for detecting and grading VUR are voiding cysto-urethrography (VCUG) and radionuclide cystography (RNC). In order to minimize radiation exposure, contrast-enhanced grey-scale voiding urosonography (CE-VUS) has been developed.

2.2.3.1
Technique

Ultrasound contrast agents are gas-filled microbubbles with a smaller mean diameter less than red blood cells, small enough to cross the lung bed [74]. The bubbles are stabilised and provide systemic vessel enhancement after intravenous injection. Levovist (Schering, Berlin, Germany), a galactose-based echo-enhancing agent, is widely used in CE-VUS. After conventional US examination of the renal tract the bladder is filled to its estimated capacity with room-temperature saline solution. Levovist is administered through the catheter at a concentration of 300 mg/ml in a volume of 8–10% of the bladder volume and the bladder, ureteral orifices and kidneys are re-evaluated with the child in the supine and prone positions before and after voiding. The contrast agent has to be injected slowly to avoid high sonographic attenuation during the initial phase of the examination.

Detection of microbubbles in the collecting system is diagnostic of VUR.

2.2.3.2
Clinical Applications

CE-VUS has been shown to have a high diagnostic value in detecting VUR and could replace VCUG and NC in the follow-up of children with previously documented reflux [10, 15, 36, 37, 101, 151]. CE-VUS can be used primarily in girls and in high-risk groups as a screening procedure [35]. In the study by Valentini et al. [151], the additional use of colour Doppler US during CE-VUS further improved detection of VUR.

2.3
Voiding Cysto-urethrography

VCUG is a fluoroscopic examination done to detect abnormalities in the lower urinary tract, especially vesicoureteral reflux (VUR). The use of appropriate techniques with special attention to fluoroscopy time will allow examinations with very low radiation exposure.

2.3.1
Technique

After thorough review of clinical data and results of prior imaging, it is essential to explain the procedure to parents and children. Current UTI with clinical symptoms is a reason for postponing this examination until up to 1 week after diagnosis [29]. A preliminary US of the genitourinary tract and a spot film of the abdomen before instillation of contrast medium provide valuable information about urine flow impairment or other genitourinary diseases and exclude bone abnormalities and calcifications. Consideration of US findings and fluoroscopic imaging together allows correct interpretation in an especially large proportion of cases and may be crucial to diagnosis.

Catheterisation of the bladder is sometimes a matter of great concern to parents and older children and must be performed atraumatically. The suprapubic approach is used only in neonates with suspected posterior urethral valves or children with malformations. In patients who are likely to be excessively frightened, oral, nasal or intrarectal midazolam provides anxiolysis and anterograde amnesia with no relevant side effects [45, 96, 138]. Numerous compli-

cations of VCUG are reported in the literature [153], but in general this technique is safe and postprocedural discomfort is rare or of minor degree.

Using a sterile technique, the intralabial region or the glans penis is generously cleansed with several swabs of an antibacterial solution. In boys, viscous lidocaine is injected in a retrograde manner several minutes before catheterisation to anaesthetise the urethra. A 8-F feeding tube (5 F for babies under 3 months of age) is inserted into the bladder and carefully taped to the inner thigh in girls and to the abdomen and penis in boys. The use of feeding tubes for catheterisation reduces the risk of injury and overdistension of the bladder. The testes should be shielded with testicular capsules wherever possible.

After a urine specimen has been taken for culture, the lower abdomen is gently pressed to empty the bladder before starting. Because of the risk of chemical irritation, the bladder is filled with relatively dilute contrast medium (150 mg I/ml) up to the estimated capacity, with the bottle at a maximum height of 70 cm above the tabletop. The bladder capacity (in millilitres) is variable, especially in children under 4 years of age, but can be roughly predicted from the following formulas [8, 166]:

Age less than 1 year:
bladder capacity = 7 × weight (kg)

Age greater than 1 year:
bladder capacity = [(age in years) + 2] × 30

In order to keep irradiation low, intermittent digital fluoroscopy and fluorography with the use of last-image-hold or video recording can significantly decrease gonadal exposure and has completely replaced film-screen systems. Further reduction of irradiation can be achieved with a low-dose VCUG. Using a tailored low-dose fluoroscopic protocol, Kleinman et al. [88] obtained diagnostically adequate images with a mean ovarian dose of 0.029 mGy, resulting in a radiation exposure comparable to that with radionuclide cystography (RNC). In a study by Hernandez and Goodsitt [63], pulsed fluoroscopy in the 7.5 pulses per second mode could reduce radiation exposure by 75% compared with conventional fluoroscopy, with only minor reduction in image quality.

At the beginning of the examination, a coned bladder film is taken during the early phase to evaluate a suspected filling defect (e.g. ureterocele) seen on previous US. Little imaging is necessary during further filling, except for another film coned to the full bladder centred on the ureterovesical junction to minimize gonadal exposure in girls. VUR is graded before and after voiding in the anterior-posterior projection according to the International Reflux Study in Children [94]. This classification is based on the extent of filling and dilatation of the ureter, the renal pelvis and the calices by VUR.

The diagnostic accuracy of the VCUG in infants less than 2 years old can be enhanced by a cyclic examination. This is done by putting the child through two or three cycles of filling and voiding before the catheter is finally removed. Evaluation of this procedure showed a discrepancy of presence and/or grade of VUR from one filling to the other in 22 (12%) of 177 patients with two cycles and in 6 (20%) of 30 patients with three cycles [75]. The authors conclude that VCUG seems less reliable for grading reflux than for documenting the absence of VUR [75].

Before micturition starts, a boy is placed in the true lateral or steep oblique and a girl in the anterior-posterior position. This is adequate to obtain a spot film during peak voiding, visualising the whole of the urethra, including the meatus. When a small feeding tube is used removal of the catheter is not always necessary and repeated filling is possible. If reflux is encountered during micturition, oblique bladder views are useful to visualise the retrovesical portion of the ureter. At the conclusion of voiding, a spot film of the bladder and the renal fossa is taken to rule out large amounts of residual urine or reflux not appreciated at fluoroscopy. In cases of high-grade reflux, a film with 5–15 min delay is helpful to evaluate concomitant obstruction at the ureteropelvic or ureterovesical junction [93]. However, the degree of bladder emptying is often limited by urethral discomfort or the unusual setting of VCUG and should be estimated by US.

2.3.2
Clinical Applications

The major indication for VCUG is detection of VUR in UTI (Fig. 10) and pre- and postnatal hydronephrosis and/or megaureter (Fig. 11) [28, 67, 165]. VCUG is appropriate for children under 5 years of age with their first documented UTI and for older children with febrile UTI or recurrent infections. According to Herndon et al. [64], VCUG or RNC is the standard procedure in the follow-up of patients with high-grade reflux undergoing medical treatment.

VCUG is usually recommended in children with ureteropelvic junction obstruction. However, Kim et al. [86] retrospectively evaluated the incidence and history of VUR in patients with this entity. All low-grade reflux coexisting with a ureteropelvic junction obstruction disappeared after pyeloplasty. They con-

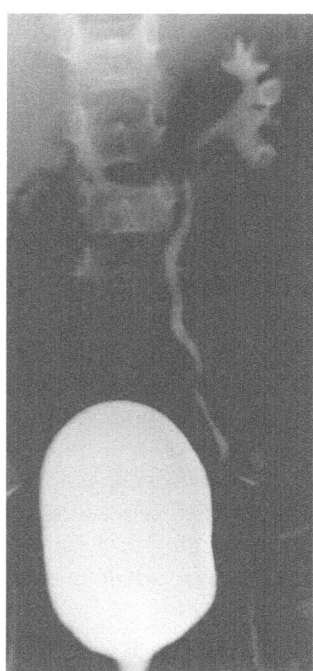

Fig. 10. Vesico-ureterorenal reflux in a 4-year-old girl with urinary tract infection (UTI). Voiding cysto-urography (VCUG) demonstrates grade 2 reflux on the left side

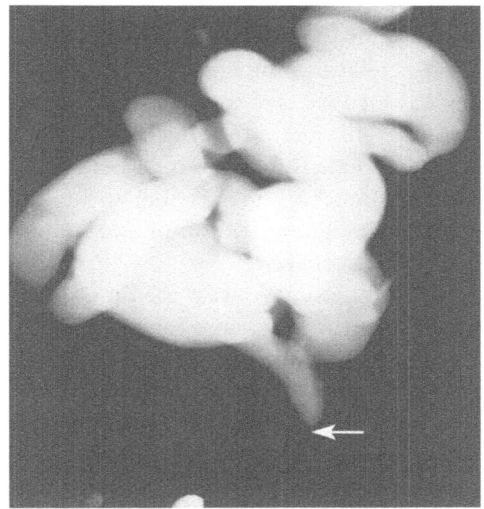

Fig. 11. Posterior urethral valve. VCUG in a newborn shows posterior urethral valve (*arrow*) and dilated posterior urethra and megaureter due to high-grade reflux

cluded that VCUG should be limited to children with megaureter on US.

VCUG is commonly used in children after uretero-cystoneostomy to evaluate for urinary tract obstruction or persistent reflux. However, a study on 153 patients with reimplantation of 267 renal units indicates that VCUG is limited in identification of patients at risk for febrile UTI [61].

VCUG can identify children with bladder instability, evaluating bladder morphology as well as filling of the posterior urethra [5], and is part of the investigative pathway in anorectal malformations and urethral trauma [13].

2.4
Intravenous Urography

Until the advent of real-time US the intravenous urography (IVU) has been the most important diagnostic modality in the assessment of urinary tract disease in childhood. Because of radiation exposure, relative invasiveness and inadequate image detail in children with diminished renal function, its impact on genitourinary imaging has been substantially diminished by US, nuclear medicine and MRI.

2.4.1
Technique

To limit radiation exposure and invasiveness of imaging procedures, the imaging sequences of IVU have to be tailored to the main clinical question [7, 79]. Keeping in mind that multiple imaging modalities can provide relevant information, the radiologist should act as a consultant to referring disciplines. A predetermined number of radiographs in IVU often provides inadequate information and entails unnecessary irradiation. This means that the radiologist has to supervise the entire examination and determine how best to proceed.

The use of nonionic contrast medium in IVU has clearly increased the safety and tolerance of contrast agents. With a lower osmolality and a higher urinary iodine concentration a denser pyelogram is achieved than with ionic agents. However, with an osmolality of 600–700 mosmol/kg they are still hyperosmolar compared with plasma. The amount of contrast medium (300 mg iodine/ml) used in paediatric IVU has to related to patient age:

- Newborns: 3 ml/kg bodyweight (minimal 15 ml, maximal 25 ml)
- Infants: 2.5 ml/kg bodyweight (maximal 25 ml)
- Older children: 1 ml/kg bodyweight (minimal 25 ml, maximal 60 ml)

Adverse contrast reactions (ACR) can be categorised as allergic, cardiovascular or toxic. Compared with ionic contrast media, nonionic contrast agents have a significantly lower incidence of ACR – lower by a factor of 4 [83] – and are well tolerated in paediatric examinations [152]. Because of complications, it seems advisable to obtain written informed consent from the parents and to be prepared to take appropriate preventive or therapeutic measures.

Recommendations for bowel preparation prior to IVU in children and adults are still a matter of debate. Different prospective studies suggest that dietary restrictions and the use of stimulant or osmotic laxatives do not improve the visualisation of the urinary tract on excretory urograms [6, 16, 139]. Therefore, vigorous bowel preparation or fluid restriction can no longer be recommended. From a practical point of view, a low-residue diet with a short fasting period of approximately 4 h before the examination seems reasonable.

In children 2–5 years old the calculated effective dose for a standard four-film IVU is 2–3 mSv [2, 146]. Like urethrocystography [168], digital radiography allows substantial dose reduction of IVU by up to 50% with no significant difference in diagnostic accuracy or image quality [73, 89] and will make repeated examinations because of exposure errors unnecessary.

After a US examination of the urinary tract the radiographic sequence starts with a supine abdominal film including the kidneys and the bony pelvis to the level of the symphysis. In the paediatric age group, preliminary or postinjection tomograms are replaced by high-resolution US. A cross-kidney collimated 5- or 7-min film usually shows sharp reproduction of calices, still providing sufficient visualisation of the nephrogram. The routine examination is completed with a full-length 15-min film in the supine position and a supine or prone full-length 30-min film, preferably after the child has voided. In order to improve the visualisation of kidneys, compression or the use of fizzy drinks is recommended to displace obscuring bowel or to create a gastric window. Delayed radiographs are obtained after 2, 4 or even 24 h in the presence of urinary obstruction.

To differentiate obstructed from nonobstructed collecting systems in suspected pelviureteric obstruction, diuretic IVU has been established for more than 20 years [161] and seems applicable to the paediatric age group [129]. After injection of frusemide (0.5 mg/kg bodyweight) increasing dilatation and poor washout of contrast medium after 20 min indicate relevant obstruction.

2.4.2
Clinical Applications

IVU has been largely supplanted in the evaluation of renal growth, abdominal masses and adrenal lesions by US, CT and MRI. In cases of renal dysplasia, IVU is

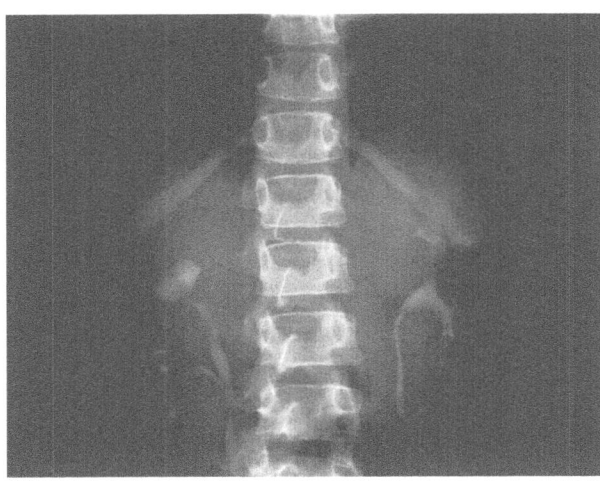

Fig. 12. Duplex kidney with partial duplication of the collecting system in an 8-year-old girl. Seven-minute cross-kidney collimated radiograph demonstrates duplication of the right collecting system with Y-shaped ureters

noncontributory owing to poor renal function. IVU can be used to provide morphological information in cases of renal duplication in order to identify an ectopic ureter or ureterocele (Fig. 12) [79, 122], but it is inferior to antero- or retrograde pyelogram in ureteric injuries [58].

IVU is no longer indicated in children with uncomplicated UTI and enuresis [3]. However, using the classic criteria for renal scarring, caliceal deformity and parenchymal reduction, IVU is able to detect reflux nephropathy or chronic atrophic pyelonephritis [68, 146, 150].

In patients with obstructive uropathy IVU should be performed after US, and only if findings of US and diuretic renography are inconclusive. IVU remains useful in the evaluation of stone diseases of the urinary tract, but could be replaced by US and CT [56, 103, 109, 140]. However, IVU remains an important part of the preoperative planning of extracorporeal shock wave lithotripsy (ESWL) in children [92, 111].

2.5
Computed Tomography

Since its inception, computed tomography (CT) has quickly become established as an important diagnostic modality. The major advantage of helical CT in paediatric imaging is the shorter examination time, with decreased image degradation from motion artefacts [143]. Contrast material-enhanced helical CT can evaluate various phases of vessel and organ enhancement and provide more extensive coverage of target areas. Other improvements are the acquisition

of near-isotropic image data with the option of true multiplanar reconstruction and the possibility of three-dimensional rendering [25, 53, 55]).

2.5.1
Technique

In order to facilitate the investigation, placement of IV lines is ideally performed before examination in an outpatient department. With either peripheral or central venous access, routine manual injection of contrast material has been partially supplanted by the use of power injectors [53, 82]. However, a complication rate of 0.4–10% was noted using central venous lines [82, 127]. Oral contrast is always preferable to delineate bowel loops from pathology using barium sulphate or water-soluble contrast medium in a dilution of 1–2%. Exceptions are patients at risk of aspiration and those with acute blunt trauma where time is insufficient for contrast administration. Depending on patient age and size, immobilisation with blankets or adhesive tapes facilitates the examination.

In the era of single-section incremental CT the long acquisition time was responsible for sedation in 8–18% of paediatric patients. With the implementation of single-slice and multislice helical CT, this rate could be significantly reduced to 3.3–10% without deterioration of image quality [117, 159]. The need for sedation has to be determined individually by the attending radiologist. For neonates and small infants, sedation can be avoided by recent breast feeding. If sedation is unavoidable and natural sleep not within reach, appropriate drugs such as chloral hydrate, midazolam and sodium pentobarbital can be used in CT and MRI examinations [12, 26, 136, 164]. Oral chloral hydrate seems to provide more effective sedation than midazolam [34, 80], but is more commonly associated with delayed side effects, e.g. motor imbalance and agitation [100].

As for IVU, nonionic iodinated contrast media are recommended. The standard amount of IV contrast material used in children has so far been 2.0–3.0 ml/kg body weight [53, 143], but lower doses of 1.0–1.5 ml/kg bodyweight with an injection rate as slow as 0.3–0.8 ml/s have also proved to be diagnostic [149]. Because of many variables (e.g. gauge and site of venous access, state of hydration and age-related changes in cardiac output) optimal enhancement in abdominal examinations is achieved with a scanning onset after all contrast material has been administered [160]. In neonates and infants, this delay may be protracted by 10 s to ensure the arrival of small contrast volumes. Recently, bolus tracking technology has allowed for determination of enhancement in regions of interest [55]. However, owing to increased radiation exposure and the lack of diagnostic value in standard situations, the bolus-tracking technique is still infrequently used in paediatric protocols [53, 160].

Radiation exposure is still an important issue in paediatric CT imaging. In a recent publication Brenner et al. [17] emphasised the association of cancer risks and low-dose radiation due to paediatric CT examinations. Effective radiation doses and radiosensitivity of organs and tissues are significantly higher in children than in adults, and highest in newborns [72, 158]. For abdominal examinations Huda et al. [72] calculated an effective dose of 5.3 mSv in newborns, 3.7 mSv in children at the age of 5 and 3.1 mSv in adults. Therefore, paediatric protocols should generally imply low milliampere settings (90–140 mA for routine body scanning, 80 mA for examination of the pelvis), adjusted collimation (3–5 mm in infants) and a high pitch up to 2 : 1 to minimise irradiation [78, 119, 160]. A recent comprehensive article on that subject proposed adjustment of tube current according to patient weight [42].

2.5.2
Clinical Applications

Although CT is widely accepted in evaluation of the abdomen and pelvis, alternative imaging modalities such as high-resolution US are commonly preferred to characterise diseases of the genitourinary tract.

The major application of spiral CT in paediatric imaging is staging and preoperative assessment of renal tumours (Figs. 13, 14) [54, 97]. Its disadvantage in this setting is the restrained differentiation between intra- and extrarenal masses owing to axial scanning and false-positive detection of vascular tumour invasion [14, 120]. Contrast-enhanced CT is superior to US in the evaluation of renal lymphoma. In abdominal trauma, it shows precisely the extent of urinoma or haematoma, renal contusion and alterations in the vascular supply to the kidney [81, 156, 164].

Unenhanced CT is superior to US and IVU for the detection of urinary tract calculi and renal scarring and can be used in paediatric patients who are well known to be allergy sufferers [103, 108, 114, 140, 147].

CT is not indicated in children with uncomplicated UTI, but may be of value in selected cases to determine the extent of an inflammatory process and to verify abscesses and calcifications [32, 104]. Contrast-

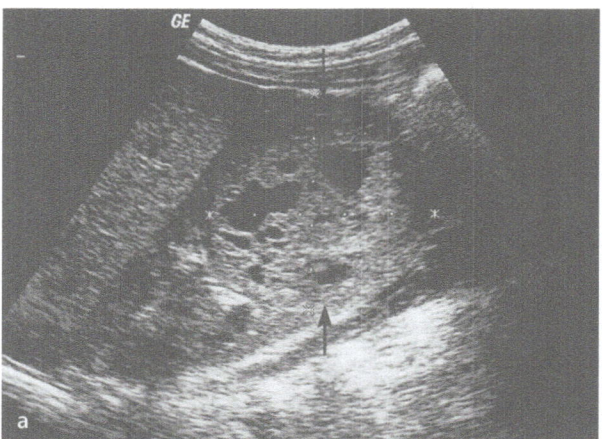

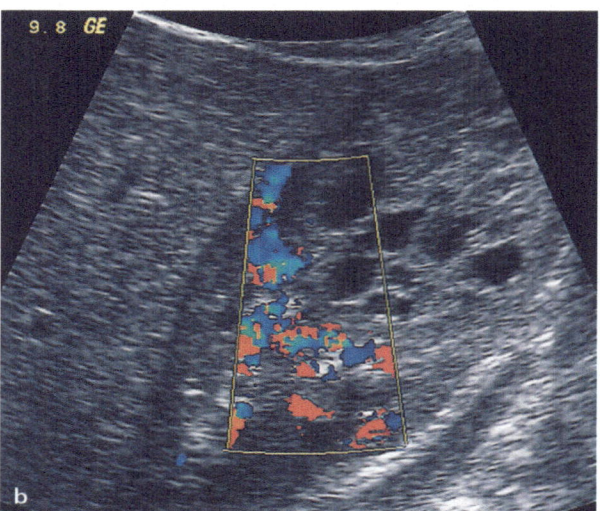

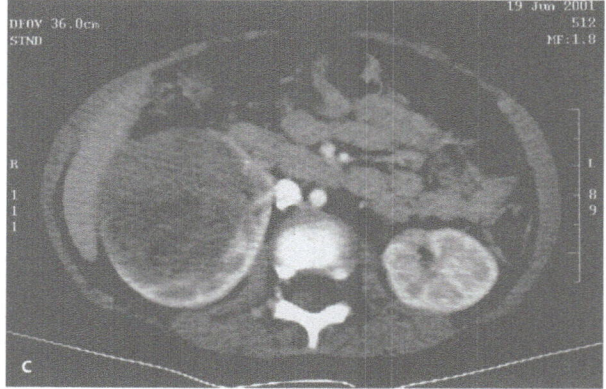

Fig. 13 a–c. Wilms' tumour. **a** Longitudinal grey-scale US shows a large, heterogeneous echogenic mass (*arrows*) with areas of necrosis in the right kidney of a 2-year-old child. **b** Colour Doppler examination demonstrates flow in the adjacent parenchyma but not in the mass. **c** Contrast-enhanced CT confirms a low-density mass compressing the surrounding cortex

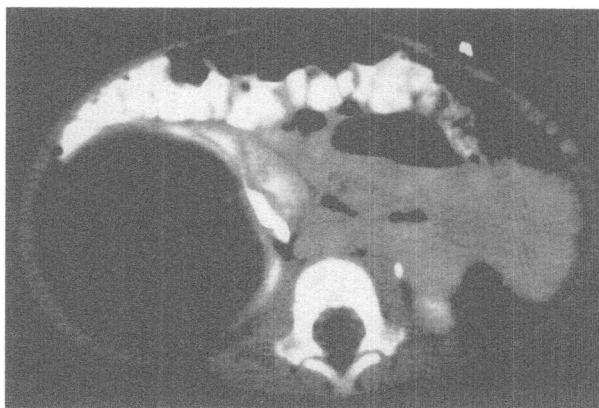

Fig. 14. Multilocular cystic nephroma. Multislice CT confirms a water attenuation mass with thin septations and a small rim of enhancing parenchyma medially

enhanced CT urography and automated measurement of renal parenchymal volume using a multislice scanner [20, 25, 109] seem inappropriate for the radiosensitive paediatric age group.

Potential applications of multiphase examinations with precontrast and postcontrast imaging in the cortical, nephrographic and excretory phase are the preoperative distinction of renal vessels from parenchymal abnormalities and improved detection of focal lesions (e.g. in nephroblastomatosis). Multiplanar imaging facilitates the depiction of vascular tumour invasion but is not superior to axial evaluation. To date, there are no routine applications for CT angiography in children. Vascular anatomy before renal transplantation and exclusion of renal artery stenosis are an indication for magnetic resonance angiography.

2.6
Magnetic Resonance Imaging

The advent of magnetic resonance imaging (MRI) has facilitated the assessment of morphology and function of the urinary tract in children. The advantage of this modality includes multiplanar imaging, high soft-tissue contrast and use of non-nephrotoxic contrast media without radiation exposure. Disadvantages are high costs and complex and time-consuming protocols. Owing to the development of MR angiography (MRA) and MR urography (MRU) it offers a one-stop imaging examination, obviating the need for conventional arteriography and IVU. The next section presents a brief survey of characteristic imaging strategies and capabilities of MRI in paediatric uroradiology.

2.6.1
Technique

As in CT examinations, appropriate and timely placement of intravenous lines, child-adapted sedation protocols and proper immobilisation are of paramount importance in MR imaging (see section on CT). If sedation is necessary, it can be safely and effectively monitored by magnetic-compatible pulse oximeters or ECG [154]. Additionally, monitoring of body temperature is advised in newborns. Coils have to be adapted to the size of the child and allow acquisition of high-resolution images.

MR imaging in paediatric urology has to be tailored to the clinical question and the age of the patient. Examination protocols for small or sedated children require respiratory triggering and have to obviate breath-hold sequences. For visualisation of kidneys and the pararenal spaces examination starts with acquisition of scout images in three orthogonal planes to ensure proper positioning. Anatomical orientation with corticomedullary differentiation can be achieved in axial and coronal planes with fat demarcating T1-weighted spin-echo (SE) sequences or gradient recalled echo sequences (GRE) during suspended respiration (e.g., FLASH, FFE). This is usually followed by a series of T2-weighted images to differentiate cystic from solid lesions and to detect parenchymal oedema or inflammatory processes. Fat-suppressed T2-weighted sequences are helpful in decreasing chemical shift artefacts and allow direct comparison with nonenhanced T1-weighted images. Fat-saturated T1-weighted dynamic sequences acquired in axial or coronal planes at different times after bolus administration of gadolinium-DTPA characterise renal disease and provide information regarding renal perfusion and filtration.

Owing to the lack of ionising radiation, the well-tolerated administration of gadolinium and obviation of arterial catheterisation, MRA offers several advantages over conventional angiography and allows multiplanar reconstruction and maximum-intensity projections (MIP). In the older and cooperative child, evaluation of renal vasculature can be achieved with axial 2D time of flight (TOF) sequences or gadolinium-enhanced 3D MRA during a breath-hold. In the absence of breath holding, the quality of MRA images remains high even in the sedated or uncooperative child. The acquisition of coronal images optimises depiction of small accessory renal arteries, which are detected with a high sensitivity.

The development of MR urography (MRU) has noticeably enriched the evaluation of the urinary tract and can supplant IVU in special cases. In order to visualise the urinary tract, T2-weighted static fluid MRU or T1-weighted contrast-enhanced (excretory) MRU can be used. Owing to the high signal, heavily T2-weighted sequences allow depiction of stationary fluid-filled spaces such as the renal collecting system, displayed in a projection comparable to standard IVU. This can be achieved with the rapid acquisition with relaxation enhancement (RARE) technique [52, 134]. RARE requires no administration of gadolinium and is independent of renal function. Inherent limitations are dependence on a dilated collecting system, the difficulty of detecting calculi and the inability to differentiate between VUR and nonrefluxing dilatation of the GU tract [144]. Further reductions in acquisition time and other improvements in relation to RARE are achieved in breathhold MRU using the half-Fourier acquisition single-shot turbo spin echo (HASTE) technique [1, 123]. HASTE reliably depicts the degree of dilatation of the collecting system and the site of obstruction [123]. In order to allow continuous breathing in small children, other techniques use respiratory-triggered T2-weighted turbo spin-echo (TSE) sequences [113, 131, 133].

Dynamic imaging after administration of gadolinium with or without a low dose of frusemide allows corticomedullary differentiation due to the first-pass effect of contrast material and enable assessment of the kidneys with differentiation between obstructive and nonobstructive diseases. In combination with static MRU it provides information about renal morphology and function [130, 148].

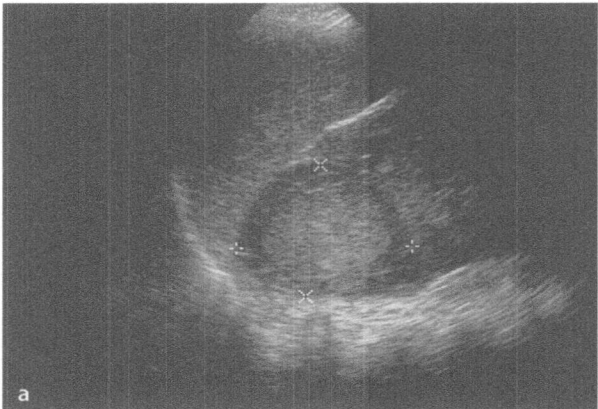

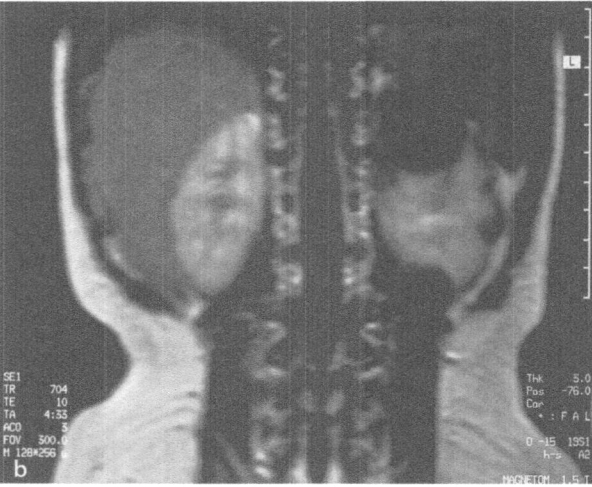

Fig. 15 a, b. Wilms' tumour. **a** Longitudinal sonogram shows an echogenic mass with a hypoechoic rim at the upper pole of the left kidney. **b** Coronal contrast-enhanced T1-weighted image demonstrates multifocal tumour development

2.6.2
Clinical Applications

MRI is well suited to differentiate benign mesenchymal masses such as haemangiomas or lipomas [38]. Contrast-enhanced MRI is the modality of choice in the preoperative staging of malignant renal tumours with its capability to depict metastatic lymph nodes as well as venous infiltration and represents an ideal technique for planning of surgical procedures (Fig. 15).

Owing to superior tissue contrast, MRI is able to detect small haemorrhages or infarctions and is as valid as other modalities in the evaluation of renal scarring [90, 128, 155]. In a study by Lonergan et al. [95], gadolinium-enhanced inversion-recovery sequences proved to be superior to cortical scintigraphy in the diagnosis of pyelonephritis. MRU provides detailed information about level and extension of the obstruction (Fig. 16) and can depict characteristic microcystic dilatation of collecting ducts in polycys-

tic kidney disease [84, 135]. MRI is an alternative to IVU in patients with renal failure, renal transplantation or previous allergic response to iodinated contrast media. In children with duplex systems and ectopic ureter MRU can be helpful in depicting renal morphology and ureteral course [148].

As it is not invasive, contrast-enhanced MRI with angiographic sequences is the modality of choice for evaluating such renovascular diseases as renal artery stenosis and can become a one-stop examination in the evaluation of prospective renal donors (Fig. 17) [120].

2.7
Conclusions

The advent of various new imaging techniques has clearly modified the diagnostic algorithms used in

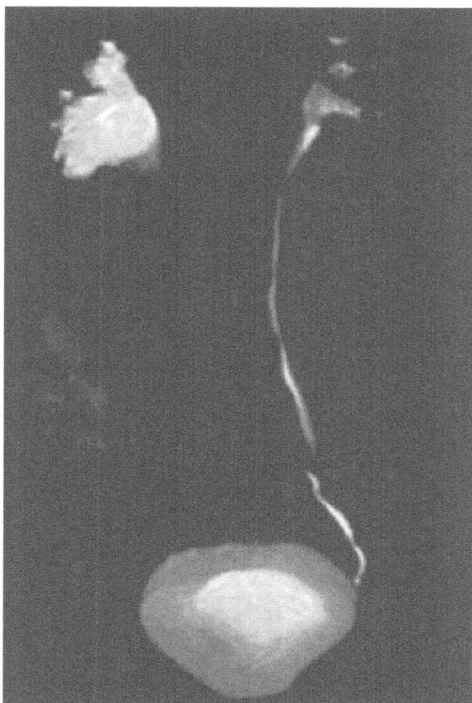

Fig. 16. Ureteropelvic junction obstruction. Gadolinium-enhanced T1-weighted excretory MRU demonstrates dilatation of the right pelvicaliceal system and the level of obstruction without identification of a ureter

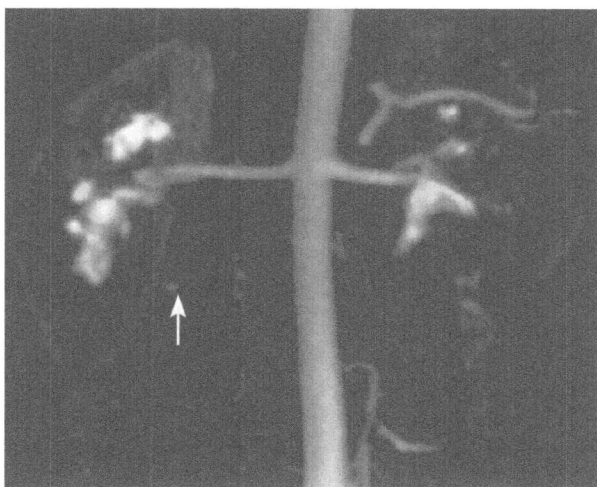

Fig. 17. Accessory renal artery. Coronal maximum-intensity projection of gadolinium-enhanced 3D MRA shows accessory renal artery (*arrow*)

paediatric uroradiology. In times when we all have to be cost conscious and increasingly sensitive to the possible dangers of low-dose radiation, paediatric radiologists have to be familiar with the strengths and weaknesses of the available modalities so as to be capable of tailoring imaging to patients' needs.

References

1. Aerts P, Van Hoe L, Bosmans H et al (1996) Breath-hold MR urography using the HASTE technique. AJR Am J Roentgenol 166:543–545
2. Almen A, Mattsson S (1995) The radiation dose to children from X-ray examinations of the pelvis and the urinary tract. Br J Radiol 68:604–613
3. Alon U, Berant M, Pery M (1989) Intravenous pyelography in children with urinary tract infection and vesicoureteral reflux. Pediatrics 83:332–336
4. Alon US, Ganapathy S (1999) Should renal ultrasonography be done routinely in children with urinary tract infection? Clin Pediatr 38:21–25
5. Bachelard M, Verkauskas G, Bertilsson M et al (2001) Recognition of bladder instability on voiding cystourethrography in infants with urinary tract infection. J Urol 166:1899–1903
6. Bailey SR , Tyrrell PN, Hale M (1991) A trial to assess the effectiveness of bowel preparation prior to intravenous urography. Clin Radiol 44:335–337
7. Ben-Ami T, Rozin M, Hertz M (1989) Imaging of children with urinary tract infection: a tailored approach. Clin Radiol 40:64–67
8. Berger RM, Maizels M, Moran GC et al (1983) Bladder capacity (ounces) equals age (years) plus 2 predicts normal bladder capacity and aids in diagnosis of abnormal voiding patterns. J Urol 129:347–349
9. Berro Y, Baratte B, Seryer D et al (2000) Comparison between scintigraphy, B-mode, and power Doppler sonography in acute pyelonephritis in children. J Radiol 81:523–527
10. Berrocal T, Gaya F, Arjonilla A et al (2001) Vesicoureteral reflux: diagnosis and grading with echo-enhanced cystosonography versus voiding cystourethrography. Radiology 221:359–365
11. Blachar A, Schachter M, Blachar Y et al (1994) Evaluation of prenatally diagnosed hydronephrosis by morphometric measurements of the kidney. Pediatr Radiol 24:131–134
12. Bluemke DA, Breiter SN (2000) Sedation procedures in MR imaging: safety, effectiveness, and nursing effect on examination. Radiology 216:645–652
13. Boemers TM, Beek FJ, Bax NM (1999) Guidelines for the urological screening and initial management for lower urinary tract dysfunction in children with anorectal malformation- the ARGUS protocol. BJU Int 83:662–671
14. Bos SD, Mensink HJ (1998) Can duplex Doppler ultrasound replace computerized tomography in staging patients with renal cell carcinoma? Scand J Urol 32:87–91
15. Bosio M (1998) Cystosonography with echocontrast: a new imaging modality to detect vesicoureteric reflux in children. Pediatr Radiol 28:250–255
16. Bradley AJ, Taylor PM (1996) Does bowel preparation improve the quality of intravenous urography? Br J Radiol 69:906–909
17. Brenner DJ, Elliston CD, Hall EJ (2001) Response to the statement by the society for pediatric radiology on radiation risks from pediatric CT scans. Pediatr Radiol 31:389–391
18. Broekhuizen-de Gast HS, Tiel-van Buul MM, Van Beek EJ (2001) Severe hypertension in children with renovascular disease. Clin Nucl Med 26:606–609

19. Brown T, Mandell J, Lebowitz RL (1987) Neonatal hydronephrosis in the era of sonography. AJR Am J Roentgenol 148:959–963
20. Brown MS, Feng WC, Hall TR et al (2001) Knowledge-based segmentation of pediatric kidneys in CT for measurement of parenchymal volume. J Comput Assist Tomogr 25:639–648
21. Brun P, Kchouk H, Mouchet B et al (1997) Value of Doppler ultrasound for the diagnosis of renal artery stenosis in children. Pediatr Nephrol 11:27–30
22. Bude RO, Rubin JM, Adler RS (1994) Power versus conventional color Doppler sonography: comparison in the depiction of normal intrarenal vasculature. Radiology 192:777–780
23. Cacciarelli AA, Kass EJ, Yang SS (1990) Urachal remnants: sonographic demonstration in children. Radiology 174:473–475
24. Carrico CW, Zerin JM (1996) Sonographic measurements of renal length in children: does the position of the patient matter? Pediatr Radiol 26:553–555
25. Chow LC, Sommer FG (2001) Multidetector CT urography with abdominal compression and three-dimensional reconstruction. AJR Am J Roentgenol 177:849–855
26. Chung T, Hoffer FA, Connor L et al (2000) The use of oral pentobarbital sodium (Nembutal) versus oral chloral hydrate in infants undergoing CT and MR imaging – a pilot study. Pediatr Radiol 30:332–335
27. Cohen HL, Cooper J, Eisenberg P et al (1991) Normal length of fetal kidneys: sonographic study in 397 obstetric patients. AJR Am J Roentgenol 157:545–548
28. Coret A, Morag B, Katz M et al (1994) The impact of fetal screening on indications for cystourethrography in infants. Pediatr Radiol 24:516–518
29. Craig JC, Knight JF, Sureshkumar P et al (1997) Vesicoureteral reflux and timing of micturating cystourethrography after urinary tract infection. Arch Dis Child 76:275–277
30. Cramer B, Husa L, Pushpanathan C (1998) Nephrocalcinosis in rabbits-correlation of ultrasound, computed tomography, pathology and renal function. Pediatr Radiol 28:9–13
31. Dacher JN, Mandell J, Lebowitz RL (1992) Urinary tract infection in infants in spite of prenatal diagnosis of hydronephrosis. Pediatr Radiol 22:401–404
32. Dacher JN, Boillot B, Eurin D et al (1993) Rational use of CT in acute pyelonephritis: findings and relationships with reflux. Pediatr Radiol 23:281–285
33. Dacher JN, Pfister C, Monroc M et al (1996) Power Doppler sonographic pattern of acute pyelonephritis in children: comparison with CT. AJR Am J Roentgenol 166:1451–1455
34. D'Agostino J, Terndrup TE (2000) Chloral hydrate versus midazolam for sedation of children for neuroimaging: a randomized clinical trial. Pediatr Emerg Care 16:1–4
35. Darge K (2002) Diagnosis of vesicoureteral reflux with ultrasonography. Pediatr Nephrol 17:52–60
36. Darge K, Troeger J, Duetting T et al (1999) Reflux in young patients: comparison of voiding US of the bladder and retrovesical space with echo enhancement versus voiding cystourethrography for diagnosis. Radiology 219:201–207
37. Darge K, Ghods S, Zieger B et al (2001) Reduction in voiding cystourethrographies after the introduction of contrast enhanced sonographic reflux diagnosis. Pediatr Radiol 31:790–795
38. Davidson AJ, Hartman DS, Choyke PL et al (1997) Radiologic assessment of renal masses: implications for patient care. Radiology 202:297–305
39. Dejter SW Jr, Gibbon MD (1989) The fate of infant kidneys with fetal hydronephrosis but initially normal postnatal sonography. J Urol 142:661–662
40. De Sanctis JT, Connolly SA, Bramson RT (1998) Effect of patient position on sonographically measured renal length in neonates, infants, and children. AJR Am J Roentgenol 170:1381–1383
41. Dinkel E, Ertel M, Dittrich M et al (1985) Kidney size in childhood. Sonographical growth charts for kidney length and volume. Pediatr Radiol 15:38–43
42. Donnelly LF, Emery KH, Brody AS et al (2001) Minimizing radiation dose for pediatric body applications of single-detector helical CT: strategies at a large children hospital. AJR Am J Roentgenol 176:303–306
43. Ebel KD (1998) Uroradiology in the fetus and newborn: diagnosis and follow-up of congenital obstruction of the urinary tract. Pediatr Radiol 28:630–635
44. Ebel KD, Bliesener JA, Gharib M (1988) Imaging of uretero-pelvic junction obstruction with stimulated diuresis. Pediatr Radiol 18:54–56
45. Elder JS, Longenecker R (1995) Premedication with oral midazolam for voiding cystourethrography in children: safety and efficacy. AJR Am J Roentgenol 164:1229–1232
46. Enriquez G, Castello F, Sousa P et al (1997) Increased cortical echogenicity of the normal kidney in infants with unilateral renal artery stenosis: report of two cases. J Ultrasound Med 16:59–63
47. Erwin BC, Carroll BA, Muller H (1985) A sonographic assessment of neonatal renal parameters. J Ultrasound Med 4:217–220
48. Evans ED, Meyer JS, Harty MP et al (1999) Assessment of increase in renal pelvic size on post-void sonography as a predictor of vesicoureteral reflux. Pediatr Radiol 29:291–294
49. Fernbach SK, Maizels M, Conway JJ (1993) Ultrasound grading of hydronephrosis: introduction to the system used by the Society for Fetal Urology. Pediatr Radiol 23:478–480
50. Foresman WH, Hulbert WC Jr, Rabinowitz R (2001) Does urinary tract ultrasonography at hospitalization for acute pyelonephritis predict vesicoureteral reflux? J Urol 165:2232–2234
51. Frauscher F, Radmayr C, Klauser A et al (1999) Assessment of renal resistance index in children with vesicoureteral reflux. Ultraschall Med 20:93–97
52. Friedburg HG, Henning J, Frankenschmidt A (1987) RARE MR urography: a fast nontomographic imaging procedure for demonstrating the efferent urinary pathways using nuclear magnetic resonance. Radiologe 27:45–47
53. Frush DP, Donnelly LF (1998) Helical CT in children: technical considerations and body applications. Radiology 209:37–48
54. Frush DP, Siegel MJ, Bisset GS III (1997) From the RSNA refresher courses. Challenges of pediatric spiral CT. Radiographics 17:939–959
55. Frush DP, Spencer EB, Donnelly LF et al (1999) Optimizing contrast-enhanced abdominal CT in infants and children using bolus tracking. AJR Am J Roentgenol 172:1007–1013

56. Gallagher HJ, Tolley DA (2000) 2000 AD: still a role for the intravenous urogram in stone management? Curr Opin Urol 10:551–555

57. Garel L, Dubois J, Robitaille P et al (1995) Renovascular hypertension in children: curability predicted with negative intrarenal Doppler results. Radiology 195:401–405

58. Ghali AM, El Malik EM, Ibrahim AI et al (1999) Ureteric injuries: diagnosis, management, and outcome. J Trauma 46:150–158

59. Goldberg SD, Witchell S, Drohomyrecky A et al (1988) Diuretic ultrasound: technique for assessment of obstructed renal unit. Urology 32:546–548

60. Grignon A, Filion R, Filiatrault D et al (1986) Urinary tract dilatation in utero: classification and clinical applications. Radiology 160:645–647

61. Grossklaus DJ, Pope JC, Adams MC et al (2001) Is postoperative cystography necessary after ureteral reimplantation? Urology 58:1041–1045

62. Han BK, Babcock DS (1985) Sonographic measurements and appearance of normal kidneys in children. AJR Am J Roentgenol 145:611–616

63. Hernandez RJ, Goodsitt MM (1996) Reduction of radiation dose in pediatric patients using pulsed fluoroscopy. AJR Am J Roentgenol 167:1247–1253

64. Herndon CD, Ferrer FA, McKenna PH (2001) Survey on medical and surgical follow-up of patients with vesicoureteral reflux from American Association of Pediatrics, Section on Urology members. J Urol 165:559–563

65. Hiraoka M, Tsukahara H, Tsuchida S et al (1993) Ultrasonographic evaluation of bladder volume in children. Pediatr Nephrol 7:533–535

66. Hiraoka M, Hori C, Tsuchida S et al (1995) Ultrasonographic evaluation of bladder volume in young children. Pediatr Nephrol 9:351–353

67. Hoberman A, Wald ER (1997) Urinary tract infections in young febrile children. Pediatr Infect Dis 16:11–17

68. Hodson CJ (1967) The radiological contribution toward the diagnosis of chronic pyelonephritis. Radiology 88:857–871

69. Homsy YL, Saad F, Laberge I et al (1990) Transitional hydronephrosis of the newborn and infant. J Urol 144:579–583

70. Hoyer PF, Schmid R, Wunsch L et al (1999) Color Doppler energy – a new technique to study tissue perfusion in renal transplants. Pediatr Nephrol 13:559–563

71. Hricak H, Slovis TL, Callen CW et al (1983) Neonatal kidneys: sonographic anatomic correlation. Radiology 147:699–702

72. Huda W, Atherton JV, Ware DE et al (1997) An approach for the estimation of effective radiation dose at CT in pediatric patients. Radiology 203:417–422

73. Hundt C, Kohz P, Leinsinger G et al (1995) The diagnostic value of digital and conventional imaging in intravenous urography. Rofo Fortschr Geb Rontgenstr Neuen Bildgeb Verfahr 163:395–399

74. Jakobsen JA, Correas JM (2001) Ultrasound contrast agents and their use in urogenital radiology: status and prospects. Eur Radiol 11:2082–2091

75. Jequier S, Jequier JC (1989) Reliability of voiding cystourethrography to detect reflux. AJR Am J Roentgenol 153:807–810

76. Jequier S, Rousseau O (1987) Sonographic measurements of the normal bladder wall in children. AJR Am J Roentgenol 149:563–566

77. Jequier S, Paltiel H, Lafortune M (1990) Ureterovesical jets in infants and children: duplex and color Doppler US studies. Radiology 175:349–353

78. Kamel IR, Hernandez RJ, Martin JE et al (1994) Radiation dose reduction in CT of the pediatric pelvis. Radiology 190:683–687

79. Kangarloo H, Gold RH, Fine RN (1985) Urinary tract infection in infants and children evaluated by ultrasound. Radiology 154:367–373

80. Kao SC, Adamson SD, Tatman LH et al (1999) A survey of post-discharge side effects of conscious sedation using chloral hydrate in pediatric CT and MR imaging. Pediatr Radiol 29:287–290

81. Karp MP, Jewett TC Jr, Kuhn JP et al (1986) The impact of computed tomography scanning on the child with renal trauma. J Pediatr Surg 21:617–623

82. Kaste SC, Young CW (1996) Safe use of power injectors with central and peripheral venous access devices for pediatric CT. Pediatr Radiol 26:499–501

83. Katayama H, Yamaguchi K, Kozuka T et al (1990) Adverse reactions to ionic and nonionic contrast media. A report from the Japanese Committee on the safety of contrast media. Radiology 175:621–628

84. Kern S, Zimmerhackl LB, Hildebrandt F et al (1999) Rare-MR-urography – a new diagnostic method in autosomal recessive polycystic kidney disease. Acta Radiol 40:543–544

85. Kessler RM, Quevedo H, Lankau CA et al (1993) Obstructive vs nonobstructive dilatation of the renal collecting system in children: distinction with duplex sonography. AJR Am J Roentgenol 160:353–357

86. Kim YS, Do SH, Hong CH et al (2001) Does every patient with ureteropelvic junction obstruction need voiding cystourethrography? J Urol 165:2305–2307

87. Kitagawa H, Pringle KC, Stone P et al (1998) Postnatal follow-up of hydronephrosis detected by prenatal ultrasound: the natural history. Fetal Diagn Ther 13:19–25

88. Kleinman PK, Diamond DA, Karellas A et al (1994) Tailored low-dose fluoroscopic voiding cystourethrography for the reevaluation of vesicoureteral reflux in girls. AJR Am J Roentgenol 162:1151–1154

89. Krug B, Harnischmacher U, Krahe T et al (1995) Digital luminescence radiography and conventional radiography in abdominal contrast examinations. Acta Radiol 36:284–289

90. Ku JH, Jeon YS, Kim ME et al (2001) Is there a role for magnetic resonance imaging in renal trauma? Int J Urol 8:261–267

91. Kuzmic AC, Brkljacic B, Ivankovic D (2000) Doppler sonographic renal resistance index in healthy children. Eur Radiol 10:1644–1648

92. Landau EH, Gofrit ON, Shapiro A (2001) Extracorporeal shock wave lithotripsy is highly effective for ureteral calculi in children. J Urol 165:2316–2319

93. Lebowitz RL, Blickman JG (1983) The coexistence of ureteropelvic junction obstruction and reflux. AJR Am J Roentgenol 140:231–238

94. Lebowitz RL, Olbing H, Parkkulainen KV et al (1985) International system of radiographic grading of vesicoureteric reflux. International Reflux Study in Children. Pediatr Radiol 15:105–109

95. Lonergan GJ, Pennington DJ, Morrison JC et al (1998) Childhood pyelonephritis: comparison of gadolinium-enhanced MR imaging and renal cortical scintigraphy for diagnosis. Radiology 207:377–388

96. Ljungman G, Kreuger A, Andreasson S et al (2000) Midazolam nasal spray reduces procedural anxiety in children. Pediatrics 105:73–78

97. Lowe LH, Isuani BH, Heller RM et al (2000) Pediatric renal masses: Wilms tumor and beyond. Radiographics 20:1585–1603

98. Maizels M, Reisman ME, Flom LS et al (1992) Grading nephroureteral dilatation detected in the first year of life: correlation with obstruction. J Urol 148:609–614

99. Majd M, Nussbaum Blask AR, Markle BM et al (2001) Acute pyelonephritis: comparison of diagnosis with 99mTc-DMSA, SPECT, spiral CT, MR imaging, and power Doppler US in an experimental pig model. Radiology 218:101–108

100. Malviya S, Voepel-Lewis T, Prochaska G et al (2000) Prolonged and delayed side effects of sedation for diagnostic imaging studies in children. Pediatrics 105: E42

101. Mentzel HJ, Vogt S, Patzer L et al (1999) Contrast-enhanced sonography of vesicoureterorenal reflux in children: preliminary results. AJR Am J Roentgenol 173: 737–740

102. Middleton WD, Kellman GM, Melson GL et al (1989) Postbiopsy renal transplant arteriovenous fistulas: color Doppler US characteristics. Radiology 171:253–257

103. Miller OF, Rineer SK, Reichard SR et al (1998) Prospective comparison of unenhanced spiral computed tomography and intravenous urogram in the evaluation of acute flank pain. Urology 52:982–987

104. Montgomery P, Kuhn JP, Afshani E (1987) CT evaluation of severe renal inflammatory disease in children. Pediatr Radiol 17:216–222

105. Mouriquand PD, Troisfontaines E, Wilcox DT (1999) Antenatal and perinatal uro-nephrology: current questions and dilemmas. Pediatr Nephrol 13:938–944

106. Mucci B, Maguire B (1994) Does routine ultrasound have a role in the investigation of children with urinary tract infection? Clin Radiol 49:324–325

107. Mutze S, Turk I, Schonberger B et al (1997) Colour-coded duplex sonography in the diagnostic assessment of vascular complications after kidney transplantation in children. Pediatr Radiol 27:898–902

108. Myers MT, Elder JS, Sivit CJ et al (2001) Unenhanced helical CT in the evaluation of the urinary tract in children and young adults following urinary tract reconstruction: comparison with sonography. Pediatr Radiol 31:135–139

109. Nolte-Ernsting CC, Wildberger JE, Borchers H et al (2001) Multi-slice CT urography after diuretic injection: initial results. Rofo Fortschr Geb Rontgenstr Neuen Bildgeb Verfahr 173:176–180

110. Oak SN, Kulkarni B, Chaubal N (1999) Color flow Doppler sonography: a reliable alternative to voiding cystourethrogram in the diagnosis of vesicoureteral reflux in children. Urology 53:1211–1214

111. Obek C, Onal B, Kantay K (2001) The efficacy of extracorporeal shock wave lithotripsy for isolated lower pole calculi compared with isolated middle and upper caliceal calculi. J Urol 166:2081–2084

112. Okada T, Yoshida H, Iwai J et al (2001) Pulsed Doppler sonography of the hilar renal artery: differentiation of obstructive from nonobstructive hydronephrosis in children. J Pediatr Surg 36:416–420

113. O'Malley ME, Soto JA, Yucel EK et al (1997) MR urography: evaluation of a three-dimensional fast spin-echo technique in patients with hydronephrosis. AJR Am J Roentgenol 168:387–392

114. O'Malley ME, Halpern E, Mueller PR et al (2000) Helical CT protocols for the abdomen and pelvis: a survey. AJR Am J Roentgenol 175:109–113

115. Palmer JM, DiSandro M (1995) Diuretic enhanced duplex Doppler sonography in 33 children presenting with hydronephrosis: a study of test sensitivity, specificity and precision. J Urol 154:1885–1888

116. Palmer JM, Lindfors KK, Ordorica RC et al (1991) Diuretic Doppler sonography in postnatal hydronephrosis. J Urol 146:605–608

117. Pappas JN, Donnelly LF, Frush DP (2000) Reduced frequency of sedation of young children with multisection helical CT. Radiology 215:897–899

118. Patel K, Mahboubi S, Sherman NH et al (1991) Diagnosis and follow-up of children with Wilms' tumor: correlative study of ultrasound and computed tomography. Report of eighteen cases. Ann Radiol 34:376–382

119. Paterson A, Frush DP, Donnelly LF (2001) Helical CT of the body: are settings adjusted for pediatric patients? AJR Am J Roentgenol 176:297–301

120. Pfluger T, Czekalla R, Hundt C et al (1999) MR angiography versus color Doppler sonography in the evaluation of renal vessels and the inferior vena cava in abdominal masses of pediatric patients. AJR Am J Roentgenol 173:103–108

121. Pietrera P, Badachi Y, Liard A et al (2001) Ultrasound for initial evaluation of post-traumatic renal lesions in children. J Radiol 82:833–838

122. Preston A, Lebowitz RL (1989) What's new in pediatric uroradiology. Urol Radiol 11:217–220

123. Regan F, Bohlman ME, Khazan R et al (1996) MR urography using HASTE imaging in the assessment of ureteric obstruction. AJR Am J Roentgenol 167:1115–1120

124. Riccabona M, Schwinger W, Ring E (1998) Arteriovenous fistula after renal biopsy in children. J Ultrasound Med 17:505–508

125. Riccabona M, Ring E, Schwinger W et al (2001) Amplitude coded-colour Doppler sonography in paediatric renal disease. Eur Radiol 11:861–866

126. Robben SG, Boesten M, Linmans J et al (1999) Significance of thickening of the wall of the renal collecting system in children: an ultrasound study. Pediatr Radiol 29:736–740

127. Roche KJ, Genieser NB, Ambrosino MM (1996) Pediatric hepatic CT: an injection protocol. Pediatr Radiol 26:502–507

128. Rodriguez LV, Spielman D, Herfkens RJ et al (2001) Magnetic resonance imaging for the evaluation of hydronephrosis, reflux and renal scarring in children. J Urol 166:1023–1027

129. Rohrschneider W, Troger J (1992) Ureteropelvic stenosis in infancy. The value of diuresis sonography compared with diuresis excretory urography. Rofo Fortschr Geb Rontgenstr Neuen Bildgeb Verfahr 157:72–78

130. Rohrschneider WK, Becker K, Hoffend J et al (2000) Combined static-dynamic MR urography for the simultaneous evaluation of morphology and function in urinary tract obstruction. II. Findings in experimentally induced ureteric stenosis. Pediatr Radiol 30:523–532

131. Rohrschneider WK, Becker K, Hoffend J et al (2000) Combined static-dynamic MR urography for the simultaneous evaluation of morphology and function in urinary tract obstruction. I. Evaluation of the normal status in an animal model. Pediatr Radiol 30:511–522

132. Rosi P, Virgili G, Di Stasi SM (1990) Diuretic ultrasound. A non-invasive technique for the assessment of upper tract obstruction. Br J Urol 65:566–569

133. Rothpearl A, Frager D, Subramanian A et al (1995) MR urography: technique and application. Radiology 194:125–130

134. Roy C, Saussine C, Jahn C et al (1994) Evaluation of RARE-MR urography in the assessment of ureterohydronephrosis. J Comput Assist Tomogr 18:601–608

135. Roy C, Saussine C, Guth S et al (1998) MR urography in the evaluation of urinary tract obstruction. Abdom Imaging 23:27–34

136. Rupprecht T, Knuth R, Bowning B et al (2000) Sedation and monitoring of paediatric patients undergoing open low-field MRI. Acta Paediatr 89:1077–1081

137. Salih M, Baltaci S, Anafarta K et al (1994) Color flow Doppler sonography in the diagnosis of vesicoureteric reflux. Eur Urol 26:93–97

138. Schmit P, Sfez M (1997) Management of anxious and painful manifestations in pediatric uroradiology. J Radiol 78:367–372

139. Schuster GA, Nazos D, Lewis GA (1995) Preparation of outpatients for excretory urography: is bowel preparation with laxatives and dietary restrictions necessary? AJR Am J Roentgenol 164:1425–1428

140. Sheley RC, Semonsen KG, Quinn SF (1999) Helical CT in the evaluation of renal colic. Am J Emerg Med 17:279–282

141. Shokeir AA, Provoost AP, EL-Azab M et al (1996) Renal Doppler ultrasound in children with obstructive uropathy: effect of intravenous normal saline fluid load and furosemide. J Urol 156:1455–1458

142. Shokeir AA, Provoost AP, El-Azab M et al (1997) Renal Doppler ultrasonography in children with equivocal obstructive uropathy: effect of intravenous normal saline fluid load and furosemide. Br J Urol 80:313–318

143. Siegel MJ, Luker GD (1995) Pediatric applications of helical (spiral) CT. Radiol Clin North Am 33:997–1022

144. Sigmund G, Stoever B, Zimmerhackl LB et al (1991) RARE-MR-urography in the diagnosis of upper urinary tract abnormalities in children. Pediatr Radiol 21:416–420

145. Slovis TL, Babcock DS, Hricak H et al (1984) Renal transplant rejection: sonographic evaluation in children. Radiology 153:659–665

146. Smellie JM (1995) The intravenous urogram in the detection and evaluation of renal damage following urinary tract infection. Pediatr Nephrol 9:213–220

147. Smergel E, Greenberg SB, Crisci KL et al (2001) CT urograms in pediatric patients with ureteral calculi: do adult criteria work? Pediatr Radiol 31:720–723

148. Staatz G, Rohrmann D, Nolte-Ernsting CC et al (2001) Magnetic resonance urography in children: evaluation of suspected ureteral ectopia in duplex systems. J Urol 166:2346–2350

149. Stoever B, Rogalla P (1999) CT studies in children. Methods and indications. Radiologe 39:455–462

150. Stokland E, Hellstrom M, Hansson S et al (1994) Reliability of ultrasonography in identification of reflux nephropathy in children. BMJ 309:235–239

151. Valentini AL, Salvaggio E, Manzoni C et al (2001) Contrast-enhanced gray-scale and color Doppler voiding urosonography versus voiding cystourethrography in the diagnosis and grading of vesicoureteral reflux. J Clin Ultrasound 29:65–71

152. Van Gessel R, Möller A, Schmiedel E (1994) Iomeprol: results of clinical trials in children with a new nonionic contrast medium. Aktuel Radiol 4:225–228

153. Vates TS, Shull MJ, Underberg-Davis SJ et al (1999) Complications of voiding cystourethrography in the evaluation of infants with prenatally detected hydronephrosis. J Urol 162:1221–1223

154. Volle E, Park W, Kaufmann HJ (1996) MRI examinations and monitoring of pediatric patients under sedation. Pediatr Radiol 26:280–281

155. Vosshenrich R, Kallerhoff M, Grone HJ et al (1996) Detection of renal ischemic lesions using GD-DTPA enhanced turbo FLASH MRI: experimental and clinical results. J Comput Assist Tomogr 20:236–243

156. Wah TM, Spencer JA (2001) The role of CT in the management of adult urinary tract trauma. Clin Radiol 56:268–277

157. Walton JM, Irwin KS, Whitehouse GH (1996) Comparison of real-time ultrasonography and magnetic resonance imaging in the assessment of urinary bladder volume. Br J Urol 78:856–861

158. Ware DE, Huda W, Mergo PJ et al (1999) Radiation effective doses to patients undergoing abdominal CT examinations. Radiology 210:645–650

159. White KS (1995) Reduced need for sedation in patients undergoing helical CT of the chest and abdomen. Pediatr Radiol 25:344–346

160. White KS (1996) Invited article: helical/spiral CT scanning: a pediatric radiology perspective. Pediatr Radiol 26:5–14

161. Whitfield HN, Britton KE, Hendry WF et al (1979) Frusemide intravenous urography in the diagnosis of pelviureteric junction obstruction. Br J Urol 51:445–448

162. Winters WD (1996) Power Doppler sonographic evaluation of acute pyelonephritis in children. J Ultrasound Med 15:91–96

163. Yamazaki Y, Yago R, Toma H (2001) Sonographic characteristics of the urinary tract in healthy neonates. J Urol 166:1054–1057

164. Zeman RK, Baron RL, Jeffrey RB Jr et al (1998) Helical body CT: evolution of scanning protocols. AJR Am J Roentgenol 170:1427–1438

165. Zerin JM, Ritchey ML, Chang AC (1993) Incidental vesicoureteral reflux in neonates with antenatally detected hydronephrosis and other renal abnormalities. Radiology 187:157–160

166. Zerin JM, Chen E, Ritchey ML et al (1993) Bladder capacity as measured at voiding cystourethrography in children: relationship to toilet training and frequency of micturition. Radiology 187:803–806

167. Zieger B, Sokol B, Rohrschneider WK et al (1998) Sonomorphology and involution of the normal urachus in asymptomatic newborns. Pediatr Radiol 28:156–161

168. Zoeller G, May C, Vosshenrich R et al (1992) Digital radiography in urologic imaging: radiation dose reduction on urethrocystography. Urol Radiol 14:56–58

J. Meller and W. Becker

3.1
Radiopharmaceuticals for Dynamic Renal Scintigraphy

Radiopharmaceuticals for dynamic renal imaging should be constantly available in every nuclear medicine department; they should offer a high photon flux, carry a low radioactive burden for any child examined with their aid, and be rapidly excreted through the kidneys to give a high renal/background ratio. Numerous tracers have been synthesised for this purpose and labelled with pure gamma emitters, such as iodine-123 (^{123}I) and ^{99m}Tc-pertechnetate (^{99m}TcO$_4^-$), but only a few are used in daily practice.

3.1.1
Iodine-123 o-Iodohippurate

Radioiodinated *o*-iodohippurate (OIH) is the prototype of a radiopharmaceutical secreted in the tubule that is suitable both for the determination of the effective renal plasma flow and for dynamic imaging with a gamma camera. Unfortunately, ^{123}I is a cyclotron product and its availability is limited.

The plasma protein binding of OIH is in the range of 65–70%, and 15% of the tracer is reversibly bound to erythrocytes. Approximately 80% of OIH is eliminated by active energy-consuming secretion in the proximal tubule and 20% by glomerular filtration. The renal extraction ratio of ^{123}I-OIH is high, approximately 85% that of paraaminohippuric acid (PAH), which is the standard substance in the determination of effective renal plasma flow (ERPF) [26]. The transtubular transport of paraaminohippuric acid (PAH), and probably also of OIH, is mediated by a basolateral and luminal transporter of the tubular cell. The basolateral transport can be competitively inhibited by probenecid, penicillin and other antibiotics [147]. Two per cent of OIH clearance is extrarenal, mainly via bile excretion [126, 129]. In patients with heavily impaired renal function biliary excretion of OIH may be even higher [27].

The clearance of OIH shows a close correlation with that of PAH but is somewhat less (85%). Differences in plasma protein binding and different affinities of the tracers to the tubular transport system have been proposed as contributory factors in this finding [108, 170].

OIH can be used in the noninvasive determination of the renal plasma flow (RPF). Renal plasma flow can be estimated by tracers that are extracted nearly completely during their first pass through the kidney. The fraction of the renal arterial blood cleared of the tracer is the extraction ratio (ER):

$$ER = (CA - CV)/CA$$

where CA is the arterial concentration of the substance, and CV is the venous concentration. Total renal plasma flow may be calculated by the equation:

$$RPF = Cl \times 1/ER$$

where Cl is the renal clearance of the tracer. If a substance is completely extracted by the kidneys in a single pass (ER = 1) the RPF can be calculated from the clearance. The extraction ratio of PAH, which is used as a reference compound to measure the RPF, is slightly lower, at about 0.8, and that of OIH is about 0.75. With these substances the real RPF can only be measured approximately and therefore the term "effective renal plasma flow" (ERPF) has been introduced to describe the clearance of these substances.

3.1.2
Technetium 99m-diethylene Triamine Pentaacetic Acid

Technetium 99m-diethylene triamine pentaacetic acid (^{99m}Tc-DTPA) has been used for renal dynamic scintigraphy since 1970 and is now replaced by technetium 99m-mercaptoacetyltriglycine (^{99m}Tc-MAG$_3$) for this purpose. ^{99m}Tc-DTPA is a metal-chelating agent which is excreted primarily by glomerular filtration. After intravenous administration, the tracer has a low plasma protein binding, which varies from 1% to 10% [148, 161]. ^{99m}Tc-DTPA, as a hydrophilic and negative charged complex, slowly enters the extracellular compartments, but does not diffuse into the cells. Negligible extrarenal excretion has been reported. DTPA is neither reabsorbed nor secreted in the tubules [127]. A high correlation between the clearance of ^{99m}Tc-DTPA and that of inulin has been noted, but the clearance of ^{99m}Tc-DTPA is slightly lower then that of inulin [27].

3.1.3
Technetium 99m-mercaptoacetyltriglycine

This tracer was introduced as a ^{99m}Tc-labelled replacement for ^{131}I-/^{123}I-OIH and is currently considered the tracer of choice for dynamic renal scintigraphy. ^{99m}Tc-MAG$_3$ is rapidly excreted in the urine, where approximately 90% of the injected activity is recovered after 3 h [86]. Approximately 90% of the tracer is excreted through active renal tubular transport. The anatomical localisation of this transport and the transporter are considered to be identical to those in the case of OIH. ^{99m}Tc-MAG$_3$ has a higher plasma protein binding (88% vs 65%) and less red blood cell (RBC) penetration than OIH and its volume of distribution is therefore lower.

A strong linear correlation between the ERPF determined by *o*-iodohippurate and the clearance of ^{99m}Tc-MAG$_3$ has been found [1, 7]. The plasma clearance of ^{99m}Tc-MAG$_3$ is approximately 250–300 ml/min, and thus 48–68% lower than the plasma clearance of ^{131}I-OIH [20, 162]. This is the consequence of a lower extraction ratio for ^{99m}Tc-MAG$_3$ than for OIH [186, 187]. Strong protein binding plus a lower affinity to the transporter may be a possible explanation for this finding. Extrarenal excretion was found to contribute 10% of the total clearance in animal studies [125]. Some biliary extraction is also present in humans, but the amount is unknown at present.

^{99m}Tc-MAG$_3$ has the advantage of more rapid excretion and thus a higher renal/background ratio than ^{99m}Tc-DTPA [50] and should therefore be preferred for dynamic renal scintigraphy.

3.2
Radiopharmaceuticals for Static Renal Scintigraphy

The first tracers used for static renal scintigraphy were radiomercury (Hg-197, Hg-203 and Hg-207)-labelled diuretics. These substances enabled imaging of the renal cortex by fixation of the tracer in the tubular cells. As radiomercury-labelled radiopharma-

ceuticals carry a relatively high radioactive burden to the patient they were abandoned in favour of other tracers in the 1970s.

3.2.1
Technetium 99m-dimercaptosuccinic Acid

This radiopharmaceutical was first introduced by Lin et al. for renal cortical imaging as a substitute to radioactive mercurial compounds [103]. Technetium 99m-dimercaptosuccinic acid (^{99m}Tc-DMSA= has high plasma protein binding of 76–90% and is mainly bound to α2-microglobulin [36, 138]. In normal volunteers the disappearance of ^{99m}Tc-DMSA from the blood follows a single exponential with a mean half-time of 56 min [49]. Compared with agents such as ^{99m}Tc-MAG$_3$, the renal clearance of ^{99m}Tc-DMSA is low, being in the range of 12 ± 3 ml/min [36]. ^{99m}Tc-DMSA is selectively taken up and fixed in the straight part of the proximal tubules. DMSA does not use the same transport mechanism as OIH or MAG$_3$, and its renal accumulation is not inhibited by PAH or probenecid. The renal uptake of ^{99m}Tc-DMSA is approximately 50% of the injected dose at 1 h after injection and 70% after 3 h and 24 h. Several studies reported good correlation between DMSA uptake and renal split function determined by ^{131}I-OIH, ^{99m}Tc-DTPA and ^{99m}Tc-MAG$_3$ [25, 113]. In an obstructed kidney, ^{99m}Tc-DMSA retained in the pelvicalyceal system may interfere with imaging of the functioning renal cortex, and therefore split function of this kidney may be overestimated. In these cases late estimation (24 h after injection) of the split function should be performed [137, 139].

Although we do not understand exactly how the kidneys handle DMSA, the uptake seems to depend mainly on the renal blood flow and the integrity of the tubular cells [34, 35]. Acidosis and dehydration are conditions that can reduce the tubular uptake of DMSA drastically [69, 209]. A small fraction of the tracer whose amount is unknown undergoes glomerular filtration and some of it may be reabsorbed [138]. Cumulative urinary excretion of 25% of ^{99m}Tc-DMSA at 14 h has been reported [36, 49]. There is negligible extrarenal biliary excretion, amounting to less than 2% of the total clearance [186].

^{99m}Tc-DMSA is currently considered the tracer of choice in static renal cortical imaging. Imaging should be preferably performed after 3–4 h post injection (p.i.). The tracer is suitable for the diagnosis of renal malformations, and highly effective in the diagnosis of pyelonephritis and renal scarring [119].

3.2.2
Technetium 99m-glucoheptonate

Following intravenous injection, only a small fraction of approximately 50% of technetium 99m-glucoheptonate (^{99m}Tc-GH) is bound to plasma proteins [5]. Uptake of ^{99m}Tc-GH appears to occur principally by active renal tubular transport and, to a lesser extent, by glomerular filtration [102]. Active transport is inhibited by PAH and probenecid, but is not influenced by acidosis [102]. Within 1 h after injection almost 40% of the dose is eliminated in the urine. Approximately 10% of the initial tracer activity is fixed in the proximal convoluted tubules and remains constant over 24 h [5]. Extrarenal clearance exists, and gallbladder and bowel activity can be noted especially in patients with renal failure.

^{99m}Tc-GH is suited to dynamic scintigraphy, but static images can also be obtained 3–4 h p.i. If an obstruction is present additional imaging 24 h p.i. should be considered for exact determination of the split function.

3.3
Dose Schedules and Radiation Burden

Recommended minimal activities are 15 MBq for ^{99m}Tc-MAG$_3$, 20 MBq for ^{99m}Tc-DTPA[1] and 10 MBq for ^{123}I-hippurate. Recommended maximum activities are 70 MBq for ^{99m}Tc-MAG$_3$, 200 MBq for ^{99m}Tc-DTPA[2] and 20–75 MBq for ^{123}I-hippurate. The doses administered should generally be based on body surface area according to the recommendations of the Paediatric Task Group of the European Association of Nuclear Medicine [140, 143].

Recent publications suggest that the radiation burden is lower than proposed earlier. For a 5-year-old child, with ^{99m}Tc-DTPA the effective dose (ED) is 0.54–0.82 mSv, the lower figure relating to a 1-h voiding interval. For ^{99m}Tc-MAG$_3$ the corresponding figures are 0.20 and 0.38 mSv, respectively. The ED to a 5-year-old when ^{123}I-hippurate is used is 0.41 mSv. The ED for ^{99m}Tc-DMSA is approximately 1 mSv per examination regardless of the age of the child, providing that the dose is adapted according to body surface [51, 177, 178].

3.4
Renal Imaging

Imaging with radioisotopes can be performed in either a static or a dynamic mode. Tracers which are readily transported through the renal parenchyma are suitable for dynamic imaging, while radiopharmaceuticals that are tubularly fixed in the renal cortex can be used for static scintigraphy. Static imaging can be performed either as planar scintigraphy or as single photon emission computed tomography (SPECT).

3.4.1
Planar Scintigraphy

If a tracer is tubularly fixed over a sufficient long time, planar scintigraphy can be performed. Planar renal imaging provides information about the size, number and position of each renal unit and an assessment of the global and regional cortical tubular function. For cortical imaging ^{99m}Tc-DMSA is administered i.v. with a minimum of 15 MBq and a maximum of 110 MBq. Scintigraphy is started 2–3 h p.i. with a gamma camera equipped with a low-energy high-resolution (LEHR) or ultra-high-resolution (LEUHR) parallel-hole collimator. Images with 250–500,000 cts. or 5- to 10-min acquisition should be obtained at least from the posterior and posterior oblique views in a 256×256 computer matrix in supine positions. The clinical value of pinhole magnification scintigraphy in small children has not been completely elucidated. If it is performed, a pinhole collimator with an internal diameter of 2 mm should be used. Each pinhole image is obtained in a 256×256 computer matrix for approximately 150,000 cts.

Ventral views are useful in horseshoe kidneys and pelvic kidney. Estimation of the split function is performed by calculating the geometric mean for each kidney from the ventral and posterior view, which can be optionally corrected for body background. Normally, the split uptake varies from 50%/50% to 45%/55%. As mentioned above, delayed estimation of the split function should be performed in patients with renal obstruction.

3.4.2
Single Photon Emission Computed Tomography

Theoretically, ^{99m}Tc-DMSA SPECT should be superior to planar cortical imaging, especially in the evaluation of small parenchymal lesions. Several experi-

---

[1] 10 MBq for ^{99m}Tc-DMSA.
[2] 100 MBq for ^{99m}Tc-DMSA.

mental and clinical publications state that SPECT is effective in disclosing more focal cortical defects than planar scintigraphy but probably increases the risk of false-positive findings [38, 82, 114, 156, 182]. In our department ^{99m}Tc-DMSA-SPECT is routinely performed following planar imaging with a three-detector system (acquisition over 360°/6° per increment/20 s per frame/128 × 128 matrix). To avoid false-positive findings raw data are carefully assessed for motion artefacts and, if possible, corrected for. Only a clear interruption of cortical uptake that is present on transverse, coronal and sagittal slices is indicative of a lesion. The knowledge of normal variants is indispensable in the correct interpretation of DMSA tomography. It has been reported that hypoactive upper poles are common, and an intrarenicular septum may produce a linear area of decreased uptake extending from the hilus to the parenchyma [38, 156].

3.4.3
Dynamic Renal Scintigraphy

Dynamic renal imaging provides information about the perfusion, relative size and position of the functional renal parenchymal units, split renal function and urine transport from the pelvicalyceal system into the bladder. For dynamic imaging a radiopharmaceutical such as ^{123}I-hippurate, ^{99m}Tc-MAG$_3$ or ^{99m}Tc-DTPA is injected i.v. as a small bolus in the antecubital vein. Following this injection, the gamma camera will detect the radioactivity in the aorta and soon afterwards in the kidneys.

Because the two kidneys normally receive approximately 20% of the cardiac output, a large fraction of the tracer reaches the kidney in the first passage through the circulation resulting in a rapid rise of activity in the kidney region. This phase reflects the speed of injection and the blood supply to the kidney and is therefore traditionally called the perfusion phase.

In the second phase, the parenchymal phase, the kidneys will continue to extract the tracer, but the increase in activity will be more gradual because the blood concentration of the tracer rapidly decreases as a consequence of its renal extraction and dilution within the vascular space. This phase represents the renal handling of the tracer.

During the third phase, usually called the drainage phase, which is mainly characterised by the efficiency of the kidney in excreting the tracer in the urine, the radiopharmaceutical is transported through the pelvicalyceal system and the ureters into the bladder.

Normally, these structures, except the bladder, are only transiently visualised.

Patient Preparation. The children should be encouraged to drink fluids, approximately 10–20 ml/kg 1 h before the scintigraphy. If possible, patients are asked to empty their bladder before the study begins. Appropriate immobilisation equipment should be available to reduce patient motion. Sedation of the children is usually not necessary. A vesical catheter should only be inserted if the patient cannot or will not void. A butterfly needle or a short intravenous catheter is used to establish intravenous access. Extravasation of the tracer compromises the quality of the study and if not recognised yields an erroneous interpretation. Children are usually examined in the supine position with the gamma camera placed underneath the examining table to view the area of the kidneys and bladder. Renal transplants are examined with the patients in the supine position, with the gamma camera viewing the kidney and the bladder from the anterior projection.

Acquisition and Analysis. If ^{99m}Tc-labelled compounds are used, dynamic imaging should be performed with a large field of view gamma camera equipped with a low-energy all-purpose (LEAP) or LEHR collimator and a 128 × 128 matrix. These collimators are also suitable for imaging ^{123}I-hippurate, but special 159-keV collimators will produce better image quality with less scatter. After the patient is positioned, the tracer is injected as a rapid i.v. bolus, and recording of the study starts simultaneously with the injection. Images are typically collected for 20–60 s within a period of 20–25 min. Many computer programs allow a higher frame rate during the initial phase shortly after i.v. injection for a more detailed analysis of the renal perfusion. For semiquantitative evaluation, regions of interest (ROIs) are placed over the kidneys, the background and the aorta. The background area must be selected with care so that the time–activity curve of the activity in the background ROI closely matches that of the over- and underlying tissue.

The time–activity curve of the first pass of the tracer through the renal region is determined mainly by the vascular supply of the kidney and can therefore be used as an estimate of its relative perfusion. The time–activity curve of the ROI over the aorta helps in assessment of the bolus quality of the injection.

During the parenchymal phase, information about overall renal morphology, position of the functional renal parenchymal units and their size can be obtained by visual interpretation of the scintigrams.

The total renal function can be qualitatively evaluated by comparing the renal uptake with the background activity from the blood pool and the liver. The higher the level of tracer activity within these regions during the parenchymal phase and the lower the renal uptake, the poorer is the renal function. Sequential images may provide important information about distinctly renal pathology. Larger scars, trauma, dysplasia and space-occupying lesions such as cysts and tumours may become apparent through reduced focal renal uptake in the early parenchymal phase. Normally, at the end of 20 min, a large propor-

tion of the radiopharmaceutical has left the renal parenchyma via the pelvicalyceal system and the ureters. At that time hydronephrosis can be assumed if persistent accumulation of the tracer is seen in the pelvicalyceal system. In addition, hydronephrosis often produces a photon-deficient area within the renal pelvis during the perfusion and the parenchymal phase.

Time–activity (renogram) curves (Figs. 1a, 2) offer the possibility of a semiquantitative analysis and should be carefully correlated with the corresponding scintigrams. If ^{99m}Tc-MAG$_3$ or ^{123}I-IOH is used,

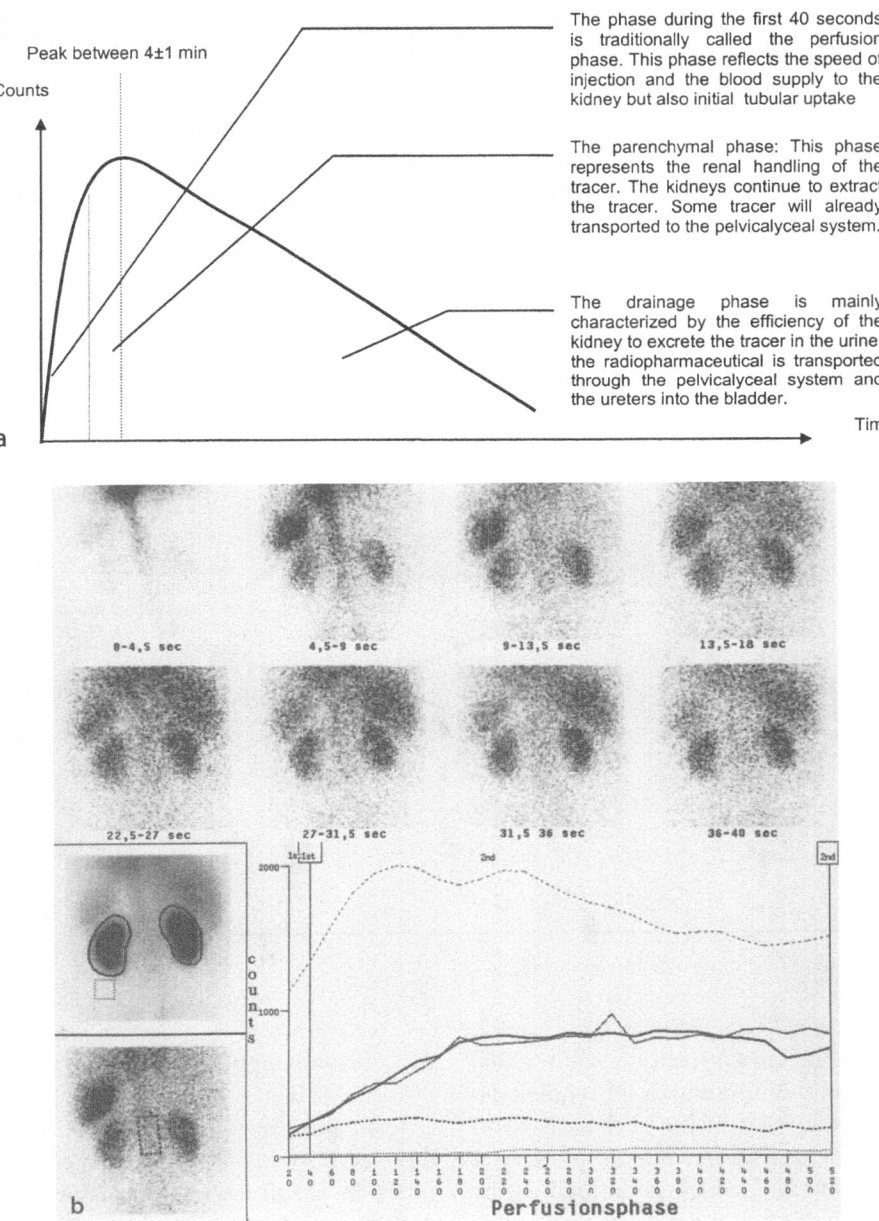

Fig. 1. a Time–activity curve of tracers secreted in the tubules like ^{99m}Tc-MAG$_3$. b Normal ^{99m}Tc-MAG3 study during the perfusion phase. c See p. 94

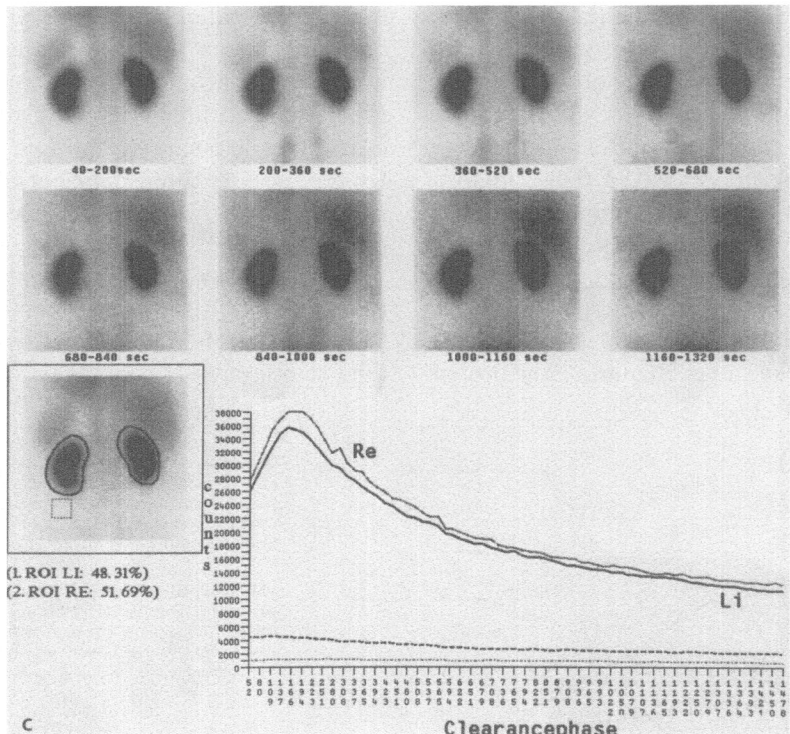

Fig. 1 (*continued*). **c** Normal ^{99m}Tc-MAG3 study during the parenchymal and drainage phase. In this example the relative function is obtained by integration of the background-subtracted renogram taken during the early parenchymal phase

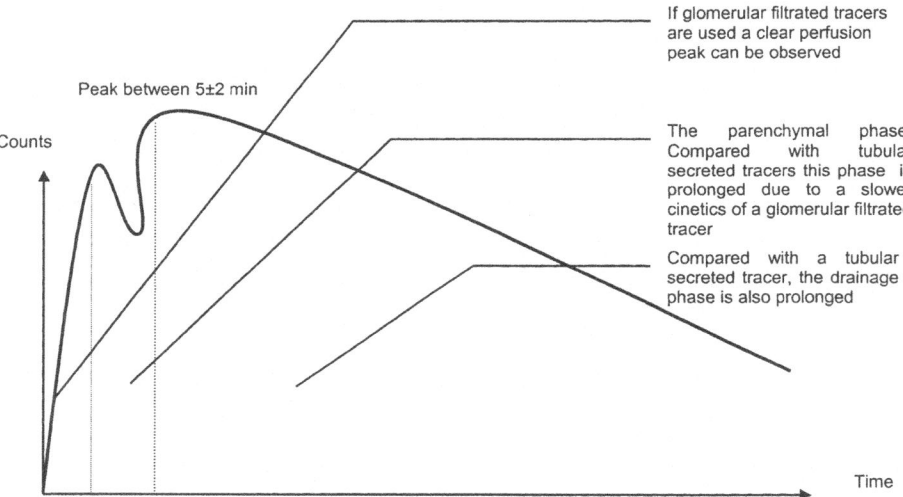

Fig. 2. Time–activity curve of glomerular filtrated tracers

the renogram curve generated from the kidney ROI reveals a peak time at 3–5 min, with a subsequent decrease to approximately 50% of the peak activity after 5–15 min (Fig. 1b). Another simple parameter is the cortical transit time, which is defined as the time between the injection of the radiopharmaceutical and its first appearance within the pelvicalyceal system. If a tracer secreted in the tubules is used it will normally appear 3–5 min after i.v. injection in the renal pelvis.

Evaluation of the slope of the second part of the time–activity curve provides an estimate of the renal function. Assuming that the kidneys are placed equidistant from the detector, activity over each kidney during the second phase will be proportional to tubular function or glomerular filtration of each kidney, depending on the tracer. The recommended method for determining relative function comprises integration of die background-subtracted renograms over 1–2 or 1–2.5 min for ^{123}I-OIH and ^{99m}Tc-MAG$_3$ (Fig. 1b) and 2–3 min for ^{99m}Tc-DTPA [135]. Alternatively, split function can be estimated either by the background-corrected mean slope of the renogram curve during a selected time interval or by the slope of the renogram corrected for the decrease in the tracer concentration in the blood, which can be measured by a ROI over the heart (Patlak-Rutland plot). For ^{99m}Tc-MAG$_3$ all these methods seem to be of equal accuracy in determination of the relative renal function [146].

3.5 Renal Clearance

Methods of Clearance Determination. The term 'clearance' describes the virtual plasma volume of a tracer that is cleared within a certain time. Ideally, a tracer used for determination of the renal clearance should eliminated exclusively by the kidneys. If the tracer is excreted by glomerular filtration, as inulin is, the clearance determined is a glomerular clearance, whereas a tubular clearance can be measured with a tracer such as PAH, which is excreted predominantly by tubular transport.

The tracer of choice for the determination of the glomerular filtration rate (GFR) is chromium-51-ethylene diamine tetraacetate (^{51}Cr-EDTA). The kinetics of this tracer, which is excreted selectively through glomerular filtration, are comparable to those of ^{99m}Tc-DTPA. Compared with ^{99m}Tc-DTPA the protein binding of which may differ from one formulation to another, ^{51}Cr-EDTA has the advantage of a extremely high chemical purity and reproducible, very low, plasma binding [23].

^{123}I- or ^{131}I-labelled IOH must be considered the preferred radiopharmaceutical for determination of the ERPF [12]. ^{99m}Tc-MAG$_3$ may be used to measure the tubular extraction rate (TER) as an estimate of the tubular function [19].

The gold standard for determination of clearance is still the use of techniques performed under steady-state conditions. These time-consuming methods require a feedback-controlled infusion and catheterisation of the urinary bladder. With such methods the clearance can be calculated from the formula:

$$Cl = U \times V/P$$

where Cl is the clearance, U is the urine concentration, V is the volume, in millilitres, of urine excreted

per minute and P is the plasma concentration of the tracer. Because the classic infusion clearance can be determined with a high degree of accuracy and reproducibility it is used as a reference method to validate single injection clearance techniques.

These techniques are based on the assumption that the tracer after a single i. v. injection is readily and homogeneously diluted within the vascular space and that the clearance can be determined from the fall of either the plasma activity or of the whole-body activity. Other methods calculate the clearance from the early renal uptake of the tracer by means of a gamma camera.

Plasma Clearance. The plasma disappearance curve of a tracer that is eliminated through the kidneys can be described by a two-compartment model [163]. In this model the first compartment is represented by the vascular space (V1), and the second corresponds to a closed extravascular space (V2). The tracer will diffuse from V1 to V2 but will also be redistributed into V1. According to this model, the clearance can be calculated as follows:

$$Cl = A \times b_1 \times b_2/a_1b_2 + a_2b_1 \ (ml/min)$$

where A is the activity injected, b_1 and b_2 are the decay constants of the compartments V1 and V2, and a_1 and a_2 correspond to the intercepts of the partial components of the curve with the y-axis. This clearance method requires six or more blood samples. Sampling has to be performed at least 3 h after injection to determine the GFR and at least 1 h after injection to determine the ERPF.

The need for simplification has led to the replacement of multicompartmental clearance methods by single-compartment techniques for which only two blood samples are necessary. Single-compartment methods rest on the assumption of a monoexponential decrease in the injected activity according to the formula:

$$Cl = A \times b/a \ (ml/min)$$

where A is the injected activity, b is the decay constant and a is the intercept of the curve with the y-axis. Blaufox and Merrill demonstrated a high correlation between the OIH clearance determined by a monoexponential approach and the classic PAH clearance if sampling is performed more than 20 min after injection [11]. Similar results were found for the GFR determined by single-compartment ^{51}Cr-EDTA clearance [23].

Further-simplified techniques requiring only one blood sample have been described. Tauxe et al. found a high degree of correlation between the ERPF determined by PAH-steady-state clearance and the reciprocal of the plasma concentration of OIH (the theoretical volume of distribution) at a certain time after a single injection [185]. Other authors have also introduced similar algorithms to determine the GFR and the TER (MAG$_3$) by single-sample methods [57, 70, 141, 190]. Ham and Piepsz demonstrated that in children the ^{51}Cr-EDTA clearance determined by a two-sample method closely correlated with the 2-h distribution volume [70]. Bubeck proposed a reliable single-sample method for the measurement of the tubular function by ^{99m}Tc-MAG$_3$, which could also be used in paediatric patients if the clearance values were normalised to a body surface of 1.73 m^2 [18].

It has to be pointed out that although single sample methods are very easy to perform, they are less accurate than multiple-sample techniques, especially if severe renal failure is present [12].

External Counting Methods. These techniques use the whole-body disappearance curve of a tracer for estimation of the clearance according to the formula:

$$-dm/dt = Cl \times C$$

Where *dm* is the amount of the substance cleared In a unit of time (dt), *Cl* is the clearance of the tracer and *C* is the plasma concentration of the tracer at the time *t* [130, 131]. One advantage of these methods is that they are independent of compartment models. Measurements of the whole-body retention curve can be performed either with a special clearance-measuring device and external collimated gamma ray probes or with a gamma camera.

In Germany, EPRF measurements with a partially shielded whole-body counter and ^{131}I-OIH were popular for many years. In its original version this system uses two probes for the measurement of the whole-body retention curve placed over the patient who is in a supine position. Activity from the urinary bladder and the kidneys is eliminated by a lead shield and therefore does not influence the whole-body measurements. The activity of each kidney can be recorded simultaneously with two separate external gamma ray probes. The split renal function can then be calculated from the area between the renogram curve in the early parenchymal phase and the retention curve projected over the renogram curve. The following equations express the relation between the two areas, AL and AR [130, 131].

$$AL = AL/AL + AR$$

$$AR = AR/AL + AR$$

where AL and AR designate the proportions of the EPRF assigned to the left and right kidney.

The Oberhausen method was later modified by replacing the gamma ray probes by a gamma camera and a connected computer [154]. This means that the renogram and a whole-body retention curve are generated by a ROI technique with the ROIs placed over the kidneys, the liver and the spleen. This modification is less accurate in determination of the EPRF than Oberhausen's original approach.

Schlegel and Hamway proposed a very simple method for determination of the global and split EPRF by measuring the renal uptake of a tubularly extracted tracer by a gamma camera between the 1st and 2nd minutes after i. v. injection corrected for kidney depth and background [167]. This method was later adapted by Gates for tracers that undergo glomerular filtration [60]. Although these algorithms are simple and have been implemented in various commercial software programs, it should be borne in mind that the measurement results exhibit standard deviations up to 20 % [10, 55]. Therefore, these methods cannot be recommended for clinical practice [12].

3.6
Diuresis Scintigraphy

Obstruction has to be differentiated from other causes of upper urinary tract dilatation, such as vesico-renal reflux, urinary inflammation, high urine flow state, relieved obstruction, congenital malformations and poorly compliant bladder. If persistent accumulation of the radiotracer is seen in the pelvicalyceal system at the end of a dynamic renal scintigraphic study, diuresis scintigraphy should be performed to differentiate these conditions.

There is no doubt that outflow obstruction will be present in a patient with loin pain associated with a dilated pelvicalyceal system and a temporary reduction in renal function. In an asymptomatic child with a dilated renal pelvis the definition of whether or not an obstruction is present is not so easy, and no gold standard can be defined.

Some authors have tried to define obstruction by pressure-perfusion studies. This technique was first proposed by Whitaker, who perfused saline or contrast media across the obstruction at a fixed flow rate, usually 10 ml/min. Obstruction is assumed if the pressure in the infusate rises above 22 cmH$_2$O, and a rise of less than 15 cmH$_2$O should exclude obstruction [204]. The predictive value of such studies has been questioned [132, 133]. Other workers have looked for histological changes in the postoperative specimens, but it is not clear whether these changes are primary or secondary to the dilatation [68].

Most authors will agree that obstruction is present if deterioration of the renal function is seen with time, or that an obstruction was present if a postoperative improvement in renal function can be noted [31]. The problem with this definition is that the diagnosis can only be made retrospectively after the renal function has already deteriorated.

Diuresis scintigraphy was developed in the late 1970s as a noninvasive technique in the prospective assessment of urinary outflow obstruction [134]. The principle of diuresis scintigraphy can be explained by the following equation [54]:

$$F = V/T$$

where F is the rate of fluid flow through the renal pelvis, V is the pelvic volume and T is the mean transit time of flow through the pelvis.

In a system that is dilated but not obstructed the flow will be unchanged. In such a system both the pelvic volume and the transit time increase. The increased transit time will be apparent as delayed washout of the tracer from the renal pelvis, so that it cannot be distinguished from obstruction.

These conditions can theoretically be differentiated by giving a diuretic (usually frusemide). If the renal pelvis is only dilated, and not obstructed, the flow rate will increase and rapid washout of the tracer will occur. In an obstructed pelvis flow will not increase sufficiently after the diuretic and therefore no washout will be observed.

This technique was first described by O'Reilly in 1978 [134]. A general description of O'Reilly's technique and his results is useful as an aid to understanding later modifications. O'Reilly investigated 52 patients with a probe system and ^{131}I-hippuran. He evaluated his patients in an upright position: they were hydrated with 500 ml oral fluid load prior to the study and 0.5 mg/kg frusemide was given 30 min after injection of the tracer. One year later Lupton et al. published similar results in 82 patients who were investigated with the same technique [106].

O'Reilly described four different response curves to frusemide and correlated these patterns with the pathological and clinical findings [132].

- The type I curve (Fig. 3) is a normal nonobstructed renogram curve.
- The type II curve represents progressive tracer accumulation in the renal pelvis without a response to frusemide (Fig. 4). This pattern is highly suggestive for obstruction.
- The type IIIa curve describes a rapid response to frusemide after initial accumulation of the radiopharmaceutical in the renal pelvis (Fig. 5). If the half-time of renal pelvic emptying (T1/2) after

frusemide injection is less than 10–15 min this pattern should exclude obstruction in the majority of cases [89].

- The type IIIb curve (Fig. 6) describes a poor response to frusemide with T1/2 greater than 15–20 min. The type IIIb curve was originally described as dilated and partially obstructed. Nowadays this pattern is rather considered as "nondiag-

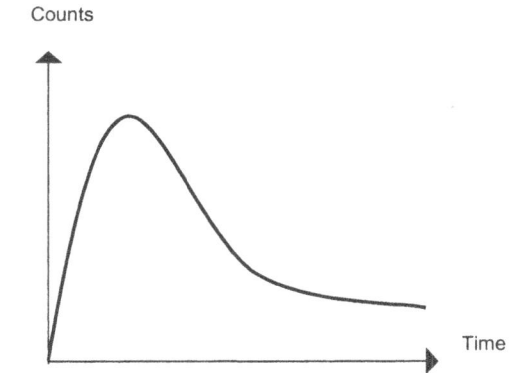

Fig. 3. Response curves to frusemide. Type I curve

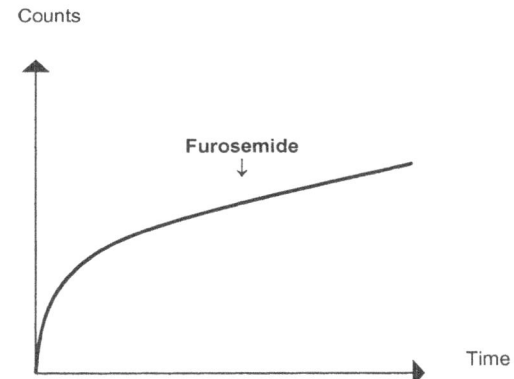

Fig. 4. Response curves to frusemide. Type II curve

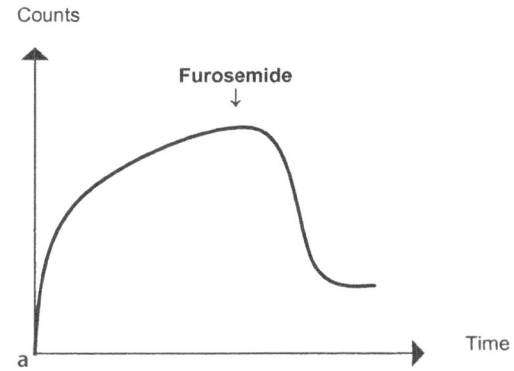

Fig. 5a–c. Response curves to frusemide. **a** Type IIIa curve. **b, c** see p. 98

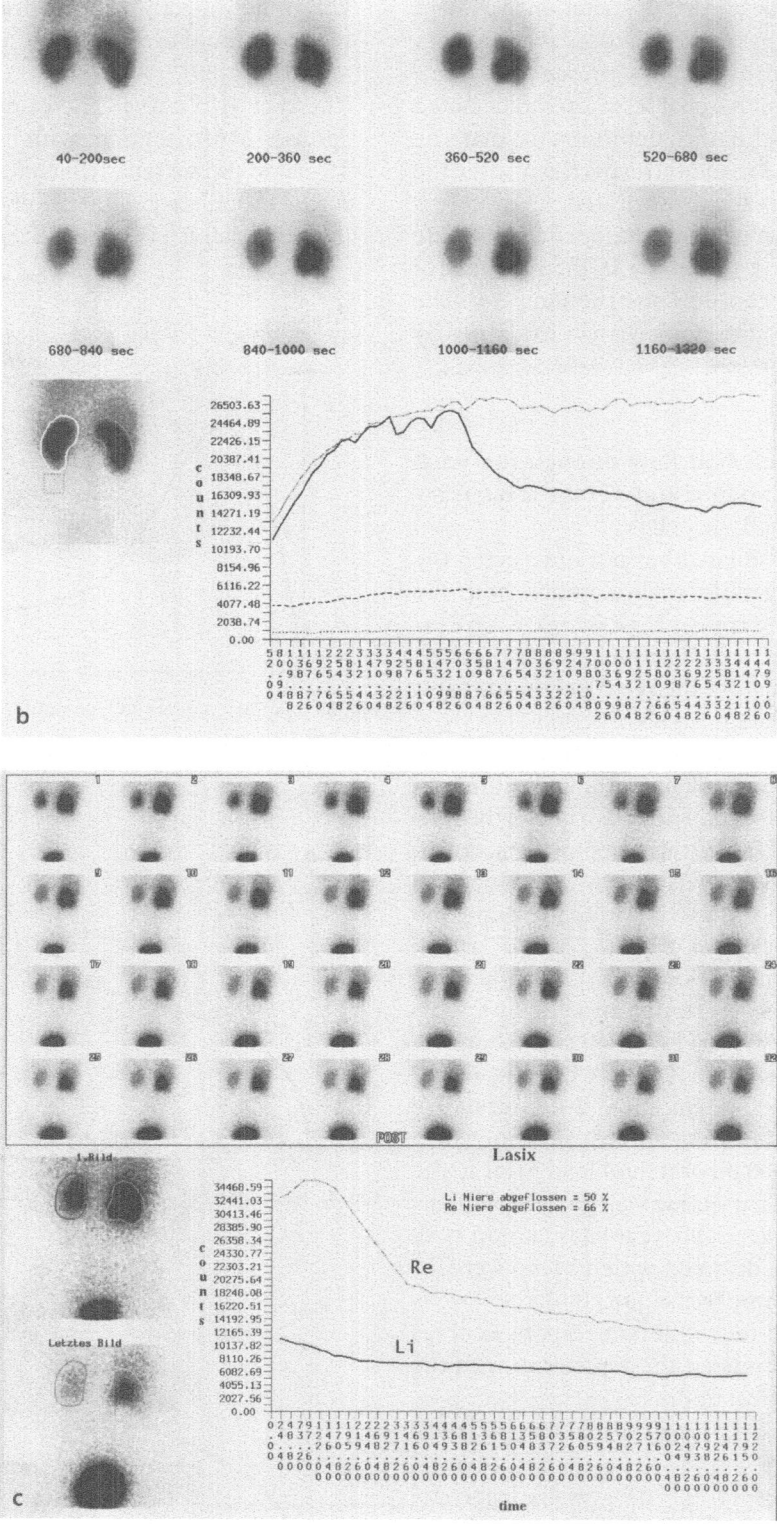

Fig. 5 (*continued*). **b** Type IIIa curve. A ^{99m}Tc-MAG3 study with accumulation of the tracer in the right drainage system during the parenchymal and drainage phase. **c** Following the injection of frusemide a significant fall of the time–activity curve (50% within 10 min) is observed

nostic" or "equivocal" [54, 89]. It often remains unclear whether this pattern reflects a good diuretic response in a obstructed system or a suboptimal diuretic response in a nonobstructed system. A T1/2 greater than 20 min should be considered to indicate that the system is obstructed [89].

– The type IV curve (Fig. 7) describes delayed decompensation. This pattern was first described by Homsy [79]. Here the initial washout in response to the diuretic is good, but at the end of the study the time–activity curve rises again. It has been hypothesised that, in an obstructed system, during the early diuretic phase the activity may be transported by the pelviureteric junction. When the flow peaks at 15 min p.i. the system can no longer transmit the urine load and the system decompensates with a consequent rise in activity in the renal pelvis.

Indirect confirmation of the validity of O'Reilly's data came from an experimental study. Bowen et al. established an animal model of chronic progressive hydronephrosis in rabbits. Experimental hydronephrosis associated with the type II drainage pattern predicted progressive deterioration of renal function, while the type IIIa pattern was associated with pre-

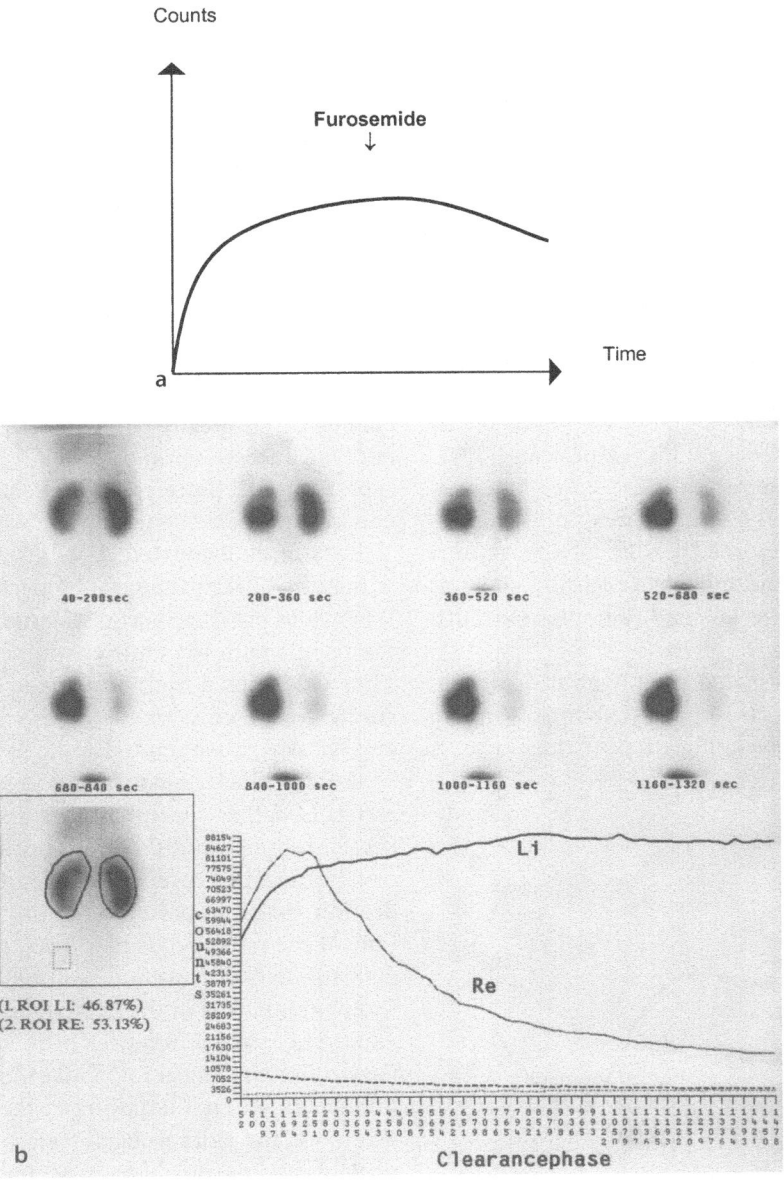

Fig. 6a–c. Response curves to frusemide. **a** Type IIIb curve. **b** A ^{99m}Tc-MAG3 study with accumulation of the tracer in the left drainage system during the parenchymal and drainage phase. **c** see p. 100

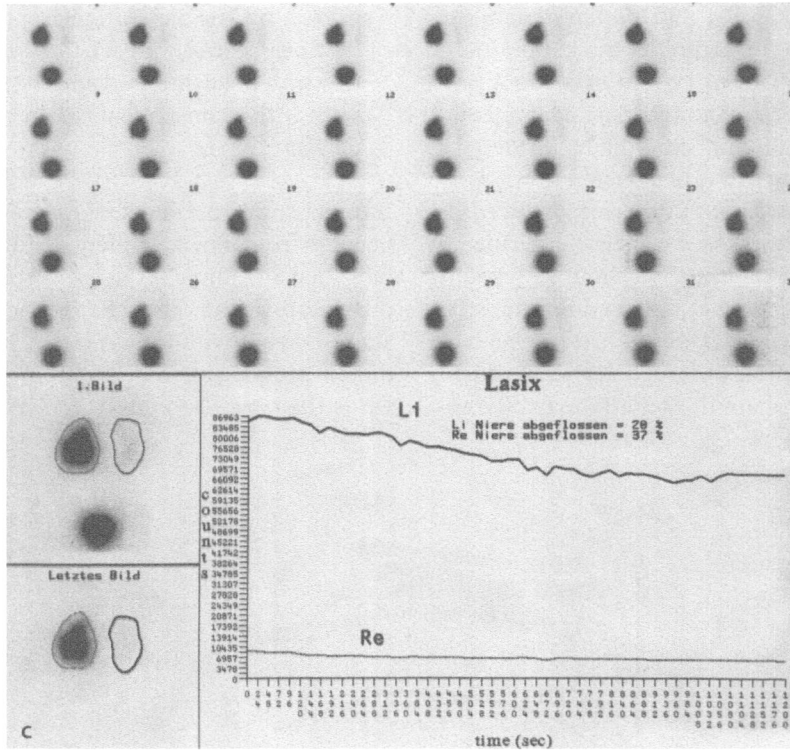

Fig. 6 (*continued*). **c** Following the injection of frusemide a nondiagnostic fall of the time–activity curve (20% within 20 min) is observed

served renal function in all cases [15]. Response curves similar to those of O'Reilly were published by Koff et al. [93], who used a gamma camera and ^{99m}Tc-DTPA for diuresis renography.

In the 1980s the probe technology and ^{131}I-hippurate were generally replaced by use of the gamma camera and other radiopharmaceuticals, such as ^{123}I-hippurate- and ^{99m}Tc-labelled radiopharmaceuticals [132].

English et al. investigated mainly adult hydronephrosis patients with ^{123}I-hippurate, giving 0.5 mg/kg frusemide 20 min after application of the tracer. A

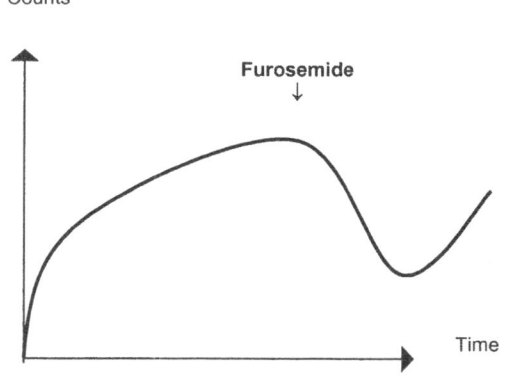

Fig. 7. Response curves to frusemide. Type IV curve

good correlation was noted between histological changes in surgically removed specimens and preoperative diuresis scintigraphy. All patients with the type II or IIIb pattern showed changes in the renal pelvis, while patients with a IIIa pattern did not [47].

Kass et al. evaluated 42 hydronephrotic kidneys with both diuresis renography, performed with ^{99m}Tc-DTPA, and pressure perfusion studies and correlated the results with the clinical course of their patients. They described a high diagnostic accuracy for both studies, with only small numbers of false-positive and false-negative scintigraphic results [89].

Besides these encouraging results, it was soon recognised that several factors could affect the diuretic response and therefore produce false-positive or false-negative results. The age of the child, the hydration status, impaired renal function and the volume of the renal pelvis have been suggested as main determinants of frusemide response [135].

Renal function in the neonate is different from the adult. There are differences in renal blood flow, urinary concentrating ability and other factors that may influence the renal handling of the radiotracer. Furthermore, the glomerular filtration rate is low in the newborn rising slowly from 40 ml min^{-1} 1.73 m^{-2} to 120 ml min^{-1} 1.73 m^{-2} at 2 years [31]. It has therefore suggested that the diuretic response will be unpredictable in the first weeks of life [94]. Recently published clinical studies refute this hypothesis and have yielded reliable results in this patient population when tubular tracers are used [44, 207, 208].

It is known that diuresis scintigraphy produces false-positive results in patients with a large dilated collecting system and in patients with poor renal function. In a massively dilated drainage system the urinary flow may be insufficient to wash out the tracer despite a normal diuretic response, and in a poorly functioning kidney adequate flow rates may never be accessed. The level of dilatation and compromised function at which the method becomes unreliable is currently unknown.

If moderately impaired function is present, a protocol according to which frusemide is injected 15 min before the tracer (F-15 method) may be more accurate than one with the diuretic given 20 min after tracer injection (F+20 technique). It has been observed that type IIIb curves (nondiagnostic) obtained with a F+20 protocol could be converted to diagnostic type I curves by the F-15 technique [197]. Similar observations were made by authors who used a volume expansion protocol [80]. On the other hand, it has been shown that regardless of hydration status and diuretic protocol, results in some kidneys with severely impaired function or hugely dilated renal pelvis will remain false positive [133].

To overcome the problems that arise in comparison of the diuretic response of kidneys with different levels of function, several authors have proposed parameters that allow normalisation of the tracer washout according to renal function. These parameters adjust the early part of the renogram to the integral of the heart curve to obtain the percentage of activity that has left the renal compartment during a predetermined time interval. These techniques have been described as output efficiency [22] or pelvic excretion efficiency [2].

Normal values for as output efficiency in children have been described, and first clinical results are already available. Saunders et al. investigated 91 hydronephrotic kidneys in 74 children with ^{99m}Tc-MAG$_3$ and a F+20 frusemide protocol. The final diagnosis was based on the clinical course or surgical findings. In this study impaired output efficiency was found to have an overall accuracy of 89% [165]. Further studies are still needed to clarify the cut-off values for good, moderate and poor drainage.

Experimental and clinical studies indicate that type I and IIIa curves will exclude obstruction with a high degree of certainty [15, 47, 89, 93, 132, 134, 197, 208], but this issue has not been completely resolved.

Hay et al. investigated 64 dilated pelvicaliceal units by diuresis renography with ^{123}I-hippuran and the Whitaker test. They used an F+13 protocol. The renographic pattern was type I or type IIIa in 45 kidneys according to O'Reilly's criteria, and 32 of these kidneys were obstructed according to Whitaker's criteria and had symptomatic improvement after pyeloplasty. Furthermore, differential function improved significantly in surgically treated patients with a IIIa pattern. The authors state that the detection of a type I or type IIIa response in a dilated, painful system cannot be taken as excluding obstruction, while type II and type IIIb patterns correlated much more closely with the results of urodynamic testing [72]. Similar results were reported by Wacksman et al. in five patients [203]. Hays and Wacksman's findings may indicate that in a noncompliant or poorly compliant system, high intrapelvic pressure may be built up in the presence of good renal function to overcome an obstruction, and the resulting renogram will appear, falsely, as normal [92]. On the other hand, we cannot confirm the frequency of false-negative diuresis renograms reported by Hay et al., which may be due in part to patient selection. In our patients false-positive findings were seen in less than 5% (Meller and Zappel, unpublished).

Since O'Reilly's initial observations, numerous modifications have been made to the performance of diuresis renography and curve interpretation. During recent years several consensus papers have been published in attempts to improve the practice of diuresis scintigraphy, and these have included proposed recommendations directed at a more standardised technique and interpretation [31, 135, 143]. Although consensus has not been reached on all issues, agreement has been found in many important areas.

Patient Position. The patient can be imaged either in a supine or in an upright position. Each of these has its specific advantages and disadvantages. In the supine position the patient is less likely to move and kidney depth variation is minimised. The advantage of an upright position lies in the hydrostatic effects on urine flow.

Patient Preparation. The child should be prepared as already described. Even in the presence of normal function, the response to frusemide may be suboptimal if the child is not adequately hydrated. If oral hydration of the child cannot be achieved, intravenous hydration (15–20 ml/kg) should be performed.

A full or rapidly filling bladder may affect upper urinary tract emptying, giving false-positive results. Effects of bladder filling on upper tract urodynamics have been found to be of clinical relevance in one third of subjects studied [86]. Older children should be asked to empty their bladder prior to imaging. Younger children cannot be expected to void on demand. However, the diuretic usually causes them to void 15–20 min after its administration. Additional data should be acquired after micturition.

Since children are usually investigated in the supine position, the tracer may be simply retained in the dilated renal pelvis by gravity. In this case it is essential that the posture of the child be changed to the erect position to improve renal drainage. After 5–10 min, 1-min dynamic imaging should be acquired to clarify postural effects. This final images have been termed post-micturition images [65, 157].

Tracer. It is generally agreed that ^{99m}Tc-MAG$_3$ is currently the agent of choice.

Frusemide Dosage and Timing. The resting flow of a single kidney is approximately 0.5 ml/min. Following the injection of 0.5 mg/kg of frusemide, the flow increases up to 25 ml/min if renal function is not impaired. It is unlikely that the urinary flow will improve any further with higher doses. The response to the diuretic becomes maximal 15–18 min p.i. [17].

The recommended dosage of frusemide should be 1 mg/kg in infants and 0.5 mg/kg in children aged 1–16 years. The technique of frusemide administration most commonly used is the F+20 method followed by 15–20 min of additional dynamic data acquisition. Some laboratories give frusemide and the radiopharmaceutical together (F+0 method) [208]. The most physiological approach is perhaps the F-15 technique. This technique seems to improve the specificity of diuresis scintigraphy in a considerable number of patients. It has been reported to reduce the 15–17% rate of equivocal results of F+20 diuresis renography to 3% [48, 197]. A nondiagnostic F+20 study should be repeated but with the F-15 method [135].

Curve Interpretation. If it is performed to evaluate pelviureteric obstruction, the renogram curve is performed with a pelvic ROI with semilunar background subtraction. This technique is not sufficient if a primary megaureter is being investigated. In such patients it is important to extend the ROI to include the whole collecting system proximal to the suspected level of obstruction to avoid false-positive results [31]. The clearance half-time (T/2) is the most common parameter used to assess drainage from the renal pelvis if an F+20 technique is performed. The ranges for obstructed, equivocal and nonobstructed

vary widely. Most investigators would agree that a T1/2>20 min is indicative of obstruction, while a half-time <10 min will exclude significant obstruction in most cases. If an F–15 technique is used the curves should be interpreted according to Figs. 8–10.

Finally, it must be stated that in our experience visual and semiquantitative evaluation will provide important diagnostic information only if the interpreta-

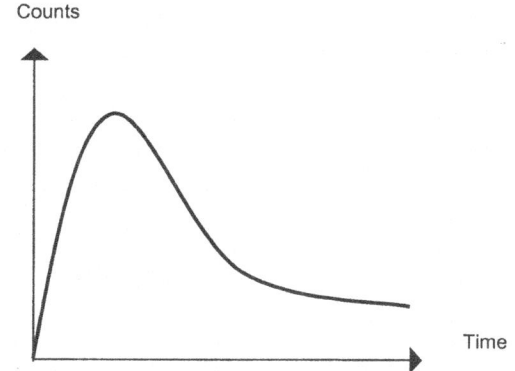

Fig. 8. F-15 renogram: nonobstructed curve

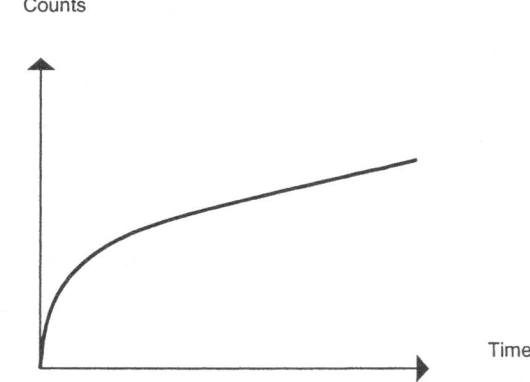

Fig. 9. F-15 renogram: obstructed curve

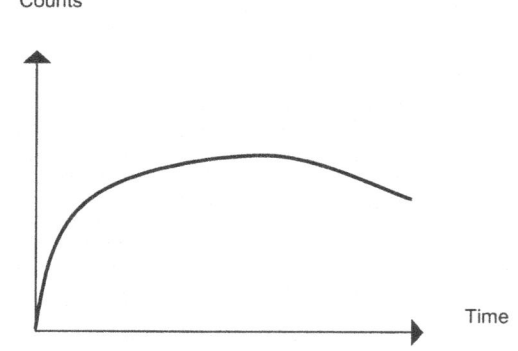

Fig. 10. F-15 renogram: equivocal result

tion of the data takes into account the child's individual clinical course, the hydration status, the volume of the renal pelvis and the level of renal function.

3.7
Renal Cortical Scintigraphy

^{99m}Tc-DMSA is the radiopharmaceutical of choice for renal cortical imaging. Introduced in the late 1970s, it was initially used mainly in the diagnosis of space-occupying lesions in the kidney, in the evaluation of renal malformations and for the assessment of split renal function. It soon became clear that the tracer was a valuable tool in the detection of pyelonephritis and renal scarring, which are the main indications for cortical imaging today. Figure 11 shows a normal scan.

3.7.1
^{99m}Tc-DMSA in the Diagnosis of Renal Malformation

Agenesis. While newborns with bilateral agenesis will not survive, children with unilateral agenesis will exhibit a contralateral hyperplastic kidney either in the typical or in an ectopic position, with normal uptake on the DMSA scan. Ectopic single kidneys in the pelvis may be difficult to visualise on intravenous urography or ultrasound and are easily imaged with ^{99m}Tc-DMSA.

Hypoplastic Kidney. Hypoplastic kidneys are rare. Because split function may be normal in bilateral hypoplasia, this condition can give a normal appearance in the DMSA scan. If unilateral hypoplasia is present, the centigram will show a diminished split function of the affected kidney without focal defects. In segmental hypoplasia (Ask-Upmark syndrome) uni- or bilateral areas of focal decreased DMSA uptake are present.

Duplication. Duplication of the ureter and the renal pelvis is one of the most common abnormalities of the urinary tract. The ureter of the lower pole, which is commonly not dysplastic, is more often refluxive. The ureter of the upper pole, which is commonly dysplastic, is more often obstructive. In our experience, the DMSA scan is neither sensitive nor specific in the diagnosis of duplication. If such complications as infection or obstruction occur and surgery is discussed, DMSA imaging is useful to evaluate the relative function of the upper and lower pole [97].

Ectopic Kidney. Renal ectopia is a congenital malposition of one or both kidneys. The most common location of unilateral ectopia is within the pelvis. Cortical imaging with DMSA is the best imaging modality to locate the ectopic kidney and to quantify its split function.

Crossed fused renal ectopia is another congenital abnormality; in this the ectopic kidney is caudal to and fused with the normal kidney. This situation can be clarified by cortical renal imaging, especially if the ^{99m}Tc-DMSA SPECT is displayed in a three-dimensional mode [3, 71].

Horseshoe Kidneys. In horseshoe kidneys, fusion is usually between the lower poles. DMSA imaging defines the anatomy of a horseshoe kidney as well as that of other malformations, such as *pancake kidney* and *sigmoidal kidney.*

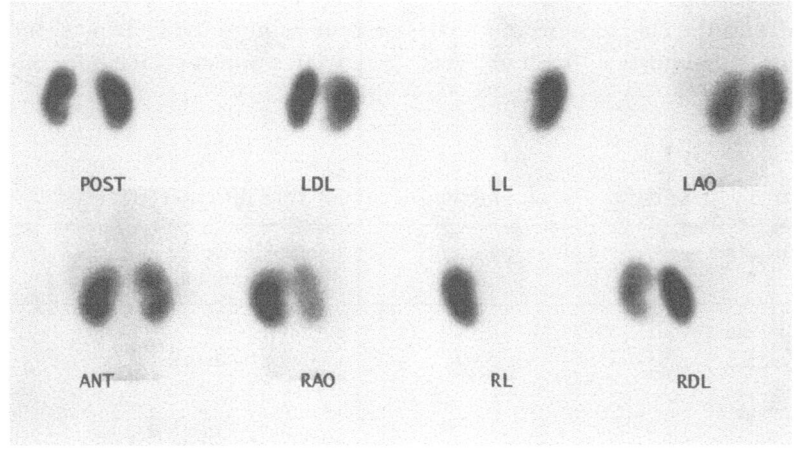

Fig. 11. Normal renal cortical scintiscan with ^{99m}Tc-DMSA

Multicystic Dysplastic Kidneys and Polycystic Renal Disease. DMSA imaging can be used in the functional assessment of these conditions. In the majority of cases no uptake will be found in the affected kidney. In other cases residual marginal renal uptake may be seen, together with multiple photopenic areas that represent cystic degeneration.

Roach et al. reviewed the ultrasound studies and ^{99m}Tc-DMSA scintigrams of 42 infants with known or suspected multicystic dysplastic kidneys. DMSA uptake was evident in 6 of the 41 (15%) dysplastic kidneys. Of the 18 patients who underwent nephrectomy, histopathological examination revealed that uptake correlated closely with the presence of mature renal cortical tissue in the affected kidney [151].

3.7.2
^{99m}Tc-DMSA in the Diagnosis of Upper Urinary Tract Infection

Pathophysiology. Urinary tract infections (UTI) can be divided into upper UTI (pyelonephritis) and lower UTI (cystitis). Renal scarring following upper UTI occurs in 10–20% of the affected children. Up to 20% of these patients will develop renal hypertension in later life, and some of them will show deterioration of renal function if bilateral scarring is present [176].

It has been shown that infected vesico-uretero-renal reflux (VUR) is one, but not the only, prerequisite for the development of pyelonephritis in siblings and children. Special virulence factors of *E. coli* and other, poorly defined, conditions may also play a part [9, 83, 152, 153, 181].

In adults pyelonephritis can easily be diagnosed by the presence of typical clinical findings (temperature >38.5°C, pain in the costovertebral angle) and laboratory tests (significant bacteriuria, leucocytosis and elevated CRP or ESR). However, siblings and children may not present with the classic signs of upper UTI, making an accurate diagnosis difficult or even impossible [21].

Reduced DMSA uptake in areas of pyelonephritis is suggested to be due to renal ischaemia and metabolic alterations of the proximal tubular cells caused by bacterial toxins [73, 87, 152, 153].

Experimental Studies. Acute upper urinary tract infection can be visualised by uni- or multifocal reduction of renal ^{99m}Tc-DMSA uptake with preservation of the normal renal contour. In some cases a global diminution of DMSA uptake can be found. The correlation between reduced ^{99m}Tc-DMSA uptake and experimental pyelonephritis in animal models has been found to be excellent [136, 158]. In experimental acute pyelonephritis in piglets, Rushton and co-workers stated a sensitivity of 87% and a specificity of 100% for the ^{99m}Tc-DMSA scan [158]. In their study only small microscopic foci of inflammation were missed on scintigraphy. Similar observations have been recorded by others [62, 111, 112].

Clinical Studies. Numerous clinical studies have investigated the diagnostic and prognostic value of ^{99m}Tc-DMSA scanning within the last decade. Tables 1 and 2 summarise the results of some larger prospective series. Although the studies are not easily comparable owing to different inclusion criteria, different imaging techniques and different time intervals between the onset of infection and scintigraphy, certain common observations emerge:

Correlation Between Clinical Findings and Scintigraphy. In children with clinical signs of pyelonephritis, diminished uptake of ^{99m}Tc-DMSA was found in 40–93% of all cases, while abnormal scans were uncommon in children with suspected lower UTI [183, 202]. Clinical parameters had 70–93% sensitivity in the prediction of an abnormal ^{99m}Tc-DMSA scan if scintigraphy was performed within the 1st week after onset of symptoms, but were not reliable in the *exclusion* of scintigraphic defects and therefore offered relatively poor specificity [8, 83–85, 100, 104, 110, 155, 202].

Table 1. Studies of children with a first episode of symptomatic urinary tract infection (UTI)

Reference	No. of patients	Positive scintigram	Interval between onset of symptoms and scintigraphy	VUR
[199]	115 renal units	33%	3 months	46%
[183]	102	21%	27 days (median)	22%
[155]	65	54%/75%	3 days	24%
[41]	193 renal units	29%	15 days	24%
[181]	175	42%	10 days (median)	27%
[100]	55	93%	Within first week	21%

Table 2. Studies of children with acute UTI

Reference	No. of patients	Positive scintigram	Interval between onset of symptoms and scintigraphy	VUR
[202]	24	54%/80%	"Early"	50%
[84]	106	78%	5 days	25%
[117]	renal units	62%	"Early"	38%

Scanning within the 1st week after the onset of symptoms seems to be more sensitive in the detection of cortical abnormalities than imaging at a later time, maybe due to a rapid reversibility of cortical defects not progressing further to renal scars. Tappin et al. investigated their patients 27 days after the clinical onset of pyelonephritis and found an abnormal scan in only 21% [183]. In other series, in which patients were investigated within the 1st week when upper UTI was suspected the sensitivity of ^{99m}Tc-DMSA scintigraphy was higher, amounting to 93% [83, 84, 100, 117, 119, 155, 183, 202].

Fever and Cortical Defects. Fever is regarded as one of the clinical features of pyelonephritis. The question remains of whether a febrile UTI predicts involvement of the renal parenchyma with certainty. Tappin and co-workers found a positive scan in only 76% of children with UTI and temperatures >38.5°C [183]. In other series, negative scintigrams were present in 24–34% of all cases with febrile UTI [8, 83, 84, 110, 117]. No correlation was found between the duration of fever and diminished ^{99m}Tc-DMSA uptake [83, 84, 110].

Leucocytosis and Cortical Defects. Leucocytosis (>10,000/mm^3) is usually considered as indicative of involvement of the renal parenchyma during a symptomatic UTI. While 58–72% of children with UTI and leucocytosis had a positive ^{99m}Tc-DMSA scan, cortical defects were also present in the absence of leucocytosis in up to 23% of the children studied during acute infection [110, 117, 119]. These findings indicate that pyelonephritis can occur without marked leucocytosis.

Elevation of CRP/ESR and Cortical Defects. In our own experience in children with a first episode of symptomatic UTI, elevation of these parameters predicted a positive scan in 78%, but in some children normal scans could be seen despite highly elevated CRP and/or ESR. In other cases cortical defects were found but the CRP and/or ESR values were within the normal range [119]. This findings are similar to the results of Benador and co-workers [8]. In a large prospective series they found that an elevation of CRP and/or ESR predicted a positive scan in 89%, while the specificity of these parameters was only 28%. Low specificity of CRP and/or ESR has also been reported in other prospective studies [110, 117].

Recently Everaert et al. reported a close correlation between urinary alpha$_1$-microglobulin and positive findings in the ^{99m}Tc-DMSA scans, indicating that alpha$_1$-microglobulin may be more specific than other laboratory tests in the evaluation of upper UTI [52]. This observation should be checked and hopefully confirmed by further studies.

Vesico-ureteral-/-renal Reflux (VUR) and Cortical Defects. Undoubtedly, intrarenal reflux of infective urine is a major risk factor for upper urinary tract infections in children. This is particularly true for kidneys with grade III-V VUR. When vesicoureteral reflux is present, 76–85% of kidneys are noted to have cortical defects in the ^{99m}Tc-DMSA scan [41, 83, 84, 100, 117, 155, 182, 184, 200, 201]. On the other hand, prospective studies with ^{99m}Tc-DMSA have shown that pyelonephritis in the absence of VUR is more common than previously suggested. In these studies VUR was usually demonstrated in less than 40% of children with a positive ^{99m}Tc-DMSA scan [8, 41, 83, 84, 100, 155].

We examined 37 children with febrile UTI with ^{99m}Tc-DMSA and micturating cysto-urethrography and found a clear correlation between the degree of VUR and the number of positive scans. In 95% of children with VUR grade III or worse findings were positive in at least one renal unit, while only 62% of children with grade II reflux had defects on the ^{99m}Tc-DMSA scan. On the other hand, 70% of the children without reflux also had a positive scan, and 41% of all positive scans occurred in children with a negative micturating cysto-urethrography [118, 119].

Comparative Imaging of Pyelonephritis. Several clinical studies have compared the diagnostic accuracy of ^{99m}Tc-DMSA imaging performed within the first 10 days after the onset of symptomatic UTI with the results of i.v. urography and sonography [5, 9, 100, 104, 181].

[99mTc]-DMSA scanning (median sensitivity: 75%) proved to be superior to urography (median sensitivity: 34%) and sonography (median sensitivity: 34%) in the diagnosis of pyelonephritis. The diagnostic accuracy of [99mTc]-DMSA imaging was comparable to that of computed tomography [43, 100]. Takeda et al. compared [99mTc]-DMSA SPECT and magnetic resonance imaging (MRI) and found comparable sensitivities for both modalities (85 vs 83.3%) [182].

SPECT vs. Planar Imaging. In the study of Giblin et al. [99mTc]-DMSA SPECT showed a 93% sensitivity and specificity in experimental pyelonephritis [62]. In another experimental study, the diagnostic accuracy of planar pinhole and SPECT imaging in the diagnosis of acute pyelonephritis was found to be similar [112]. Several authors reported that DMSA SPECT detected 16–22% more abnormalities than planar imaging in acute pyelonephritis and claimed a higher diagnostic performance for this method [114, 122, 182]. Unfortunately, it is not clear whether these findings should really be taken to reflect an increase in sensitivity or rather an increase in the proportion of false-positive results. At present there is no consensus about the usefulness of SPECT for DMSA scintigraphy in children. In the performance of SPECT, special attention must be paid to the avoidance of motion artefacts, and therefore to the necessity for heavy sedation in young children.

3.7.3
[99mTc]-DMSA in the Diagnosis of Renal Scarring

Pathophysiology. The role of vesicoureteral reflux in the pathogenesis of pyelonephritis and renal scarring is not fully understood. Hodson et al. were the first to demonstrate the formation of renal scars in the upper and lower poles of refluxing pigs [74]. It has been shown that reflux per se does not produce scars, but only intrarenal reflux of infective urine. Further evidence for the importance of reflux comes from clinical studies which have shown that patients with higher grades of reflux are more likely to have renal damage than those with moderate grades of reflux [41, 83, 84, 100, 107, 117, 155, 182, 184, 200, 201].

For many years the emphasis on the investigation of the child with UTI centred on the diagnosis of reflux. At this time the formation of renal scars was considered to be due exclusively to VUR. It has since been recognised that many children with reflux will not develop scars and that many scars will develop following renal infection without the presence of a demonstrable VUR [85, 100, 120, 121, 155, 159, 160, 181, 199].

Experimental Studies. Renal scars detected by the DMSA scan appear as focal or generalised areas of reduced uptake associated with loss or contraction of functioning renal cortex. The correlation between reduced [99mTc]-DMSA uptake and experimental scars has been found to be higher than 90%. In the publication of Arnold et al., the sensitivity is given as 85% and the specificity as 97% those of histology [4].

Risdon et al. reported the effects of 3 weeks' antimicrobial treatment on the pathology and appearance of the [99mTc]-DMSA renal image in piglets with pyelonephritis induced by a combination of VUR and urinary infection. While almost all of the areas of slightly reduced uptake in the DMSA scan resolved with treatment, photon-absent scintigraphic abnormalities usually persisted after treatment and were always associated with significant scarring confirmed by histology [150].

Clinical Studies. Several clinical studies have shown, that 32–54% of lesions that were seen during a first acute pyelonephritis on the [99mTc]-DMSA scan persisted during a 3-month to 2-year follow-up. The sites of new renal scarring corresponded exactly to the sites of pyelonephritis during the first DMSA scan. In other kidneys the initial defect completely resolved [85, 100, 120, 121, 155, 158, 199]. These data support the hypothesis that the first upper UTI is highly important for the development of later renal scarring and therefore for the prognosis of the affected child.

The number of defects in the DMSA scans correlates well with the number of further recurrences. In a series seen in our own institution, 66% of children had normal scans after their first episode of febrile UTI. Conversely, 92% of the children with three or more episodes had a positive scan during follow-up [119].

We do not know exactly how long a DMSA defect caused by an episode of acute pyelonephritis can persist without irreversible renal damage, but 6 months seems to be an acceptable period after acute infection before abnormalities are seen as permanent sequelae.

Risk Factors of Renal Scarring. In the study by Stokland et al. renal damage seen on the DMSA scan 1 year after a first UTI was significantly correlated with initial elevation of CRP and fever. [181]. This observation was not confirmed by others [85, 159, 160]. When children with and without renal scars after upper UTI were compared, no significant difference could be observed in race, gender, duration of fever, elevation of the white blood cell count (WBC) or the ESR during the initial infection [85, 159, 160]. Children who developed new renal scars were significantly older at the time of acute upper UTI than children those renal function was preserved [85]. This is consistent with our experience that older children, mostly those between 1 and 3 years of age, will develop renal scarring after pyelonephritis more often than siblings [118, 119].

Another independent risk factor for the evolution of renal scarring is an associated bladder pathology, regardless of whether reflux is present or not [159, 160].

VUR was identified early on as an important risk factor for renal damage after a first episode of pyelonephritis. The risk of renal infection and subsequent scarring has been found to be substantially lower in children with mild reflux than in those with moderate or severe reflux [83, 84, 110].

In the European limb of the "International Reflux Study in Children", 287 children with grade II–V VUR were prospectively followed up with ^{99m}Tc-DMSA scans for 5 years. During entry into the study most of the children with severe reflux (82%) had some abnormality on the DMSA scan or differential isotope uptake. During follow-up 48 children (17%) developed new areas of reduced renal DMSA uptake regardless of whether they were treated conservatively or by surgery. Deterioration was more frequent in children with grade IV reflux than in children with grade III reflux [142].

In Stokland's study the relative risk for the development of renal scars in children with dilating VUR combined with high fever and CRP during their first pyelonephritis was tenfold that in children without these features [181].

Merrick and co-workers reported data recorded on more than 600 children during follow-up after UTI. No single investigation at presentation was able to predict subsequent deterioration, but the use of a combination of imaging investigations made it possible to distinguish groups with high or low probability of progressive damage. In the low-risk group without reflux and without a defect revealed by the DMSA scan at initial presentation, the incidence of progressive damage was 0.2%. If a positive scintigram was present during initial presentation a 6.9-fold increase in the relative risk of progressive renal damage was found, indicating that the initial DMSA scan gives independent information about the later outcome of a child with pyelonephritis. The combination of both defects in the DMSA scan and reflux at presentation, or one of them but accompanied by subsequent documented UTI, was associated with a 17-fold increase in the relative risk of progressive renal damage compared with children without these features [121].

Although dilating VUR, if present, is a major risk factor for renal scarring, many scars develop without reflux. Studies including children with initially abnormal ^{99m}Tc-DMSA scans, irrespectively of whether or not VUR was present, demonstrated that up to 60% of scars were not related to a demonstrable reflux [85, 100, 120, 121, 155, 159, 160, 200]. This observation provides evidence that infection of the renal parenchyma, rather than VUR, is the essential condition for postnatal renal scarring in children.

Comparative Imaging of Renal Scarring. Clinical studies that compared ^{99m}Tc-DMSA imaging with pyelography and ultrasound demonstrated that the DMSA scan is superior in the diagnosis of renal scarring.

Goldraich et al. compared ^{99m}Tc-DMSA scans of 202 children with 299 refluxing renal units with the results of IV urography [64]. Concordance between the two imaging procedures was noted in 88% of the kidneys. In 34 kidneys with a normal pyelogram, the DMSA scan showed one or more defects. During a follow-up of 1–3 years 30 of these kidney exhibited evidence of scarring. These findings indicate that abnormalities detected on a DMSA scan precede the changes on a pyelogram.

In another series of 208 patients the IV pyelogram showed focal scarring in 50 kidneys, and the DMSA scan, in 96 kidneys. All the patients with scarring on the pyelogram also had corresponding defects on the DMSA scan [45]. Similar results were published by Shanon et al. [171].

Tasker et al. performed ultrasound and DMSA scans in 100 children with a proven UTI and found 19 scarred kidneys in 17 children, whereas ultrasound detected only 7 of the scarred kidneys [184].

Mucci and Maguire examined 193 children with urinary tract infection. In this study ultrasound was able to detect only 3 kidneys among 21that showed defects or a pathological split function on the DMSA scan [124]. Similar findings have also been published by others [171].

These publications underline the fact that DMSA scanning may serve as a gold standard in the diagnosis of renal scarring. It has to be stressed that lesions seen on the DMSA scan are nonspecific and that it is not possible to differentiate between scarring and infectious lesions if the child concerned is evaluated during acute UTI. Furthermore, similar lesions can be found in renal abscess, cyst, duplex kidney, and hydronephrosis. In these clinical situations the combination of ultrasound and DMSA scintigraphy will allow a better differentiation [144].

3.7.4
Cortical Scintigraphy: Conclusion

Scintigraphy with ^{99m}Tc-DMSA is a simple and highly effective method in the diagnosis of renal malformations, pyelonephritis and renal scarring. It offers important information about the further prognosis of a child with UTI. In upper UTI ^{99m}Tc-DMSA scintigraphy may be more specific than the clinical tests available. In the diagnosis of pyelonephritis and renal scarring DMSA imaging has been confirmed to be more sensitive than pyelography and ultrasound, and its diagnostic power is at least equal to that of computed topography.

Therefore, DMSA scintigraphy can be recommended as the technique of choice for the evaluation of renal infection and sequelae. Although it seems to be debatable whether a DMSA scan should be performed during a first febrile UTI, since half of the acute lesions are transitory and will have disappeared at follow-up, scanning after 6 months seems to be useful, in order to evaluate if scarring has occurred.

Since reflux is seen in less than 40% of children with a pathologic DMSA scan and the prognosis of children with a UTI without a pathologic DMSA scan is usually good, the question arises of whether a micturating cysto-urethrography is necessary in the diagnostic work-up of children with symptomatic UTI and a normal DMSA scan.

According to the guidelines of the European Society of Nuclear Medicine (EANM), the correct indications for ^{99m}Tc-DMSA imaging are [144]:
1. Detection of focal renal parenchymal abnormalities.
2. Detection of renal sequelae, 6 months after acute infection.
3. Detection of acute pyelonephritis.
4. Detection of associated abnormalities: abnormal duplex kidney, small kidney, dysplastic tissue.
5. Detection of ectopic kidney.
6. Confirmation of nonfunctional multicystic kidney.

3.8
Radionuclide Cystography

Cystography is an essential procedure in the diagnosis of vesico-ureteral/renal reflux (VUR). The generally accepted gold standard in the diagnosis of VUR is the radiological micturating cystogram (MCU). It not only detects reflux with high sensitivity, but also provides detailed anatomical information and grading of VUR. While the MCU is indispensable in the initial diagnosis, radionuclide cystography can be used in the follow-up and has become the procedure of choice for this purpose in our institution within the last decade.

Two forms of radionuclide cystography have been described: a direct and an indirect method. Each of these techniques has its own advantages and disadvantages.

Direct radionuclide cystography requires catheterisation of the urinary bladder, with the risk of catheter-induced UTI; it is uncomfortable for the child, but seems to be more sensitive than the indirect method [37].

3.8.1
Direct Radionuclide Cystography

This method was first described by Conway 1976 [30]. Slight modifications were later proposed by Willi and Treves [206]. Our technique for performing the scan is very similar and is described in detail below.

Patient Preparation. It is essential to prepare the child and their parents for the examination. Full explanation of the procedure allays much of the anxiety accompanying the procedure in most cases. The study should be performed in a quiet atmosphere in the presence of the parents. During the study every single step of the test is again explained to the child. A physician or technologist should talk to the patient almost continuously to reduce the child's anxiety. Sedation of the child is usually not required [43].

Before the study, the child is asked to void in the bathroom. For catheterisation and radionuclide imaging the child lies supine on the examination table. The urinary bladder is catheterised under aseptic conditions by an experienced physician using a catheter 1.5.–2.5 mm in diameter. A sample of urine is obtained and cultured. In our opinion a balloon catheter, as advocated by some groups, is not necessary. The catheter is fixed with adhesive surgical tape, in girls to the inner thigh, and in boys to the dorsal shaft of the penis. The child can void around the catheter whenever desired.

Filling. To prepare the radiotracer solution for the next step, 37 MBq of ^{99m}Tc-Sn-colloid is mixed with sterile isotonic saline solution. We do not use free pertechnetate, because systemic absorption and renal excretion may occur, with a consequent false-positive diagnosis of vesico-renal reflux [43]. A saline bag larger than the patient's suggested bladder capacity is hung approximately 1 m above the table.

Although the relationship between normal bladder capacity and age in children follows a nonlinear curve, it can be described by two practical linear equations: 2 × age (years) + 2 = capacity (ounces, 1 ounce = 30 ml) for children less than 2 years old, and age (years) ÷ 2 + 6 = capacity (ounces) for those 2 years old or older [88].

The bladder is now gradually filled with the radio-tracer solution under hydrostatic pressure (70–90 cmH$_2$O). The operator monitors the cystogram with the aid of a persistence oscilloscope. The bladder should be filled at least to capacity, and preferably beyond. In a cooperative child, the end of the filling phase is indicated by the decreasing rate of flow of the infusate.

Voiding. With filling of the bladder to capacity the child is allowed to void. In our institution the patient voids with the catheter still in place. The majority of children will expel the catheter with the initiation of voiding. In the case of any who do not, the catheter is gently withdrawn. In this phase the patient may be either in a supine position or sitting upright voiding into a bedpan.

Imaging and Analysis. Dynamic imaging is performed from the beginning of the filling phase until the end of voiding. A large field of view gamma camera equipped with a highly sensitive collimator is positioned below the child, who is lying supine on the examination table. For the acquisition we use a framing rate of 6 frames/min and a 128 × 128 matrix. The sequential images of the cystogram are displayed in a cine-mode technique on a computer monitor (Fig. 12). Contrast enhancement is used to detect small volumes of reflux.

If reflux can be identified, regions of interest (ROIs) are drawn over the kidneys/ureters and the urinary bladder. A background region is advocated by others, but seems not to be necessary as virtually no background is present. Time–activity curves are generated for each ROI.

If we assume that the tracer is homogeneously distributed in the saline, that the attenuation the gamma-radiation of ^{99m}Tc is always the same and that negligible amounts of urine will be excreted via the kidney during the study, the counts will be proportional to the volume [192].

$$V = R \times C$$

where *V* is the volume, R is a constant and *C* is the count.

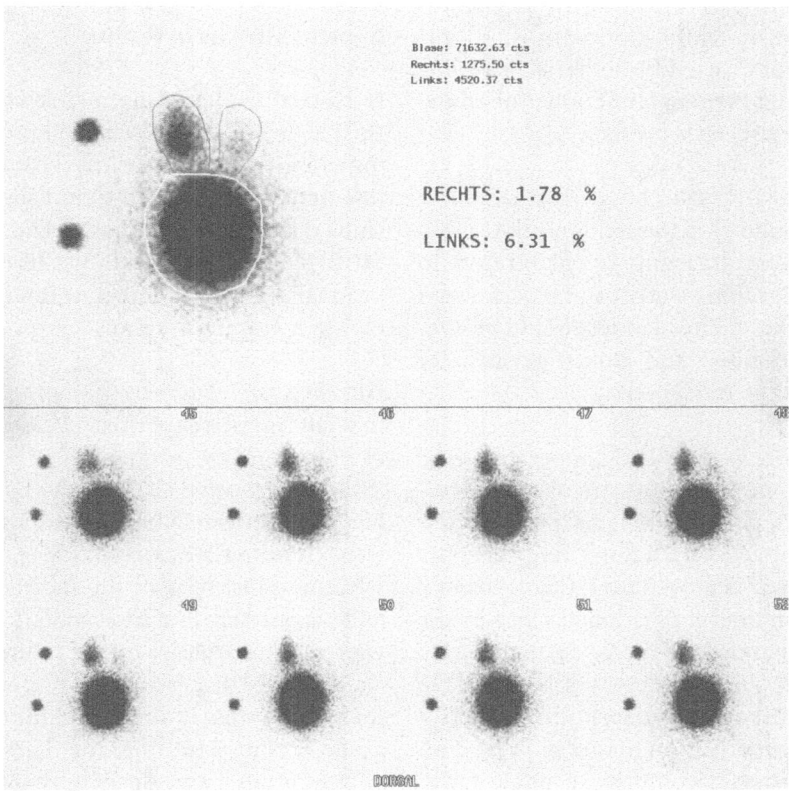

Fig. 12. Shows a bilateral VUR during the filling phase of a direct voiding scintigram. The reflux of the right side is very small (1.78 % of bladder filling), while on the right side a moderate reflux (6.31 % of the bladder filling) is present

R can be calculated by relating the voided volume to the decrease in total counts during the voiding phase. At the beginning of voiding the volume is V_o and the count is C_o. At the end of voiding the volume is V_e and the count is C_e. Therefore $V_o = R \times C_o$ and $V_e = R \times C_e$ and $R = (V_o - V_e)/(C_o - C_e)$. R can be simply expressed as: R = change in volume/change in count.

Once the constant has been calculated, any desired volume or change of volume over the time of the study can be determined:

1. Volume of the bladder during the first occurrence of reflux
2. Maximum bladder volume
3. Volume of reflux
4. Residual bladder volume
5. Average voiding flow rate

3.8.2
Indirect Radionuclide Cystography

Indirect radionuclide cystography (IRC) can be obtained as a part of a normal dynamic renal scintigraphy, is noninvasive and allows micturition to be studied under physiological conditions. Moreover, the technique provides information about the renal function. One major drawback of ICR is the higher radioactive burden on the child than with direct radionuclide cystography. In addition, reliable results can only be obtained if the renal function is obtained and no upper urinary stasis is present.

Patient Preparation. IRC can be performed after MAG$_3$ renography. Following the renogram the child returns to the waiting area and is encouraged to drink freely. A scintigraphic study can be performed if the child wants to void. The bladder should be adequately at that time, filled and almost no activity should be present in the renal pelvis.

Imaging and Analysis. During IRC cooperative girls can be seated on a commode. Boys are usually investigated in a standing position. A large field of view gamma camera equipped with a low-energy all-purpose (LEAP) collimator is moved from the horizontal to a vertical position and is positioned close to the child's back. The dynamic study is performed with a framing rate of 4–5 s/frame. A 64×64 or 128×128 computer matrix is used. Data acquisition starts 30 s before spontaneous micturition and should be continued until micturition is complete. If quantitative analysis of the study is considered the volume voided should be measured.

If the micturition is incomplete with tracer left in the collecting system, the child should encouraged to drink again, and if the child wants to void the complete procedure can be repeated.

For qualitative analysis the sequential images are displayed in a cine-mode technique. Contrast enhancement should used to detect small volumes of reflux. The investigator should make a careful comparison of the activity in the pelvicalyceal systems during the study against the activity before micturition. For quantitative analysis ROIs are drawn over the bladder and kidneys. A background region should be used. If reflux is present the renal time–activity curve will rise, while the bladder activity falls. Residual bladder activity and the volume of the reflux can be easily calculated if the voided volume has been collected and measured using the same equations as described for direct cystographic studies.

In contrast to direct cystography, where no activity in the kidney and no background is present at the start of the study, diagnosis of vesico-renal reflux by the indirect technique requires both the visual impression of the investigator that reflux is present and typical time–activity curves for the bladder and the affected kidney.

3.8.3
Clinical Studies in Reflux

In clinical studies radionuclide cystography (DIC or IRC) have been used in the follow-up of patients during their spontaneous clinical course or after surgical intervention. Many of the published study reports include data on the accuracy of DIC and IRC relative to MCU. Methodological studies have addressed the reproducibility of radionuclide imaging and tried to establish a grading system.

Direct Versus Indirect Cystography. Early evidence that DIC may be superior to ICR came from the study of Bower and co-workers. Of 54 renal units assessed, 21 ureters showed VUR on the DIC. All these ureters had been proven to be refluxive by means of MCU or were draining a scarred kidney. Relative to that of DIC, the sensitivity of the indirect studies was only 68%: six ureters that showed VUR on the direct study were read as negative on the indirect cystogram [16].

In a study that compared ICR with DIC, Majd et al. found that the indirect technique missed 67% of grade I reflux, 61% of grade II, 39% of grade III, and 12% of grade IV, while all grade V refluxes were correctly diagnosed by both techniques [109]. Compared with MCU, no false-negative DIC studies were found. Similar results were published by Corso et al., who found that ICR had a sensitivity of 32% relative to the direct technique [33].

De Sadeleer reported data about children who were investigated with IRC during acute UTI and with MCU 6 weeks later (group 1; $n = 40$). Another group (group 1; $n = 42$) underwent both ICR and DIC in the follow-up of known reflux. In this study ^{99m}Tc-MAG$_3$ ICR missed two-thirds of the refluxing kidneys that were diagnosed by means of any cystographic technique. Not only were most of the small refluxing volumes missed, but also 50% even of major refluxes [37].

In view of these data, the guidelines on IRC from the paediatric committee of the EANM state that ICR is only contributory to the diagnosis of reflux if positive, while a negative ICR cannot exclude VUR [144].

The higher sensitivity of the direct cystogram may be due to the absence of body background, which permits imaging of very small refluxing volumes as small as 0.2 ml [206]. In addition, indirect scintigraphy can only be performed in a cooperative child who voids at a required time and will not void before adequate drainage of the upper urinary tract is achieved. In the study of Majd and co-workers 21 (17.5%) of the 120 indirect cystograms lost their value for these reasons [109].

DIC Versus MCU. Nasrallah et al. demonstrated at an early stage that the sensitivity of DIC may be at least as high as, or even higher than, that of conventional MCU. In his study, 17.4% (15 of 86) of refluxing renal units were seen only on DIC but not on MCU. On the other hand, 4 patients had reflux seen only on MCU, all of which were unilateral and low–grade, and all these resolved spontaneously [128]. Similar evidence came from the study of Fretzayas and co-workers [58].

In a large series, Saraga et al. compared the results of MCU and DIC in 131 patients with recurrent UTI. VUR was present according to DIC in 9 renal units in which MCU failed to detect the reflux. In 17 renal units a grade I reflux was diagnosed by MCU, whereas DIC revealed backflow from the bladder up to the renal pelvis [164].

Dikshit et al. reported the results of comparative imaging in 92 kidney–ureter units, with similar results. MCU detected VUR in 20 units, whereas 22 units were positive on DIC, which revealed reflux up to the renal pelvis [40].

One advantage of DIC over MCU is its ability to assess bladder filling and emptying continuously with a considerable saving in radiation dose. Continuous monitoring by DIC may therefore allow the diagnosis of intermittent refluxes that otherwise would be missed on the MCU. The accuracy of DIC can be further improved if the scintigraphy is repeated immediately following a negative scan. This method has been called cyclic DIC. Fettich and al. reported that within the first cycle 29% of VUR I, 36% of VUR II and 9% VUR III were missed, which were detected in the second cycle [53]. This study clearly demonstrated the variable nature of reflux, whose severity can change from one examination to another. This should be kept in mind especially in serial assessment of children with VUR who receive prophylactic antibiotic treatment before the medication is discontinued. Perhaps two consecutive normal scintigraphic studies are more reliable than a single one to confirm that VUR has disappeared [193].

Early studies suggested that IRC may offer sensitivity equal to [24] or even higher than that of conventional MCU [145] in the diagnosis of VUR. This could not be confirmed in later series. Again in contrast to the high accuracy of DIC, indirect radionuclide scintigraphy revealed lower sensitivities which were in the range of 50–75% relative to radiological MCU [33, 37, 67].

Scintigraphic Grading of Reflux. The radiological grading proposed by the International Reflux Study Committee (IRSC) is widely used in the description of VUR [81]. Grade I reflux is into the ureter only. Grade II reflux is vesico-renal without dilatation of the ureter and pelvicalyceal system. Grade III reflux is vesico-renal with mild dilatation or tortuosity of the ureter and pelvicalyceal system. In grade IV moderate dilatation and tortuosity of these structures is present. In grade V gross dilation and tortuosity of these structures is present and papillary impressions are no longer visible in the majority of calyces.

Analysis of comparative studies should take into account that reflux exhibits a high degree of variability and may be of different grade on subsequent studies. This holds especially true for low-grade reflux [53]. In addition, qualitative grading is operator and technique dependent and subjective to some degree.

Skoog et al. visually graded radionuclide cystograms according to the radiological grading system and found 6.6% grade I, 54.2% grade II, 31.6% grade III, 5.7% grade IV and 1.9% grade VURs. With the exception of a low frequency of grade I refluxes the severity of reflux in this study were similar to those previously reported in series that were graded by MCU [175].

Zhang and co-workers compared visual grading of MCU and radionuclide cystography of 31 nephro-ureteral units in 25 patients [211]. They reported a tendency of radionuclide cystography to overgrade grade II and IV refluxes. However, when grades II and III were combined into a single category of low-grade reflux and grades IV and V into a category of high-grade reflux, the correlation between the two techniques was 100%.

Fretzayas et al. used direct radionuclide cystography and quantitative parameters in the grading of reflux. In this study the volume of refluxing urine and the duration of reflux were positively correlated with radiographic reflux grade. Residual urine was found to be higher in children with VUR than in those without reflux [58]. Similar observations have been recorded by our own group [210].

Mozley et al. demonstrated that quantitative parameters can be used in the assessment of prognosis in children with VUR who are treated medically. They found that children who did not begin to reflux until their bladders had been filled up to more than 60% total bladder capacity had a lower risk of needing surgery. The same hold true for patients with a refluxive volume of lower than 2% their of total bladder capacity [123].

3.8.4
Radiation Burden

Radiation dosimetry for direct radionuclide cystography proves that there is very little radiation exposure for the patient, the radiation dose being at least one tenth that needed for conventional MCU. For children between 1 and 10 years old, the absorbed radiation dose estimates are 0.18–0.27 mGy for the bladder wall, 10–20 mGy for the ovaries, and < 10–20 mGy for the testes, while the dose to the kidneys has been calculated to be 0.0002–0.0004 mGy/ml of reflux per min of residence in the pelvicalyceal system [193, 206].

3.9
Meta-iodobenzylguanidine in Neuroblastoma

Radiolabelled meta-iodobenzylguanidine (MIBG) was developed and described by a group working at the University of Michigan in 1980 [205] as an in vivo tracer for the sympathetic nervous system and tumours derived from it. Labelling can be performed either with the β and γ-emitter ^{131}I for diagnostic and therapeutic use or with the γ-emitter ^{123}I for imaging.

Radioiodinated MIBG has been extensively studied in the diagnosis and treatment of phaeochromo-

cytoma and paraganglioma in adults. Pooled results of a total of 562 cases imaged with ^{131}I-MIBG revealed a sensitivity of 88% and a specificity 97%. Similar results have been obtained with ^{123}I-MIBG (monographic review: [56]).

The first report on imaging of neuroblastoma with MIBG dates back to 1984 [90]. Since then the tracer has been widely used for this purpose. Furthermore, MIBG has great potential as a therapeutic agent in children with neuroblastoma.

3.9.1
Pharmacology

MIBG is structurally similar to norepinephrine and the neurosecretory granule-depleting agent guanethidine. MIBG shares the same uptake mechanism with norepinephrine and is taken up presynaptically at sympathetic nerve endings and stored in neurosecretory granules. Like other catecholamines, MIBG is released to the synaptic gap and then reabsorbed and stored again.

Active presynaptic transport (uptake I mechanism) is thought to be due to the sodium- and energy-dependent, saturable and high-affinity human norepinephrine transporter (hNET) [63, 116]. Uptake II mechanism is due to passive diffusion and is independent of sodium- and energy [63]. The clinical significance of uptake II remains unclear [63].

MIBG uptake can be found in various tissues. The highest uptake is seen in the adrenal medulla. Other organs with sympathetic innervation, such as the heart, the salivary glands, the basal parts of the lung and, infrequently, the spleen, are also visualised. Uptake in the liver is partly attributable to the deiodination of the compound. MIBG is not degraded by catechol-*o*-methyltransferase (COMT) or by monoamine oxidase (MAO). Of the activity given, 64% is excreted, mainly unmetabolised, via the kidney within 24 h [98]. Some gastrointestinal uptake due to hepatobiliary excretion is always present.

Tumours of the neuronal crest, such as phaeochromocytoma, paraganglioma and neuroblastoma, can usually be imaged with radioiodinated MIBG. A direct proportional correlation was found between the percentage uptake of ^{123}I-MIBG by these tumours and the number of neurosecretory granules [13]. In normal adrenal medullary tissue and phaeochromocytomas the tracer is preferentially stored within the granules. In contrast, up to 90% of MIBG uptake in neuroblastomas is extravesicular and therefore essentially different from the uptake in normal sympathetic tissue [6, 29]. It is essential to discontinue sub-

Table 3. Drugs known or expected to affect the uptake of MIBG

MIBG uptake decreased
Adrenergic blocking agents e.g. bretylium, guanethidine
α-Agonists
Propranolol
Labetalol
Reserpine
Guanethidine
Phenylephrine
Ephedrine
Terbutaline
Pseudoephedrine
Phenylpropanolamine
Cocaine
MAO-blocking substances
Phenothiazines
Thiothixines
Tricyclic antidepressants
Calcium channel-blocking agents

stances that may interfere with MIBG for at least several days before administering MIBG [179] (Table 3). Most of these drugs inhibit uptake type 1 or provoke depletion of granules.

3.9.2
Scintigraphy with ^{131}I-Meta-iodobenzylguanidine

Scintigraphy with ^{131}I-labelled MIBG has been used for many years as the standard procedure in neuronal crest tumour imaging, but in Europe it has been widely replaced by ^{123}I-MIBG scintigraphy.

Patient Preparation. The thyroid should be blocked with potassium iodine [100 mg] from 1 day before until at least 4 days after i.v. injection of 18–37 MBq ^{131}I-MIBG/1.7m^2 body surface area. The tracer should be injected slowly within 30–40 s to prevent such sympathicoadrenergic side effects as flushing and hypertension.

Imaging. Scintigraphy is performed 24, 48 and 72 h p.i. A large field of view gamma camera fitted with a high-energy collimator and a 64×64 computer matrix is used. Ventral and dorsal spot views of the whole body with 100 000 cts. each are acquired. Alternatively, imaging can be performed with a preset time of 20 min.

3.9.3
Scintigraphy with ^{123}I-Meta-iodobenzylguanidine

[123]I has many potential advantages over ^{131}I as a radiolabel for MIBG. It offers a higher photon flux, a photon energy better suited to modern gamma cameras (159 vs 364 keV) and greater ease of collimation with less septal penetration. The mode of decay yields no particulate emission, and this, together with a short half-time of approximately 13 h yields, a far more favourable radiation dosimetry. High photon flux together with suitable photon energy permits the performance of SPECT up to 24 h p.i.

Patient Preparation. The thyroid should be blocked with potassium iodine (100 mg) from 1 day before until 3 days after i.v. injection of 185–300 MBq/1.7m^2 body surface area ^{123}I-MIBG. Precautions during injection are the same as described for ^{131}I-MIBG.

Imaging. Scintigraphy is performed 4 and 24 h p.i. A large field of view gamma camera fitted with a low-energy high-resolution (LEHR) collimator and a 256×256 computer matrix is used. Ventral and dorsal spot views of the whole body with 200–400 kcts. each are acquired. Alternatively, imaging can be performed with a preset time of 10 min. SPECT is performed preferably 6 h p.i.

3.9.4
The ^{123}I-MIBG Scan in Neuroblastoma

The normal distribution of ^{123}I-MIBG includes salivary glands, myocardium, liver, the kidneys, and urinary bladder. If the thyroid is adequately blocked only faint thyroid uptake should be observed. The lung base and the spleen are infrequently seen. Uptake in the adrenal medulla is visualised in almost all cases, especially if SPECT performed. On normal scans no bone uptake is detectable. Usually the colonic excretion is well visualised.

Bonnin et al. described a number of particularities and pitfalls related to paediatric MIBG imaging, which have to be considered in the interpretation of scans [14]. Bilateral upper thoracic uptake is common in children and should not be misinterpreted as metastatic disease. The uptake in the salivary glands and radioactive salvia can be very intense and may mimic mandibular bone marrow involvement. In this situation repeated and delayed views are recommended. Every uptake in the bone marrow has to be considered as metastatic. After unilateral adrenalectomy the uptake in the contralateral gland may increase to a degree that makes it indistinguishable from contralateral tumour involvement. In such cases correlative imaging is indispensable. Retrocardial tumour involvement can be missed on planar scans due to cardiac uptake, and therefore lateral views or SPECT should be performed.

Previous studies have shown that computed tomography (CT), magnetic resonance imaging (MRI) and scintigraphy with radioiodinated MIBG are complementary procedures in the staging and restaging of neuroblastoma. CT and MRI are sensitive in the detection of the primary tumour and metastases. Radiographic techniques provide superior anatomical detail and are somewhat more accurate in the diagnosis of the primary tumour and small metastatic sites. MIBG provides more specific functional information, is the most specific test and can be used as a whole-body screening procedure, especially in the postoperative situation [32, 115, 198].

In neuroblastoma the sensitivity of MIBG imaging in the diagnosis of the primary tumour is about 90%, or even higher [42, 61, 76, 83, 174, 194, 195].

False-negative results of MIBG scanning for the primary tumour are rare and due either to small tumour volumes or to loss of specific uptake in some neuroblastomas [172].

Some MIBG-negative tumours express somatostatin type 2 receptors [149], and somatostatin receptor scintigraphy with In-111 pentetreotide may therefore be useful in neuroblastoma patients with a normal MIBG scan [96].

False-positive results have been described in some nonneuronal crest tumours, such as Wilms' tumour [168]. Other tumours of the neuronal crest (paragangliomas, phaeochromocytomas) can be confused with neuroblastoma due to their MIBG uptake [95], but they are extremely rare during childhood.

Conflicting results have been reported with the scintigraphy in the diagnosis of liver metastases. Dessner et al. reported a low sensitivity for the method due to a low target-to-background ratio between tumour involvement and physiologic liver uptake [39]. In another study, Lastoria et al. compared ^{131}I-MIBG scintigraphy with CT in 28 children with neuroblastoma. MIBG scintigraphy detected nine out of ten liver metastases, while the sensitivity of CT was only 60% [99]. These data indicate that radiological and scintigraphic techniques should be used to complement each other.

Lymph node metastases are common in neuroblastoma and can be visualised sensitively by ^{123}I-MIBG, but small metastases (< 1,5 cm) may be missed [42, 61, 76, 83, 99, 174, 194, 195].

MIBG is not taken up in the bone marrow and therefore metastases at this site can readily be recognised. However scintigraphic differentiation between bone marrow and bone metastases is not possible with MIBG. Sensitivity levels between 81% and 86% have been reported for MIBG scintigraphy in the diagnosis of bone marrow involvement [28, 115].

MIBG scanning is superior to bone scintigraphy with ^{99m}Tc-labelled diphosphonates and reveals more sites of tumour involvement. In addition, MIBG is more specific than bone scintigraphy because it does not accumulate at sites of bone repair of healing metastases. In one study the results of the bone scan and of MIBG imaging of 77 patients with confirmed neuroblastoma were compared. In all patients the two modalities were concordant for the presence or absence of skeletal metastases but MIBG diagnosed almost twice as many skeletal lesions [173]. In another series MIBG revealed 161 positive sites while the ^{99m}Tc-MDP scan showed only 100 positive sites [66].

Some series included a moderate number of patients with skeletal metastases that were positive on bone scan but negative on MIBG scintigraphy [66, 166]. These data suggest that the bone scan may be a valuable adjunct to MIBG scintigraphy, especially if there is clinical suspicion of skeletal involvement without demonstrable bone marrow metastases on the MIBG scan.

Following therapy MIBG can be used in the early identification of children with progressive disease or relapse. Persistent or new pathologic uptake strongly suggests a viable neuroblastoma [46]. Unfortunately, some tumour sites lose their ability to store MIBG and subsequently become negative on the scan [46]. Lebtahi et al. compared MRI with MIBG scintigraphy in the follow-up of children with bone marrow metastases after chemotherapy. They showed that normalisation of bone marrow uptake on the MIBG scan excluded persistent tumour involvement, while a hypointense signal on T1-weighted MRI persisted in these cases for as long as 2 years or even longer after the end of chemotherapy [101].

Because a negative MIBG scan does not exclude persistent disease and persistent changes on MRI does not confirm the viability of bone marrow metastases after therapy, only multimodal imaging together with laboratory testing and the clinical evaluation of the child will allow a proper follow-up of neuroblastoma.

3.9.5
^{131}I-MIBG Therapy in Neuroblastoma

In neuroblastomas disseminated disease is present in up to 70% of cases at diagnosis. Metastatic spread usually involves bone and bone marrow, liver and lymph nodes. The prognosis of these children is poor, but conventional strategies such as chemotherapy, external total-body beam radiation and bone marrow reinfusion will be beneficial for some children in this situation. Therapy with ^{131}I-MIBG has been proven to be safe, and less toxic than but at least as effective as chemotherapy.

Radiobiology of ^{131}I-MIBG. [131]I decays with a physical half live of 8.1 days by β^- transition to [131]Xe. Most – 90% – of the radiation effects of ^{131}I-MIBG result from the beta radiation, which has a mean range in tissue of about 0.5 mm. This short range leads to destruction of tumour cells, which selectively take up the tracer by the human norepinephrine transporter [hNET], but ensures that the extratumoral radiation exposure is limited and side effects are therefore few. High target doses to the tumour can only be expected in foci with high target-to-nontarget ratios, which can be evaluated on a diagnostic MIBG-scan.

Indications for ^{131}I-MIBG Therapy. Most experience with ^{131}I-MIBG has been recorded in patients with TNM stage III and IV neuroblastoma in recurrent or progressive disease following surgery and chemotherapy [75]. Within recent years encouraging results have been obtained with ^{131}I-MIBG as a first-line therapy prior to surgery in stage III and IV disease. [75, 78].

Contraindications for ^{131}I-MIBG Therapy. Contraindications for ^{131}I-MIBG therapy are severe myelosuppression and renal failure. A relative contraindication is the presence of unstable clinical conditions which do not allow isolation of the patient in a specific unit.

Patient Preparation and Therapy. In children with tumoral bone marrow involvement harvesting of bone marrow prior to ^{131}I-MIBG therapy should be considered. Medication that is known or thought to interfere with the uptake and/or retention of ^{131}I-MIBG should be withdrawn for at least 2 weeks prior to therapy. If necessary, propranolol should be used to control hypertension. Thyroid blockade is performed by daily oral administration of 100 mg potassium iodide for 2 weeks starting 1 day before therapy.

After insertion of a short intravenous catheter a fixed dose of 3.7–7.4 GBq (100–200 mCi) of ^{131}I-MIBG with a high specific activity (up to 1.48 GBq/mg) is usually infused within 30–60 min.

Results. Different small series of patients treated with ^{131}I-MIBG have been published [59, 75, 77, 91, 105, 194–196]. In these patients with stage III and IV neuroblastoma and relapse or progressive disease after conventional therapy regimens an overall response rate of 35% has been observed (pooled results of a total of 273 treated patients).

The therapy is generally well tolerated. Nausea and vomiting may occur during the first 2 days after administration. A mild and temporary myelosuppression can typically be seen 4–6 weeks after therapy. Thrombocytopenia may selectively occur due to radiation of the bone marrow and/or due to selective uptake of MIBG in platelets. In patients with bone marrow involvement, extensive prior chemotherapy, a history of prior myeloablative therapy with stem cell support or delayed renal clearance of MIBG severe haematotoxicity can be expected. In this situation the use of stem cells or bone marrow for transplantation is advisable. Occasionally hypertensive crises may be evoked by MIBG-induced release of catecholamines, requiring alpha-blockade [194–196].

The objective of introducing ^{131}I-MIBG therapy as the first-line therapy was to reduce the tumour volume, making adequate surgical resection possible, and to avoid toxicity and the induction of early drug resistance. An additional advantage of such an approach is that the child's general condition is unaffected or even improved before surgery. In this approach chemotherapy is reserved for the treatment of minimal residual disease.

In their initial results, Hoefnagel et al. demonstrated that the objective response rate was better than after conventional treatment: in 70% of patients complete or >95% resection of the primary tumour was achieved or surgery was not required at all [78]. The only toxicities after such a first-line therapy were mild thrombocytopenia and moderate myelosuppression. In conclusion, first-line treatment with ^{131}I-MIBG is at least as effective as when it is combined with chemotherapy but involves significantly less toxicity.

3.9.6
Radiation Burden of MIBG Scintigraphy and Therapy

For a 5-year-old child the effective dose (ED) is 3.7 mSv if 96 MBq ^{123}I-MIBG is given. If ^{131}I-MIBG is used the effective dose per MBq is 19- 27-fold this, depending on the age of the child [180].

References

1. Abdel Dayem HM, Sadek S, al-Bahar R et al (1989) Comparison of 99Tcm-mercaptoacetyltriglycine and 131I-orthoiodohippurate in determination of effective renal plasma flow (ERPF). Nucl Med Commun 10:99–107
2. Anderson PJ, Rangarjan V, Gordon I (1997) Assessment of drainage in PUJ dilatation: pelvic excretion efficiency as an index of renal function. Nucl Med Commun 18:823–826
3. Applegate K, Connolly L, Treves ST (1995) Tc-99 m DMSA imaging of crossed fused renal ectopia. Clin Nucl Med 10:947–948
4. Arnold AJ, Brownless SM, Carty HM et al (1990) Detection of renal scarring by DMSA scanning-an experimental study. J Pediatr Surg 25:391–339
5. Arnold RW, Subramanian G, McAfee JG et al (1975) Comparison of Tc-99 m complexes for renal imaging. J Nucl Med 16:357–367
6. Babich JW, Graham W, Fischman AJ (1997) Effect of adrenergic receptor ligands on meta-iodobenzylguanidine uptake and storage in neuroblastoma cells. Eur J Nucl Med 24:538–543
7. Bagni B, Portaluppi F, Montanari L et al (1990) 99mTc-MAG3 versus 131I-orthoiodohippurate in the routine determination of effective renal plasma flow. J Nucl Med Allied Sci 34:67–70
8. Benador D, Benador N, Slosman DO et al (1994) Cortical scintigraphy in the evaluation of renal parenchymal changes in children with pyelonephritis. J Pediatr 124:17–20
9. Bjorgvinsson E, Majd M, Eggli KD (1991) Diagnosis of acute pyelonephritis in children: comparison of sonography and 99mTc-DMSA scintigraphy. AJR 157:539–543
10. Blaufox MD (1991) Procedures of choice in renal nuclear medicine. J Nucl Med 32:1301–1309
11. Blaufox MD, Merrill JP (1966) Simplified hippuran clearance. Measurement of renal function in man with simplified hippuran clearances. Nephron 3:274–281
12. Blaufox MD, Aurell M, Bubeck B et al (1996) Report of the Radionuclides in Nephrourology Committee on Renal Clearance. Nucl Med 1883–1890
13. Bomanji J, Levison DA, Flatman WD et al (1987) Uptake of iodine-123 MIBG by pheochromocytomas, paragangliomas, and neuroblastomas: a histopathological comparison. J Nucl Med 28:973–978
14. Bonnin F, Lumbroso J, Tenenbaum F et al (1994) Refining interpretation of MIBG scans in children. J Nucl Med 35:803–810
15. Bowen J, Sharma H, Gough DCS (1994) Chronic hydronephrosis: renographic drainage patterns and renal morphology in an animal model. Br J Urol 74:26–30
16. Bower G, Lovegrove FT, Geijsel H et al (1985) Comparison of "direct" and "indirect" radionuclide cystography. J Nucl Med 26:465–468
17. Brown SCW, Upsdell SM, O'Reilly PH (1992) The importance of renal function in the interpretation of diuresis renography. Br J Urol 69:121–125
18. Bubeck B (1993) Renal clearance determination with one blood sample: improved accuracy and universal applicability by a new calculation principle. Semin Nucl Med 23:73–86
19. Bubeck B, Brandau W, Eisenhut M et al (1987) The tubular extraction rate (TER) of Tc-99 m MAG$_3$: a new quantitative parameter of renal function. Nucl Compact 18:260–267
20. Bubeck B, Brandau W, Steinbächer M et al (l988) Technetium-99 m labeled renal function and imaging agents. II. Clinical evaluation of ^{99m}Tc MAG3 (^{99m}Tc mercaptoacetylglycylglycylglycine). Nucl Med Biol l5:109–118
21. Busch R, Huland H (1984) Correlation of symptoms and results of direct bacterial localization in patients with urinary tract infections. J Urol 132:281–285
22. Chaiwatanarat T, Padhy AK, Bomanji JB et al (1993) Validation of renal output efficiency as an objective quantitative parameter in the evaluation of upper urinary tract obstruction. J Nucl Med 34:845–848
23. Chantler C, Garnett ES, Parsons V et al (1969) Glomerular filtration rate measurement in man by die single injection method using ^{51}Cr-EDTA. Clin Sci 37:169–180
24. Chapman SJ, Chantler G, Haycock GB et al (1988) Radionuclide cystography in vesicoureteric reflux. Arch Dis Child 63:650–651
25. Chevet D, Moisan A, Le Pogamp P et al (1984) Quantification of separate renal function using Tc 99 m DTPA and Tc 99 m DMSA. Correlations between individual isotopic data and creatinine clearance. Nephrologie 5:21–25
26. Chervu LR, Freeman LM, Blaufox MD (1974) Radiopharmaceuticals for renal studies. Semin Nucl Med 4:3–22
27. Chervu LR, Blaufox MD (1989) Radiopharmaceuticals for the measurement of glomerular filtration rate and renal plasma flow. In: Blaufox MD (ed) Evaluation of renal function and disease with radionuclides. Karger, Basel, pp 28–59
28. Claudiani F, Stimamiglio P, Bertolazzi L et al (1995) Radioiodinated meta-iodobenzylguanidine in the diagnosis of childhood neuroblastoma. Q J Nucl Med 39 [Suppl 1]:21–24
29. Clerc J, Halpern S, Fourre C et al (1993) SIMS microscopy imaging of the intratumor biodistribution of metaiodobenzylguanidine in the human SK-N-SH neuroblastoma cell line xenografted into nude mice. J Nucl Med 34:1565–1570
30. Conway JJ, Kruglik GD (1976) Effectiveness of direct and indirect radionuclide cystography in detecting vesicoureteral reflux. J Nucl Med 17:81–83
31. Conway JJ, Maizels M (1992) The "well tempered" diuretic renogram: a standard method to examine the asymptomatic neonate with hydronephrosis or hydroureteronephrosis. A report from combined meetings of The Society for Fetal Urology and members of The Pediatric Nuclear Medicine Council – The Society of Nuclear Medicine. J Nucl Med 33:2047–2051

32. Corbett R, Olliff J, Fairley N et al (1991) A prospective comparison between magnetic resonance imaging, meta-iodobenzylguanidine scintigraphy and marrow histology/cytology in neuroblastoma. Eur J Cancer 12:1560–1564

33. Corso A, Ostinelli A, Trombetta MA (1989) "Indirect" radioisotope cystography after the furosemide test: its diagnostic efficacy compared to "direct" study. Radiol Med Torino 78:645–648

34. Daley JJ, Jones WA, Rudd TG et al (1977) Differential 99mTc dimercaptosuccinic acid (DMSA) renal localization: correlations with renal function. J Nucl Med 18:594–595

35. Daley JJ, Jones W, Rudd TG et al (1979) Differential renal function using technetium-99 m dimercaptosuccinic acid (DMSA): in vitro correlation. J Nucl Med 20:63–66

36. De Lange MJ, Piers-DA, Kosterink JG et al (1989) Renal handling of technetium-99 m DMSA: evidence for glomerular filtration and peritubular uptake. J Nucl Med 30:1219–1223

37. De Sadeleer C, De Boe V, Keuppens F et al (1994) How good is technetium-99 m mercaptoacetyltriglycine indirect cystography? Eur J Nucl Med 21:223–227

38. De Sadeleer C, Bossuyt A, Goes E et al (1996) Renal technetium-99m-DMSA SPECT in normal volunteers. J Nucl Med 37:1346–1349

39. Dessner DA, DiPietro MA, Shulkin BL (1993) MIBG detection of hepatic neuroblastoma: correlation with CT, US and surgical findings. Pediatr Radiol 23:276–280

40. Dikshit MP, Acharya VN, Shikare S et al (1993) Comparison of direct radionuclide cystography with micturating cystourethrography for the diagnosis of vesicoureteric reflux, and its correlation with cystoscopic appearances of the ureteric orifices. Nephrol Dial Transplant 8:600–602

41. Ditchfield MR, de Campo JF, Nolan TM et al (1994) Risk factors in the development of early renal cortical defects in children with urinary tract infection. AJR Am J Roentgenol 162:1393–1397

42. Edeling CJ, Frederiksen PB, Kamper J et al (1987) Diagnosis and treatment of neuroblastoma using meta-iodobenzylguanidine. Clin Nucl Med 12:632–637

43. Eggli DF, Tulchinsky M (1993) Scintigraphic evaluation of pediatric urinary tract infection. Semin Nucl Med 23:199–218

44. Eising EG, Bonzel KE, Zander C et al (1997) Value of diuresis renography in the post-natal period of assumed physiological renal immaturity. Nucl Med Commun 18:1008–1016

45. Elison BS, Taylor D, Van der Wall H et al (1992) Comparison of DMSA scintigraphy with intravenous urography for the detection of renal scarring and its correlation with vesicoureteric reflux. Br J Urol 69:294–302

46. Englaro EE, Gelfand MJ, Harris RE et al (1992) ^{131}I-MIBG imaging after bone marrow transplantation for neuroblastoma. Radiology 182:515–520

47. English PJ, Testa HJ, Gosling JA et al (1982) Idiopathic hydronephrosis in childhood-a comparison between diuresis renography and upper urinary tract morphology. Br J Urol 54:603–607

48. English PJ, Testa HJ, Lawson RS et al (1987) Modified method of diuresis renography for the assessment of equivocal pelviureteric junction obstruction. Br J Urol 59:10–14

49. Enlander D, Weber PM, dos Remedios LV (1974) Renal cortical imaging in 35 patients: superior quality with [99 m]Tc-DMSA. J Nucl Med 15:743–749

50. Eshima D, Taylor A (1992) Technetium-99 m (99mTc) mercaptoacetyltriglycine: update on the new [99mTc] renal tubular function agent. Semin Nucl Med 22:61–73

51. Evans K, Lythgoe MF, Anderson PJ et al (1996) Biokinetic behavior of technetium-99m-DMSA in children. J Nucl Med 37:1331–1335

52. Everaert K, Raes A, Hoebeke P et al (1998) Combined use of urinary alpha1-microglobulin and 99mTc DMSA scintigraphy in the diagnosis and follow-up of acute pyelonephritis and cystitis in children. Eur J Urol 34:486–491

53. Fettich JJ, Kenda RB (1992) Cyclic direct radionuclide voiding cystography: increasing reliability in detecting vesicoureteral reflux in children. Pediatr Radiol 22:337–338

54. Fine EJ (1991) Interventions in renal scintigraphy. Semin Nucl Med 21:116–127

55. Fine EJ, Axelrod M, Gorkin J et al (1987) Measurement of effective renal plasma flow: a comparison of methods. J Nucl Med 8:1393–1400

56. Fischer M, Gross MD, Shapiro B et al (1993) Nebenniere-Nuklearmedizinische Diagnostik und Therapie. Springer, Berlin Heidelberg New York

57. Fisher M, Veall N (1975) Glomerular filtration rate estimation based on a single blood sample. Br Med J 2:542

58. Fretzayas A, Karpathios T, Dimitriou P et al (1984) Grading of vesicoureteral reflux by radionuclide cystography. Pediatr Radiol 14:148–150

59. Garaventa A, Bellagamba O, Lo Piccolo MS et al (1999) 131I-metaiodobenzylguanidine (131I-MIBG) therapy for residual neuroblastoma: a mono-institutional experience with 43 patients. Br J Cancer 81:1378–1384

60. Gates GF (1982) Glomerular filtration rate: Estimation from fractional renal accumulation of ^{99m}Tc DTPA (stannous). AJR Am J Roentgenol 138:565–570

61. Geatti O, Shapiro B, Sisson JC et al (1985) Iodine-131 metaiodobenzylguanidine scintigraphy for the location of neuroblastoma: preliminary experience in ten cases. J Nucl Med 26:736–742

62. Giblin JG, O'Connor KP, Fildes RD et al (1993) The diagnosis of acute pyelonephritis in the piglet using single photon emission computerized tomography dimercaptosuccinic acid scintigraphy: a pathological correlation. J Urol 150:759–762

63. Glowniak JV, Kilty JE, Amara SG et al (1993) Evaluation of metaiodobenzylguanidine uptake by the norepinephrine, dopamine and serotonin transporters. J Nucl Med 34:1140–1146

64. Goldraich NP, Ramos OL, Goldraich IH (1989) Urography versus DMSA scan in children with vesicoureteric reflux. Pediatr Nephrol 3:1–5

65. Gordon I, Mialdea Fernandez RM, Peters AM (1988) Pelviuretic junction obstruction: The value of post micturition view in Tc99 m DTPA diuretic renography. Br J Urol 61:409–412

66. Gordon I, Peters AM, Gutman A, Morony S et al (1990) Skeletal assessment in neuroblastoma–the pitfalls of iodine-123-MIBG scans J Nucl Med 31:129–134

67. Gordon I, Peters AM, Morony S (1990) Indirect radionuclide cystography: a sensitive technique for the detection of vesico-ureteral reflux. Pediatr Nephrol 4:604–606

68. Gosling JA, Dixon JS (1978) Functional obstruction of the ureter and renal pelvis. A histological and electron microscopic study. Br J Urol 50:145–152

69. Green DA, Davies SG (1997) Dimercaptosuccinic acid distribution in renal tubular acidosis. Br J Radiol 70: 1291–1292

70. Ham HR, Piepsz A (1991) Estimation of glomerular filtration rate in infants and in children using a single-plasma sample method. J Nucl Med 32:1294–1297

71. Harvey CJ, Buscombe JR, Hilson AJ (1998) 3-D display of Tc-99 m DMSA SPECT in crossed fused renal ectopia. Clin Nucl Med 23:399–340

72. Hay AM, Norman WJ, Rice ML et al (1984) Comparison between diuresis renography and the Whitaker test in 64 kidneys. Br J Urol 56:561–564

73. Hill GS, Clark RL (1972) A comparative angiographic, microangiographic and histologic study of experimental pyelonephritis. Invest Radiol 7:33–47

74. Hodson CJ, Maling TMJ, Mc Manaman PJ et al (1975) The pathogenesis of reflux nephropathy (chronic atrophic pyelonephritis). Br J Radiol 48 [Suppl 13]:1–26

75. Hoefnagel CA (1999) Nuclear medicine therapy of neuroblastoma. Q J Nucl Med 43:336–343

76. Hoefnagel CA, Voute PA, de Kraker J et al (1985) Total-body scintigraphy with ^{131}I-meta-iodobenzylguanidine for detection of neuroblastoma. Diagn Imaging Clin Med 54:21–27

77. Hoefnagel CA, Voute PA, de Kraker J, Valdes Olmos RA (1991) [131I] metaiodobenzylguanidine therapy after conventional therapy for neuroblastoma. J Nucl Biol Med 35:202–206

78. Hoefnagel CA, de Kraker J, Valdes Olmos RA et al (1994) 131I MIBG as a first line treatment in high risk neuroblastoma patients. Nucl Med Commun 15:712–717

79. Homsy YL, Mehta PH, Huot D, Danais S (1988) Intermittent hydronephrosis: a diagnostic challenge. J Urol 140:1222–1226

80. Howman-Giles R, Uren R, Roy LP, Filmer RB (1987) Volume expansion diuretic renal scan in urinary tract obstruction. J Nucl Med 28:824–828

81. International Reflux Study Committee (1981) Medical versus surgical treatment of primary vesicoureteral reflux. Pediatrics 67:392–400

82. Itoh K, Yamashita T, Tsukamoto E et al (1995) Qualitative and quantitative evaluation of renal parenchymal damage by 99mTc-DMSA planar and SPECT scintigraphy. Ann Nucl Med 9:23–28

83. Jakobsson B, Nolstedt L, Svensson L et al (1992) 99mTechnetium-dimercaptosuccinic acid scan in the diagnosis of acute pyelonephritis in children: relation to clinical and radiological findings. Pediatr Nephrol 6:328–334

84. Jakobsson B, Soderlundh S, Berg U (1992) Diagnostic significance of 99mTc-dimercaptosuccinic acid (DMSA) scintigraphy in urinary tract infection. Arch Dis Child 67:1338–1342

85. Jakobsson B, Berg U, Svensson L (1994) Renal scarring after acute pyelonephritis. Arch Dis Child 70:111–115

86. Jones DA, Lupton EW, George NJR (1990) Effect of bladder filling on upper tract urodynamics in man. Br J Urol 65:492–496

87. Kaak MB, Dowling KJ, Patterson GM et al (1986) Immunology of pyelonephritis VIII: E. coli causes granulocytic aggregation and renal ischemia. J Urol 136:1117–1122

88. Kaefer M, Zurakowski D, Bauer SB et al (1997) Estimating normal bladder capacity in children. J Urol 158: 2261–2264

89. Kass EJ, Majd M, Belman AB (1985) Comparison of the diuretic renogram and the pressure perfusion study in children. J Urol 134:92–96

90. Kimmig B, Brandeis WE, Eisenhut (1984) Scintigraphic diagnosis of neuroblastoma with [131]MIBG. J Nucl Med 25:773–775

91. Klingebiel T, Feine U, Treuner J, Reuland P et al (1991) Treatment of neuroblastoma with [^{131}I]metaiodobenzylguanidine: long-term results in 25 patients. J Nucl Biol Med 35:216–219

92. Koff SA (1987) Problematic ureteropelvic junction obstruction. J Urol 138:390

93. Koff SA, Thrall JH, Keyes JW (1979) Diuretic radionuclide urography: a noninvasive method for evaluating nephroureteral dilatation. J Urol 122:451–454

94. Koff SA, Mc Dowell GC, Byard M (1988) Diuretic radionuclide assessment of obstruction in the infant: guidelines for successful interpretation. J Urol 140: 1167–1168

95. Krenning EP, Kwekkeboom DJ, Bakker WH et al (1993) Somatostatin receptor scintigraphy with In-111 DTPA-D-Phe1-and ^{123}I-Tyr-octreotide: the Rotterdam experience with more than 1000 patients. Eur J Nucl Med 20:716–731

96. Kropp J, Hofmann M, Bihl H (1997) Comparison of MIBG and pentetreotide scintigraphy in children with neuroblastoma. Is the expression of somatostatin receptors a prognostic factor? Anticancer Res 17:1583–1588

97. Kullendorff CM, Wallin L (1993) DMSA scintigraphy in renal duplex system. Eur J Pediatr Surg 3:83–86

98. Lashford LS, Moyes J, Ott R et al (1988) The biodistribution and pharmacokinetics of meta-iodobenzylguanidine in childhood neuroblastoma. Eur J Nucl Med 13:574–577

99. Lastoria S, Maurea S, Caraco C et al (1993) Iodine-131 metaiodobenzylguanidine scintigraphy for localization of lesions in children with neuroblastoma: comparison with computed tomography and ultrasonography. Eur J Nucl Med 20:1161–1167

100. Lavocat MP, Granjon D, Allard D et al (1997) Imaging of pyelonephritis. Pediatr Radiol 27:159–165

101. Lebtahi N, Gudinchet F, Nenadov-Beck M et al (1997) Evaluating bone marrow metastasis of neuroblastoma with iodine-123-MIBG scintigraphy and MRI. J Nucl Med 38:1389–1392

102. Lee HB, Blaufox MD (1985) Mechanism of renal concentration of technetium-99 m glucoheptonate. J Nucl Med 26:1308–1313

103. Lin TH, Khentigan A, Winchell HS (1974) A Tc-99 m chelate substitution for organomercurial agents. J Nucl Med 15:34–35

104. Linne T, Fituri O, Escobar-Billing R (1994) Functional parameters and 99mtechnetium-dimercaptosuccinic acid scan in acute pyelonephritis. Pediatr Nephrol 8: 694–699

105. Lumbroso J, Schlumberger M, Tenebaum F et al (1991) 131I-metaiodobenzylguanidine therapy in 20 patients with malignant pheochromocytoma. J Nucl Med Biol 35:288–291

106. Lupton EW, Testa HJ, Lawson RS et al (1979) Diuresis renography and the results of pyeloplasty for idiopathic hydronephrosis. Br J Urol 51:449–453

107. MacKenzie JR (1996) A review of renal scarring in children. Nucl Med Commun 17:176–190
108. Maher FT, Tauxe WN (1969) Renal clearance in man of pharmaceuticals containing radioactive iodine. Influence of plasma binding. JAMA 207:97
109. Majd M, Kass EJ, Belman AB (1985) Radionuclide cystography in children: comparison of direct (retrograde) and indirect (intravenous) techniques. Ann Radiol Paris 28:322–328
110. Majd M, Rushton HG, Jantausch B et al (1991) Relationship among vesicoureteral reflux, P-fimbriated *Escherichia coli*, and acute pyelonephritis in children with febrile urinary tract infection. J Pediatr 119: 578–585
111. Majd M, Rushton HG (1992) Renal cortical scintigraphy in the diagnosis of acute pyelonephritis. Semin Nucl Med 22:98–111
112. Majd M., Rushton HG, Chandra R et al (1996) Technetium-99m-DMSA renal cortical scintigraphy to detect experimental acute pyelonephritis in piglets: comparison of planar (pinhole) and SPECT imaging. J Nucl Med 37:1731–1734
113. Mariss P, Thiede GI (1977) Estimation of individual renal function by Tc-DMSA-uptake. Rofo Fortschr Geb Rontgenstr Nuklearmed 126:442–446
114. Mastin ST, Drane WE, Iravani A (1995) Tc-99m DMSA SPECT imaging in patients with acute symptoms or history of UTI. Comparison with ultrasonography. Clin Nucl Med 407–412
115. Maurea S, Cuocolo A, Reynolds JC, Tumeh SS et al (1993) Iodine-131-metaiodobenzylguanidine scintigraphy in preoperative and postoperative evaluation of paragangliomas: comparison with CT and MRI. J Nucl Med 34:173–179
116. McEwan AJ, Shapiro B, Sisson JC et al (1985) Radioiodobenzylguanidine for the scintigraphic location and therapy of adrenergic tumors. Semin Nucl Med 15:231–135
117. Melis K, Vandevivere J, Hoskens C et al (1992) Involvement of the renal parenchyma in acute urinary tract infection: the contribution of 99mTc dimercaptosuccinic acid scan. Eur J Pediatr 151:536–539
118. Meller J, Zappel H, Conrad M et al (1999) 99mTc-DMSA-scintigraphy in the diagnosis and risk stratification in urinary tract infections in children. Nuklearmedizin 38:A93
119. Meller J, Zappel H, Becker W (2000) Indications for pediatric 99mTc-dimercaptosuccinic-scintigraphy. Nuklearmediziner 23:237–254
120. Merrick MV, Notghi A, Chalmers N et al (1995) Long term follow up to determine the prognostic value of imaging after urinary tract infections. 1. Reflux. Arch Dis Child 72:388–392
121. Merrick MV, Notghi A, Chalmers N et al (1995) Long term follow up to determine the prognostic value of imaging after urinary tract infections. 2. Scarring. Arch Dis Child 72:393–396
122. Mouratidis B, Ash JM, Gilday DL (1993) Comparison of planar and SPECT 99Tcm-DMSA scintigraphy for the detection of renal cortical defects in children. Nucl Med Commun 14:82–86
123. Mozley PD, Heyman S, Duckett JW et al (1994) Direct vesicoureteral scintigraphy: quantifying early outcome predictors in children with primary reflux. J Nucl Med 35:1602–1608
124. Mucci B, Maguire B (1994) Does routine ultrasound have a role in the investigation of children with urinary tract infection? Clin Radiol 49:324–325
125. Müller-Suur R, Müller-Suur C (1986) Renal and extrarenal handling of a new imaging compound (99m-Tc-MAG-3) in the rat. Eur J Nucl Med 12:438–442
126. Müller-Suur R, Müller-Suur C (1989) Glomerular filtration and tubular secretion of MAG-3 in the rat kidney. J Nucl Med 30:1986–1991
127. Müller-Suur R, Gutsche HU (1995) Tubular reabsorption of technetium-DMSA. J Nucl Med 36:1654–658
128. Nasrallah PF, Sreeramulu N, Crawford J (1982) Clinical applications of nuclear cystography. J Urol 128:550–553
129. Nordyke RA, Tubis M. Bladh WH (1960) Use of radioiodinated hippuran for individual kidney function tests. J Lab Clin Med 56:438–445
130. Oberhausen E, Romahn A (1968) Bestimmung der Nierenclearance durch externe Gammastrahlenmessung. In: Hoffmann G, Höfer R (eds) Radionuklide in Kreislaufforschung und Kreislaufdiagnostik. Schattauer, Stuttgart, pp 323–326
131. Oberhausen E, Kirsch W, Emrani I (1972) Measurement of unilateral renal plasma flow by combination of clearance determination and renograms. In: Blaufox MD, Funck-Brentano JL (eds) Radionuclides in nephrology. Grune and Stratton, New York, pp 233–239
132. O'Reilly PH (1986) Diuresis renography 8 years later: an update. J Urol 136:993–999
133. O'Reilly PH (1990) Investigations of obstructive uropathy. In: O'Reilly PH, George NJ, Weiss RM (eds) Diagnostic techniques in urology. Saunders, Philadelphia, pp 401–425
134. O'Reilly PH, Testa HJ; Lawson RS et al (1978) Diuresis renography in equivocal urinary tract obstruction. Br J Urol 50:76–80
135. O'Reilly PH, Aurell M, Britton K et al (1996) Consensus on diuresis renography for investigation of the dilated upper urinary tract. J Nucl Med 37:1872–1876
136. Parkhouse HF, Godley ML, Cooper J et al (1989) Renal imaging with 99Tcm-labelled DMSA in the detection of acute pyelonephritis: an experimental study in the pig. Nucl Med Commun 10:63–70
137. Pauwels EK, Lycklama A, Nijeholt AA et al (1987) The determination of relative kidney function in obstructive uropathy with 99Tcm-DMSA. Nucl Med Commun 8:865–867
138. Peters AM, Jones DH, Evans K, Gordon I (1988) Two routes for 99mTc-DMSA uptake into the renal cortical tubular cell. Eur J Nucl Med 14:555–561
139. Piepsz A, Ham HR, Roland JH et al (1986) Technetium-99 m DMSA imaging and the obstructed kidney. Clin Nucl Med 11:389–391
140. Piepsz A, Hahn K, Roca I et al (1990) A radiopharmaceuticals schedule for imaging in paediatrics. Paediatric Task Group European Association Nuclear Medicine. Eur J Nucl Med 17:127–129
141. Piepsz A, Gordon I, Hahn K et al (1993) Determination of the technetium-99 m mercaptoacetyltriglycine plasma clearance in children by means of a single blood sample: a multicentre study. The Paediatric Task Group of the EANM. Eur J Nucl Med 20:244–248
142. Piepsz A, Tamminen-Mobius T, Reiners C et al (1998) Five-year study of medical of surgical treatment in children with severe vesico-ureteral reflux dimercaptosuc-

cinic acid findings. International Reflux Study Group in Europe. Eur J Pediatr 157:753–758

143. Piepsz A, Blaufox MD, Gordon I et al (1999) Consensus on renal cortical scintigraphy in children with urinary tract infection. Scientific Committee of Radionuclides in Nephrourology. Semin Nucl Med 29:160–174

144. Piepsz A, Colarinha P, Gordon I et al (2001) Guidelines on ⁹⁹ᵐTc-DMSA scintigraphy in children. Eur J Nucl Med (in press)

145. Pollet JE, Sharp PF, Smith FW et al (1981) Intravenous radionuclide cystography for the detection of vesicorenal reflux. J Urol 125:75–78

146. Prigent A, Cosgriff P, Gates GF et al (1999) Consensus report on quality control of quantitative measurements of renal function obtained from the renogram: International consensus committee from the scientific committee of radionuclides in nephrourology. Semin Nucl Med 29:146–159

147. Rantz LA, Kirby WMM (1944) Absorption and excretion of penicillin following continuous intravenous and subcutaneous administration. J Clin Invest 23:789

148. Rehling M, Nielsen LE, Marqversen J (1997) Protein binding of ⁹⁹ᵐTc DTPA, ⁵¹Cr-EDTA and ¹²⁵I-iothalamate. Nucl Med Commun 18:324

149. Reubi JC (1995) Neuropeptide receptors in health and disease: The molecular basis for in vivo imaging. J Nucl Med 36:1825–1835

150. Risdon RA, Godley ML, Gordon I et al (1994) Renal pathology and the ⁹⁹ᵐTc-DMSA image before and after treatment of the evolving pyelonephritic scar: an experimental study. J Urol 152:1260–1266

151. Roach PJ, Paltiel HJ, Perez-Atayde A et al (1995) Renal dysplasia in infants: appearance on ⁹⁹ᵐTc DMSA scintigraphy. Pediatr Radiol 25:472–475

152. Roberts JA (1991) Etiology and pathophysiology of pyelonephritis. Am J Kidney Dis 17:1–9

153. Roberts JA, Roth JK Jr, Domingue G et al (1982) Immunology of pyelonephritis in the primate model. V. Effect of superoxide dismutase. J Urol 128:1394–1400

154. Rohlof R, Hast B, Leisner B et al (1974) Determination of 131-J-hippuran clearance in renal camera functional scintigraphy using simplified Oberhausen's method. Nuklearmedizin 13:303–320

155. Rosenberg AR; Rossleigh MA, Brydon MP et al (1992) Evaluation of acute urinary tract infection in children by dimercaptosuccinic acid scintigraphy: a prospective study. J Urol 148:1746–1749

156. Rossleigh MA (1994) The interrenicular septum. A normal anatomical variant seen on DMSA SPECT. Clin Nucl Med 19:953–955

157. Rossleigh MA, Leighton DM, Farnsworth RH (1993) Diuresis renography. The need for an additional view after gravity-assisted drainage. Clin Nucl Med 18:210–213

158. Rushton HG, Majd M, Chandra R et al (1988) Evaluation of 99 m Technetium-dimercaptosuccinic acid renal scans in experimental acute pyelonephritis in piglets. J Urol 140:1169–1174

159. Rushton HG, Majd M (1992) Dimercaptosuccinic acid renal scintigraphy for the evaluation of pyelonephritis and scarring: a review of experimental and clinical studies. J Urol 148:1726–1732

160. Rushton HG, Majd M, Jantausch B et al (1992) Renal scarring following reflux and nonreflux pyelonephritis in children: evaluation with 99mtechnetium-dimercaptosuccinic acid scintigraphy. J Urol 147:1327–1332

161. Russell CD, Rowell KL, Scott JW (1986) Quality control of technetium-99 m DTPA: correlation of analytic test with in vivo protein binding in man. J Nucl Med 27:560–562

162. Russell CD, Taylor A, Eshima D (1989) Estimation of technetium-99m-MAG3 plasma clearance in adults from one or two blood samples. J Nucl Med 30:1955–1959

163. Sapirstein LA, Vidt DG, Mandel MJ et al (1955) Volumes of distribution and clearances of intravenously injected creatinine in the dog. Am J Physiol 181:330–336

164. Saraga M, Stanicic A, Markovic V (1996) The role of direct radionuclide cystography in evaluation of vesicoureteral reflux. Scand J Urol Nephrol 30:367–371

165. Saunders CAB, Choong KKL, Larcos G et al (1997) Assessment of pediatric hydronephrosis using output efficiency. J Nucl Med 38:1483–1486

166. Sautter-Bihl ML, Bihl H, Heinze HG (1991) The place of 99mTc-MDP skeletal scintigraphy in neuroblastoma. Is a new assessment necessary? Nuklearmedizin 30:7–12

167. Schlegel JU, Hamway SA (1976) Individual renal plasma flow determination in 2 minutes. J Urol 116:282–285

168. Schmiegelow K, Simes MA, Agertoft L et al (1989) Radio-iodobenzylguanidine scintigraphy of neuroblastoma: conflicting results, when compared with standard investigations. Med Pediatr Oncol 17:127–130

169. Schofer O, König G, Bartels U, Bockisch A et al (1995) Technetium-99 m mercaptoacetyltriglycine clearance: reference values for infants and children. Eur J Nucl Med 22:1278–1281

170. Schwartz FD, Madeloff MS (1961) Simultaneous renal clearances of radiohippuran and PAH in man. Clin Res 9:208

171. Shanon A, Feldman W, McDonald P, Martin DJ et al (1992) Evaluation of renal scars by technetium-labeled dimercaptosuccinic acid scan, intravenous urography, and ultrasonography: a comparative study. J Pediatr 120:399–403

172. Shapiro B, Gross MD (1987) Radiochemistry, biochemistry, and kinetics of ¹³¹I-metaiodobenzylguanidine (MIBG) and ¹²³I-MIBG: clinical implications of the use of 123I-MIBG. Med Pediatr Oncol 15:170–177

173. Shulkin BL, Shapiro B, Hutchinson RJ (1992) Iodine-131-metaiodobenzylguanidine and bone scintigraphy for the detection of neuroblastoma. Nucl Med 33:1735–1740

174. Shulkin BL, Shapiro B (1998) Current concepts on the diagnostic use of MIBG in children. J Nucl Med 39:679–688

175. Skoog SJ, Belman AB, Majd M (1987) A nonsurgical approach to management of vesicoureteral reflux. J Urol 138:941–946

176. Smellie J, Norman IC (1975) Bacteriuria, reflux and renal scarring. Arch Dis Child 50:581–585

177. Smith T, Evans K, Lythgoe MF et al (1996) Radiation dosimetry of Tc-99 m DMSA in children. J Nucl Med 37:1336–1342

178. Smith T, Gordon I (1998) An update of radiopharmaceutical schedules in children. Nucl Med Commun 19:1023–1036

179. Solanki KK, Bomanji J, Moyes J et al (1992) A pharmacological guide to medicines which interfere with the biodistribution of radiolabelled meta-iodobenzylguanidine (MIBG). Nucl Med Commun 13:513–521

180. Stabin MG, Gelfand MJ (1998) Dosimetry of pediatric nuclear medicine procedures. Q J Nucl Med 42:93–112

181. Stokland E, Hellstrom M, Jacobsson B et al (1996) Renal damage one year after first urinary tract infection: role of dimercaptosuccinic acid scintigraphy. J Pediatr 129:815–820

182. Takeda M, Katayama Y, Tsutsui T et al (1994) Value of dimercaptosuccinic acid single photon emission computed tomography and magnetic resonance imaging in detecting renal injury in pediatric patients with vesicoureteral reflux. Comparison with dimercaptosuccinic acid planar scintigraphy and intravenous pyelography. Eur Urol 25:320–325

183. Tappin DM, Murphy AV, Mocan H et al (1989) A prospective study of children with first acute symptomatic E. coli urinary tract infection. Early ^{99m}technetium dimercaptosuccinic acid scan appearances. Acta Paediatr Scand 8:923–929

184. Tasker AD, Lindsell DR, Moncrieff M (1993) Can ultrasound reliably detect renal scarring in children with urinary tract infection? Clin Radiol 47:177–179

185. Tauxe WN, Dubovsky EV, Kidd TE (1984) Comparison of measurement of effective renal plasma flow by single plasma sample and plasma disappearance slope/volume methods. Eur J Nucl Med 9:443–445

186. Taylor A, Lallone RL, Hagan PL (1980) Optimal handling of dimercaptosuccinic acid for quantitative renal scanning. J Nucl Med 21:1190–1193

187. Taylor A, Eshima D, Fritzberg AR, Christian PE et al (1986) Comparison of iodine-131 OIH and technetium-99 m MAG3 renal imaging in volunteers. J Nucl Med 27:795–803

188. Taylor A, Eshima D, Alazraki N (1987) ^{99m}Tc-MAG3, a new renal imaging agent: preliminary results in patients. Eur J Nucl Med 12:510–514

189. Taylor A, Nally J, Aurell M et al (1996) Consensus report on ACE inhibitory renography for detecting renovascular hypertension. J Nucl Med 37:1876–1882

190. Tepe PG, Tauxe WN, Bagchi A et al (1987) Comparison of measurement of glomerular filtration rate by single sample, plasma disappearance slope/intercept and other methods. Eur J Nucl Med 13:28–31

191. Treves ST (1994) The ongoing challenge of diagnosis and treatment of urinary tract infection, vesicoureteral reflux and renal damage in children. J Nucl Med 35:1608–1611

192. Treves ST, Majd M, Kuruc A et al (1995) Kidneys. In: Treves ST (ed) Pediatric nuclear medicine, 2nd edn. Springer, Berlin Heidelberg New York, pp 339–499

193. Treves ST, Gelfand M, Willi UV (1995) Vesicoureteric reflux and radionuclide cystography. In: Treves ST (ed) Pediatric nuclear medicine, 2nd edn. Springer, Berlin Heidelberg New York, pp 411–429

194. Troncone L, Rufini V, Danza FM et al (1990) Radioiodinated metaiodobenzylguanidine (*I-MIBG) scintigraphy in neuroblastoma: a review of 160 studies. J Nucl Med Allied Sci 34:279–288

195. Troncone L, Rufini V, Montemaggi P et al (1990) The diagnostic and therapeutic utility of radioiodinated metaiodobenzylguanidine (MIBG). 5 years experience. Eur J Nucl Med 16:325–335

196. Troncone L, Galli G (1991) The role of ^{131}I-metabenzylguanethidine in the treatment of neural crest tumors. J Nucl Biol Med 35:177–362

197. Upsdell SM, Testa HJ, Lawson RS (1992) The F-15 diuresis renogram in suspected obstruction of the upper urinary tract. Br J Urol 69:126–131

198. Velchik MG, Alavi A, Kressel HY et al (1989) Localization of pheochromocytoma: MIGB, CT, and MRI correlation. J Nucl Med 30:328–336

199. Verber IG, Strudley MR, Meller ST (1988) ^{99m}Tc dimercaptosuccinic acid (DMSA) scan as first investigation of urinary tract infection. Arch Dis Child 63:1320–2325

200. Verber IG, Meller ST (1989) Serial ^{99m}Tc dimercaptosuccinic acid (DMSA) scans after urinary infections presenting before the age of 5 years. Arch Dis Child 64:1533–1537

201. Verboven M, Ham HR, Josephson S et al (1987) 99Tcm-DMSA uptake in obstructed kidneys. How inaccurate are the 5 h measurements? Nucl Med Commun 8:45–48

202. Verboven M, Ingels M, Delree M et al (1990) ^{99m}Tc-DMSA scintigraphy in acute urinary tract infection in children. Pediatr Radiol 20:540–542

203. Wacksman J, Brewer E, Gelfand MJ, Towbin R et al (1986) Low grade pelviureteric junction obstruction with normal diuretic renography. Br J Urol 58:364–367

204. Whitaker RH (1973) Methods of assessing obstruction in dilated ureters. Br J Urol 45:15–22

205. Wieland DM, Wu JL, Brown LE et al (1980) Radiolabeled adrenergic neuron blocking agent: adrenomedullary imaging with [131] iodobenzylguanidine. J Nucl Med 21:349–353

206. Willi U Treves S (1983) Radionuclide voiding cystography. Urol Radiol 5:161–173

207. Wong JCH, Rossleigh A, Farnworth RH (1995) Utility of Technetium-99m-MAG3 diuretic renography in the neonatal period. J Nucl Med 36:2214–2219

208. Wong DC, Rossleigh MA, Farnsworth RH (1999) F+0 diuresis renography in infants and children. J Nucl Med 40:1805–1811

209. Yee CA, Lee HB, Blaufox MD (1981) Tc-99 m DMSA renal uptake: influence of biochemical and physiologic factors. J Nucl Med 22:1054–1058

210. Zappel HF, Meller J, Zöller G et al (1997) Diagnostic significance of sonography, radiology and scintigraphy in vesico renal reflux. Monatsschr Kinderheilkd 145:SP 730

211. Zhang G, Day DL, Loken M et al (1987) Grading of reflux by radionuclide cystography. Clin Nucl Med 12:106–109

Case Reports

H. Zappel and J. Meller

Introduction

Interdisciplinary conferences can be extremely useful procedures for qualified diagnostic and therapeutic decisions in daily practice. Typical case reports presented in this chapter demonstrate how decisions both about the most common and also about rare diseases of the urinary tract in childhood are made in this context.

The scope of these reports is focused more on how a correct diagnosis of complex conditions can be established by using different imaging techniques than on a complete overview of the whole spectrum of diseases that might occur in daily practice.

Several of these cases demonstrate that in some urological diseases in childhood diagnosis and risk stratification can be improved by the use of molecular genetic methods. In the diagnosis of urological diseases ultrasonography has a major role and has replaced older radiological procedures. The importance of functional scintigraphic imaging has increased in the past 15 years. New radiological techniques such as MRI and MR angiography will further improve the diagnostic accuracy.

Our experience has made it obvious that only a constructive multidisciplinary approach will enable successful diagnosis and therapy of urological diseases in childhood.

CASE 1 ▶ *Bilateral Renal Hypoplasia*

Clinical Course: Both kidneys appeared to be very small during sonographic screening in a 6-week-old boy (Fig. 1.1). Their volume was clearly below the weight-adjusted normal range (Fig. 1.2). The corticomedullary differentiation was well preserved, the drainage systems were not dilated, and the renal cortex showed a slightly enhanced echogenicity. These findings were diagnostic for bilateral renal hypoplasia.

In children with bilateral renal hypoplasia, kidney volumes do not increase adequately during their further clinical course, and progressive deterioration of the global renal function associated with growth retardation can often be observed. In this child growth was also retarded, but due to a relatively well-preserved renal function, the boy developed within the upper range of the percentile curve of patients with hypo- and dysplastic kidneys (Fig. 1.3). Our patient is now 7 years old, and his renal insufficiency is compensated up to now (Fig. 1.4). At the moment he is being successfully treated with cholecalciferol and phosphate binder, and slowly restricted protein intake.

Comment: The diagnosis of bilateral renal hypoplasia can be established by ultrasound alone. Further investigations are usually not necessary. Early symptomatic theray helps to prevent the complications of renal failure (growth retardation, hypertension, and osteopathy).

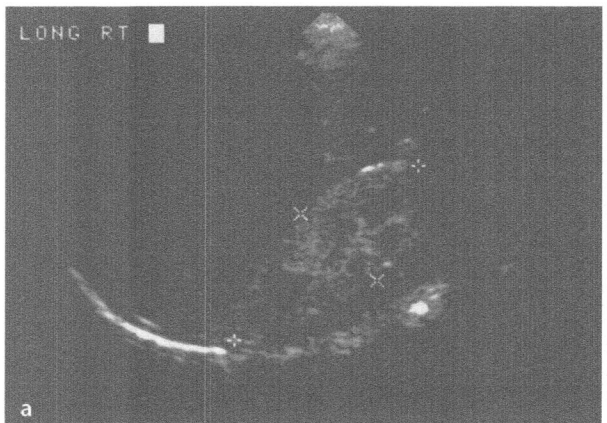 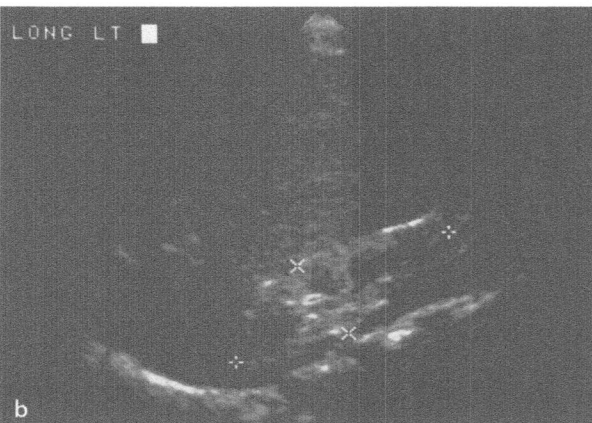

Fig. 1.1 a, b. Sonography of **a** the left and **b** the right kidney (longitudinal sections) with typical features of renal hypoplasia

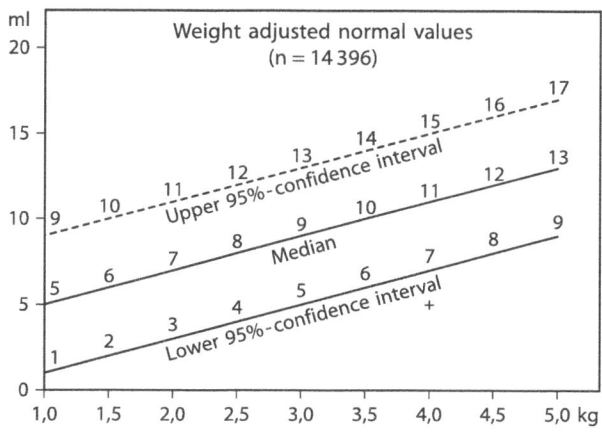

Fig. 1.2. Weight-adjusted normal ranges of renal volume. The kidney volume of this child (5 ml) is clearly below the 5th percentile

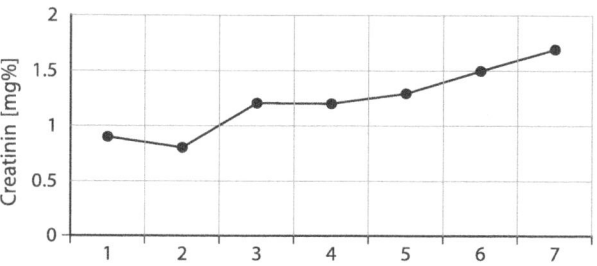

Fig. 1.4. Development of the boy's serum creatinine within the last 7 years

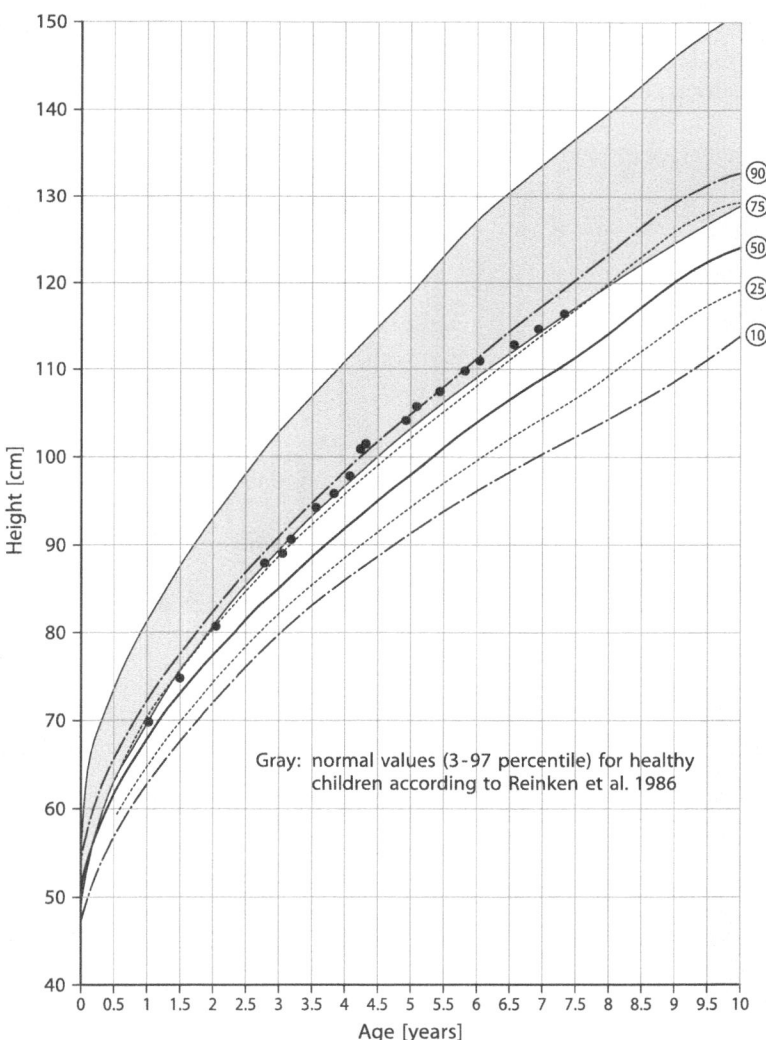

Fig. 1.3. Growth curve of our patient compared with the growth curve of a collective of normally developed children (*shaded*) and patients with a glomerular filtration rate smaller than 25 ml min^{-1} 1.73 m^{-2}

CASE 2 ▶ *Unilateral Renal Agenesis Combined with VUR on the Contralateral Side*

Clinical Course: A first febrile urinary tract infection occurred in a 5-month-old boy. On the initial sonography (Fig. 2.1) the left kidney was not seen. The right kidney appeared to be hypertrophic (volume: 30 ml), showing increased parenchymal echogenicity together with poor corticomedullary differentiation suggestive of pyelonephritis. The right renal pelvis and the distal ureter were moderately dilated. Although antibiotic prophylaxis was immediately started, the child developed a second febrile urinary tract infection.

Voiding cysto-urethrography (Fig. 2.2) demonstrated grade-IV VUR on the right side. The urogram showed a single right kidney, and dilatation of the right ureter without normal or ectopic renal parenchyma contralaterally.

On the planar ^{99m}Tc-DMSA scan (Fig. 2.3) there were no signs of scarring on the right kidney. In addition, ^{99m}Tc-DMSA excluded the presence of a functioning renal parenchyma elsewhere.

Unfortunately, the child's parents refused consent for operative therapy until a third febrile urinary tract infection occurred. The reimplantation of the refluxing ureter was performed according to Papin's method. No complications occurred during the further clinical course of the child.

Six months after surgery we performed direct voiding scintigraphy (Fig. 2.4), which showed no evidence of persisting reflux. Sonography at this time showed a hypertrophic single right kidney without scarring. The dilatation of the ureter and the renal pelvis hat completely resolved.

Comment: Agenesis of the kidney is often combined with other malformations of the urinary tract. In our patient we found a high-grade dilating reflux associated with a single kidney. Surgical correction became necessary because antibiotic prophylaxis failed. Renal scarring was prevented by early correction of the reflux.

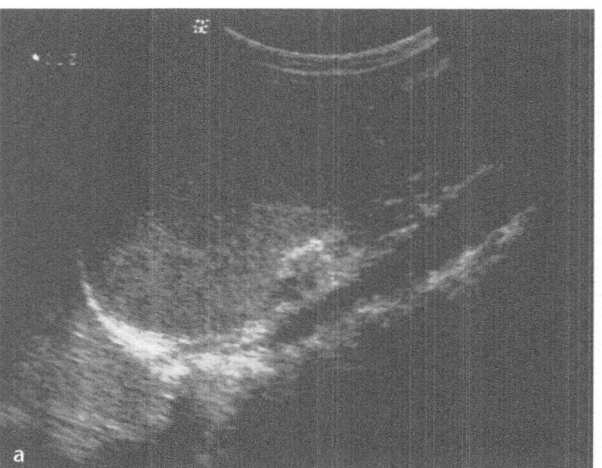

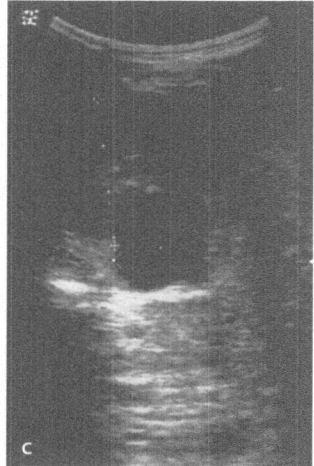

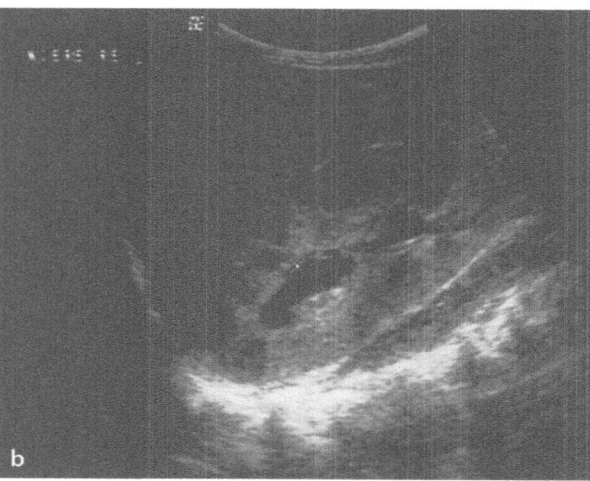

Fig. 2.1 a–f. The initial sonography shows **a** left renal agenesis (longitudinal section) and **b, c** an enlarged right kidney (37 ml) with hyper echoic parenchyma (**b** longitudinal section; **c** transverse section). **d–f** see p. 127

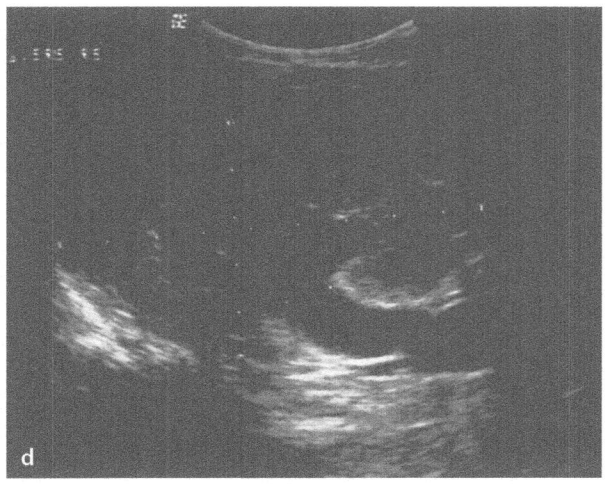

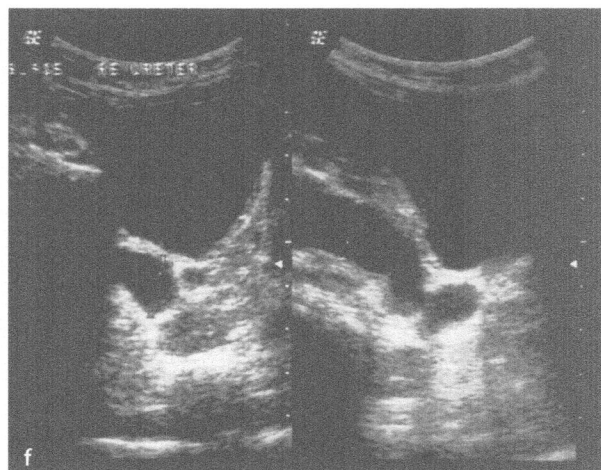

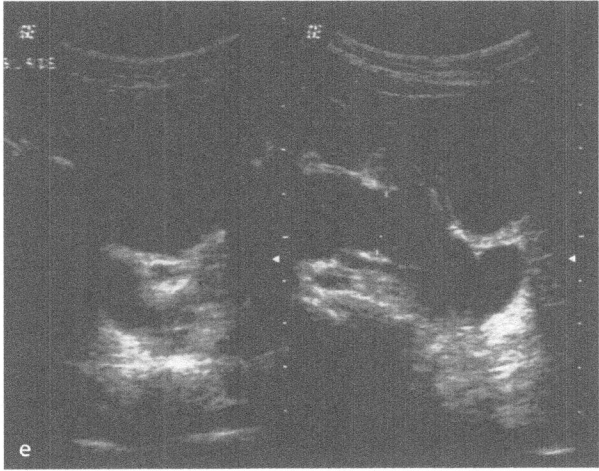

Fig. 2.1 (*continued*). **d** Dilatation of the renal pelvis (longitudinal section) and **e, f** a paravesical megaureter are present

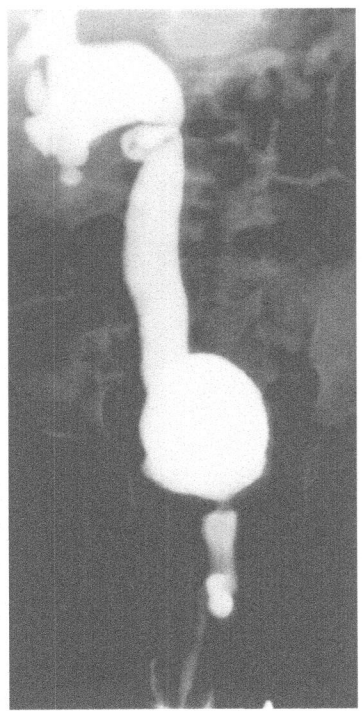

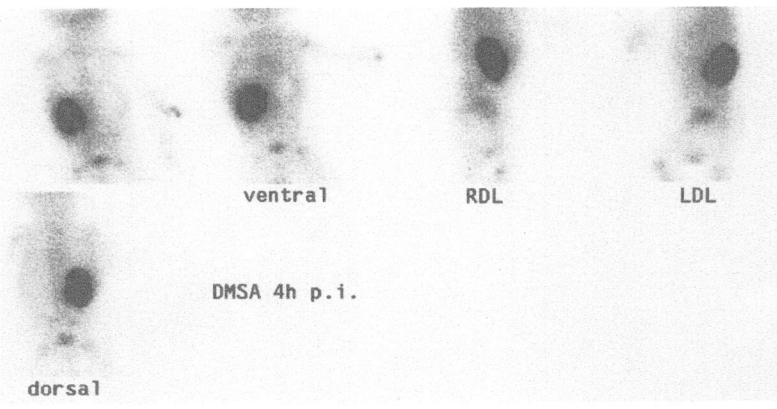

▲ **Fig. 2.3.** On the planar 99mTc-DMSA scan there are no signs of scarring on the right kidney. In addition 99mTc-DMSA also excludes the presence of a functioning renal parenchyma elsewhere

◄ **Fig. 2.2.** Voiding cysto-urethrography demonstrating a grade-IV VUR on the right side

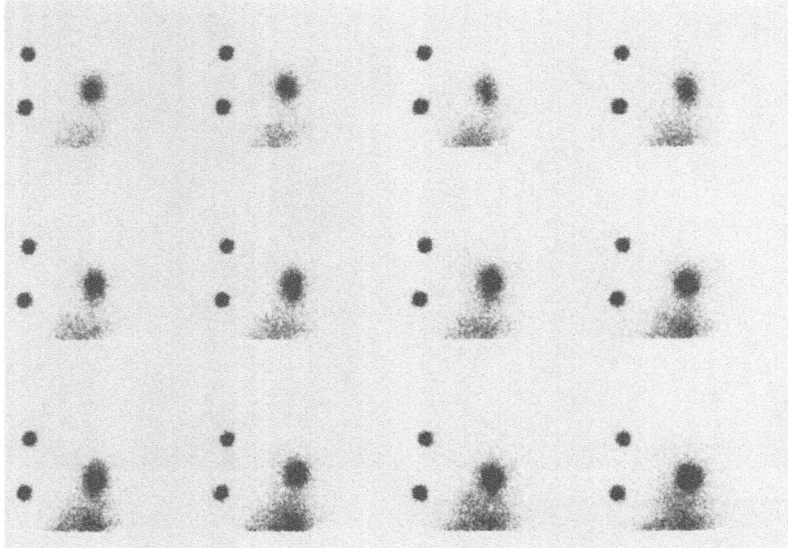

Fig. 2.4. Postoperative direct voiding scintigraphy; the highgrade reflux has completely resolved. Note the radioactive markers placed 10 cm apart on the left side

CASE 3 ▶ *Pancake Kidney*

Clinical Course: Renal dystopia and unilateral agenesis are often incidental sonographic findings and may be detected during early screening procedures of the newborn. In this male newborn, sonography demonstrated a solitary pancake-like kidney in the left pelvis combined with a dilated ureter (Fig. 3.1). On the intravenous pyelogram an ectopic and malrotated kidney was found (Fig. 3.2). No reflux was present during voiding cysto-urethrography (Fig. 3.3).

The boy remained symptom free during an 8-year-follow-up. Up to now the creatinine clearance and the blood pressure are still within the normal range.

Comment: Owing to the availability of facultative neonatal sonographic screening, asymptomatic malformations of the urinary tract can be detected early. In asymptomatic patients there is no need for invasive diagnostic procedures. Risk-adapted guidance of the child, which includes yearly ultrasonography and measurements of the retention parameters, is sufficient in most cases.

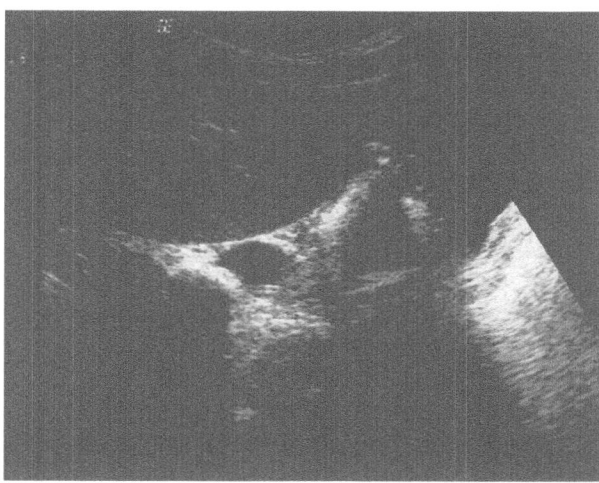

Fig. 3.1. Sonography of a single pancake-like kidney in the left pelvis (transverse section). Normal echogenicity and dimensions of the renal parenchyma. No dilatation of the pelvicalyceal system is present. The dilated ureter is clearly visualized

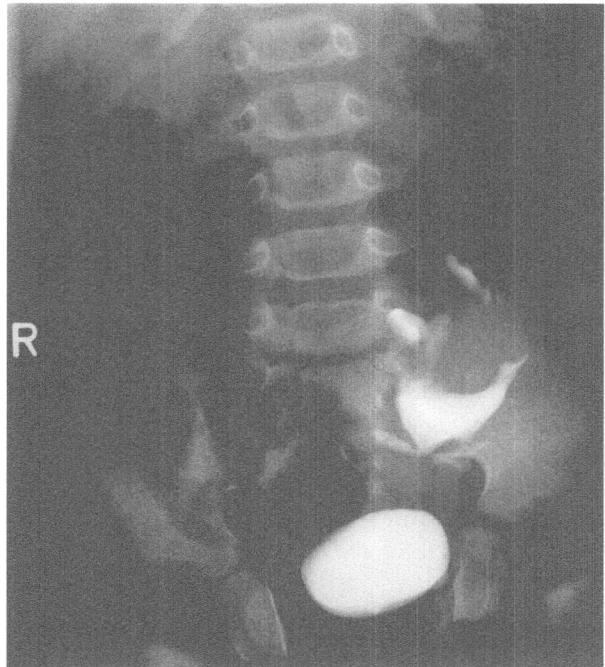

Fig. 3.2. On the intravenous pyelogram an ectopic and malrotated kidney can be found in the left hemipelvis. The ureter is only slightly dilated

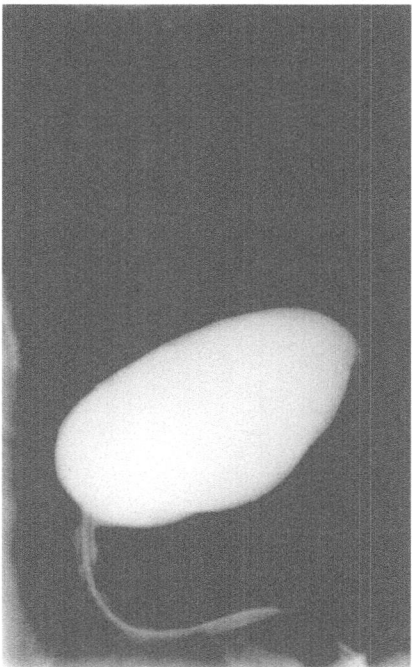

Fig. 3.3. No reflux can be demonstrated on the voiding cystourethrogram

CASE 4 ► *Unilateral Renal Dysplasia with Contralateral Subpelvic Obstruction*

Clinical Course: Surgery of a diaphragmatic hernia was performed in a male preterm newborn within the 1st day of life. During preoperative sonography left pyeloectasia associated with a normal-sized kidney and a relatively small right kidney were noted (Fig. 4.1). Intravenous and retrograde pyelography were highly suggestive of a subpelvic intrinsic obstruction on the left kidney (Fig. 4.2). During sonographic follow-up, the right kidney exhibited a progressive volume reduction and confirmed increasing massive dilatation of the left renal pelvis.

Repeat ^{99m}Tc-MAG$_3$ diuretic scintigraphy revealed an obstructive pattern on the left side and showed progressive deterioration of the right kidney function (Figs. 4.3, 4.4).

It was decided that surgical correction (Anderson-Hynes method) should be performed. During surgery the radiological and scintigraphic tentative diagnosis of intrinsic obstruction of the proximal ureter was confirmed. Postoperative MAG, scintigraphy revealed better excretion of the left kidney, but the function of the right dysplastic kidney had deteriorated further (Fig. 4.5).

Comment: In this child clinical, scintigraphic and radiological findings were indicative of obstructive uropathy of the left kidney. After surgery the function of this kidney remained stable, while sonographic and scintigraphic findings showed continuous deterioration of function in the contralateral dysplastic kidney.

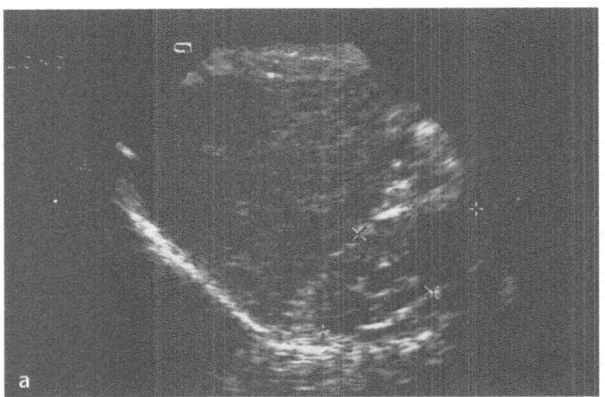

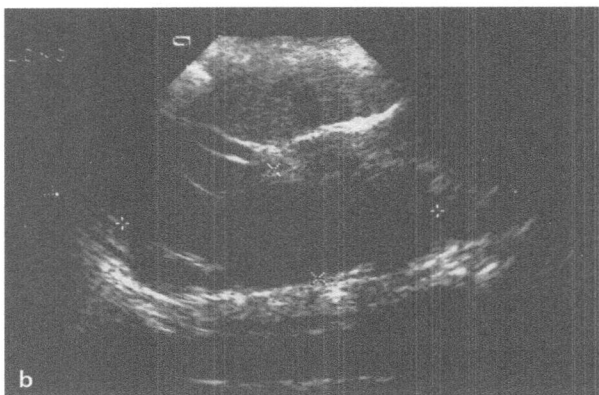

Fig. 4.1. a The initial sonography shows a hyperechoic small right kidney without a corticomedullary differentiation. **b** In addition, there is marked pelvicalyceal dilatation of the left kidney without dilation of the ureter

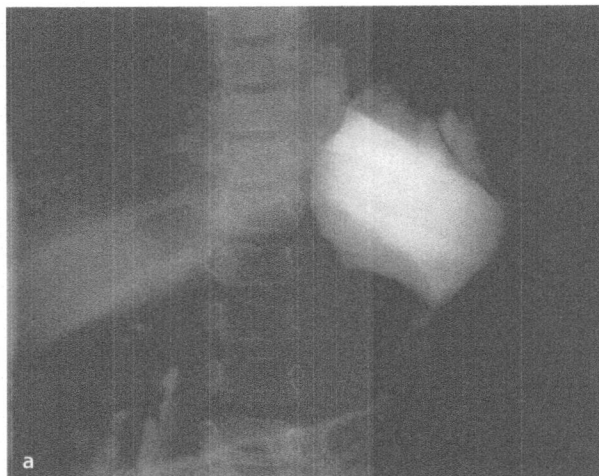

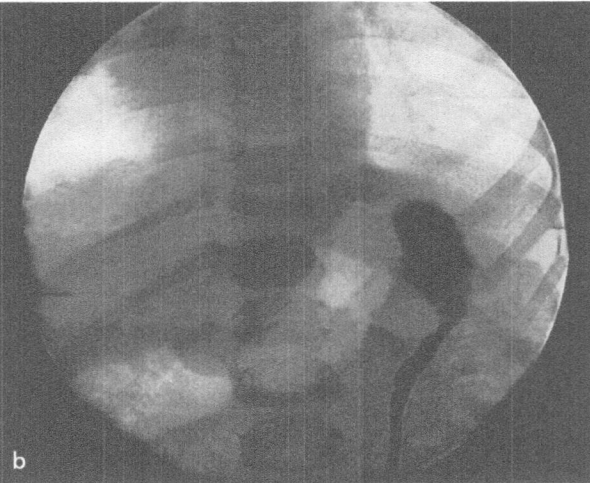

Fig. 4.2. a On the late radiograms 140 min after injection delayed excretion to the right renal pelvis is seen. On the left side there is a huge dilated and deformed collecting system. **b** On the retrograde urogram an intrinsic narrowing in the proximal ureter can be diagnosed

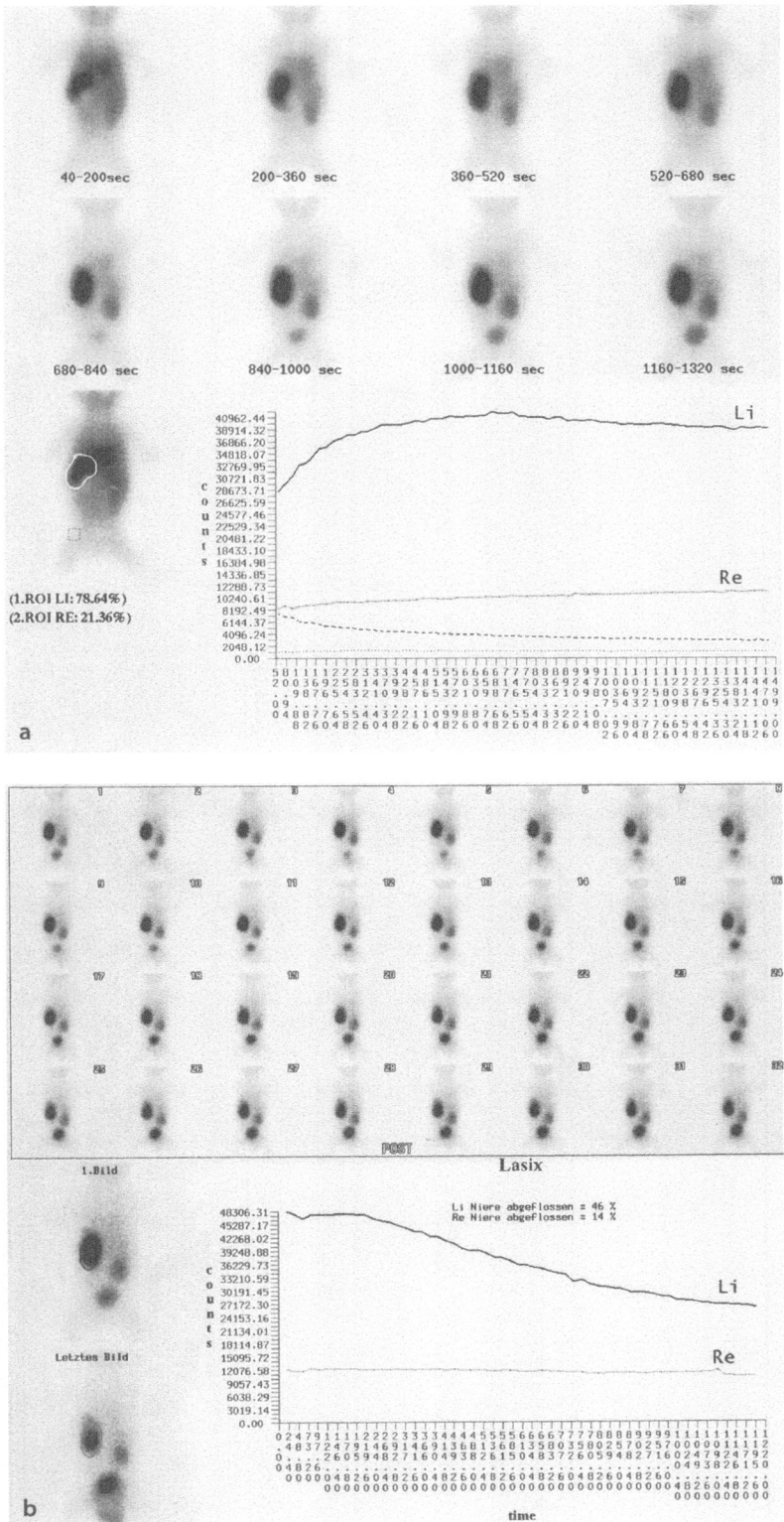

Fig. 4.3. a On the initial MAG₃ study the function of the left kidney is preserved. **b** After frusemide a decline in activity of less than 50% within 20 min can be noted. The function of the right kidney is impaired (split function: 21%)

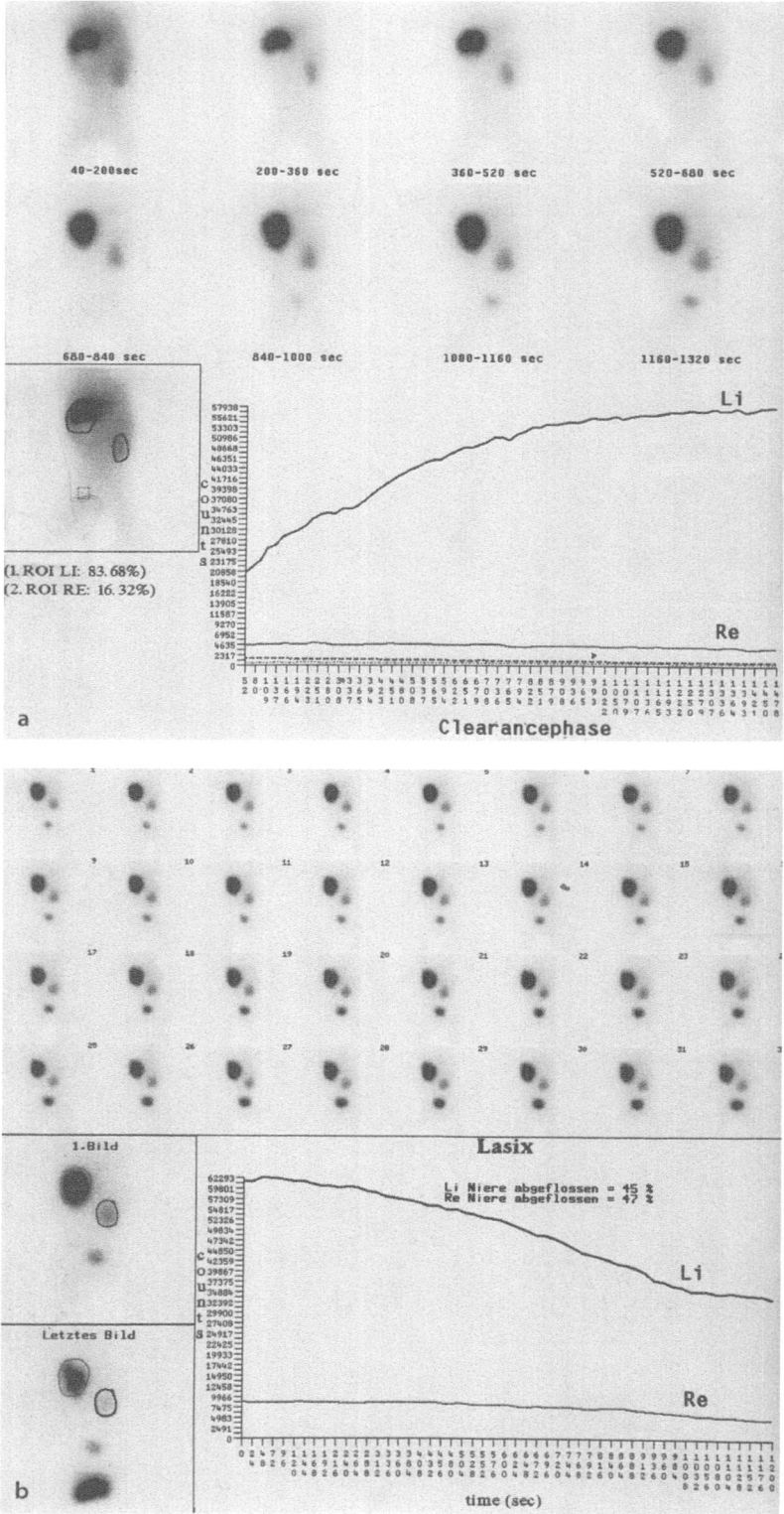

Fig. 4.4. a During scintigraphic follow-up progressive deterioration of the function of the right kidney (split function: 16%) is seen. **b** Left-sided obstruction confirmed by diuretic scintigraphy

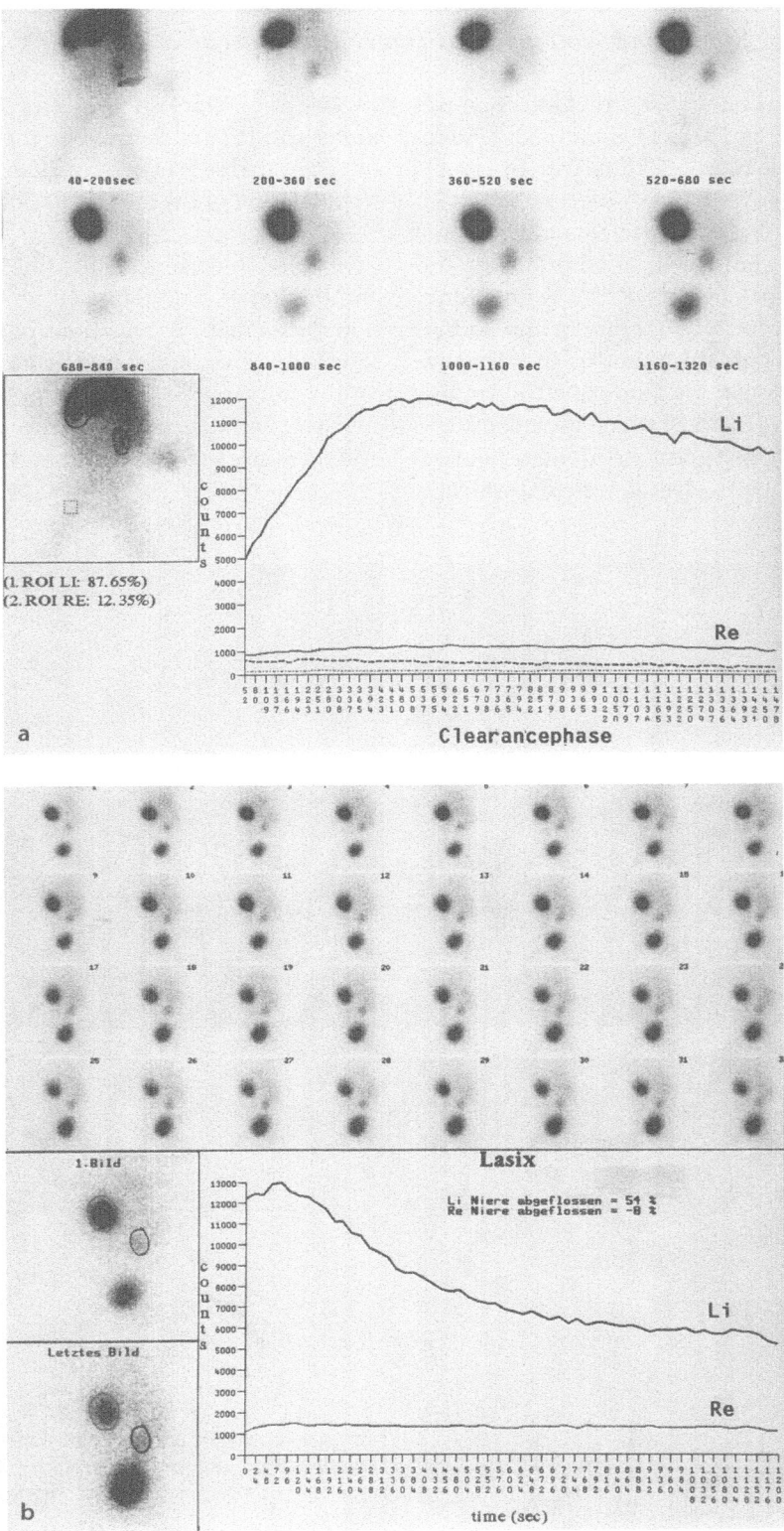

Fig. 4.5 a, b. The postoperative scan shows improve excretion of the tracer during the parenchymal phase. **a** Only residual function (12% split function) of the dysplastic right kidney is present. **b** After frusemide a decline of activity of 50% within 10 min can be observed on the left side

CASE 5 ► *Horseshoe Kidney and Symptomatic Urinary Tract Infections*

Clinical Course: The first urinary tract infection was diagnosed when the girl was 11 months old. Sonography revealed a smaller left kidney in an ectopic position in the pelvis. After a second urinary tract infection the sonography was repeated and ectopia of the left kidney was confirmed. In addition, a paravertebral parenchymal bridge to the right kidney was observed, suggestive of a horseshoe kidney (Fig. 5.1 a–c). Although dilatation of the drainage system was not present, we performed a voiding cysto-urethrography (Fig. 5.2) which excluded VUR. On the intravenous pyelogram we found a bilateral 90° rotation of the pelvicalyceal systems, which is typical for a horseshoe kidney (Fig. 5.3). The left ureter was located laterally to the renal pelvis, while the right ureter was seen medial to the renal pelvis. No dilatation of the ureters was observed.

Comment: Recurrence of urinary tract infections and the initial sonographic findings were an indication for further investigations in this child. A horseshoe kidney was diagnosed by its typical appearance on the intravenous pyelogram. Reflux and obstruction were excluded during further diagnostic work-up and therefore surgical correction was not necessary.

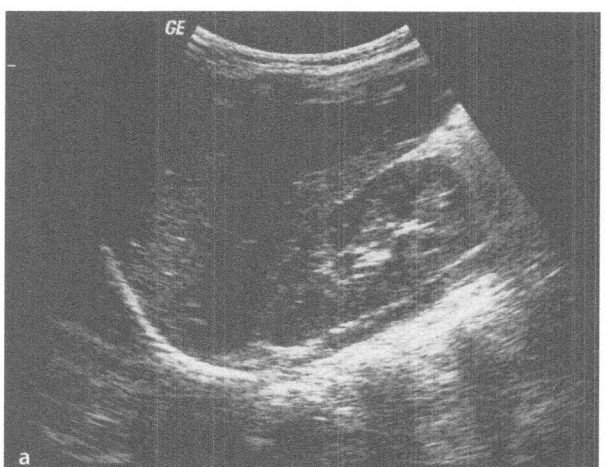

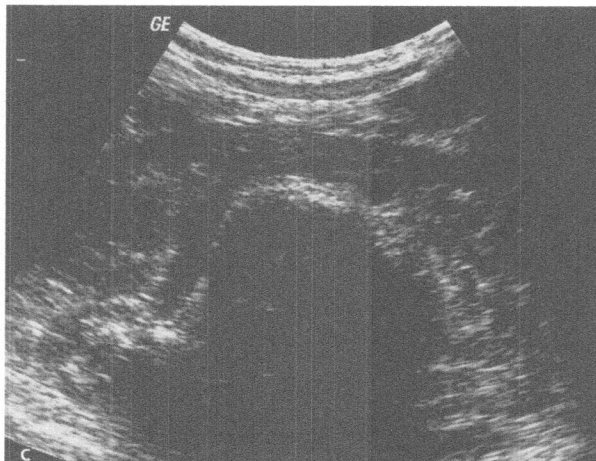

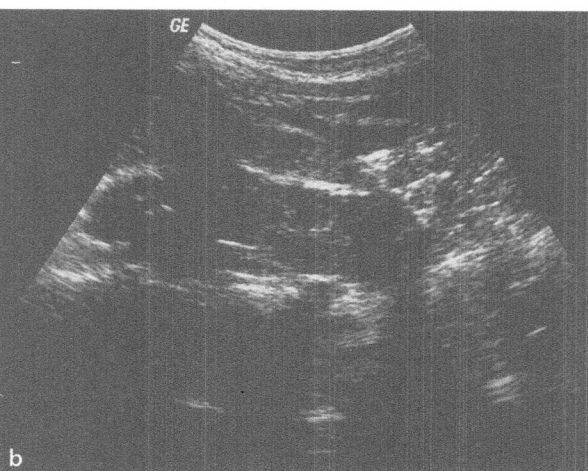

Fig. 5.1 a – c. Sonography. **a** Right kidney (longitudinal section). **b** Ectopic and smaller left kidney. **c** Parenchymal bridging between the two kidneys, suggestive of a horseshoe kidney

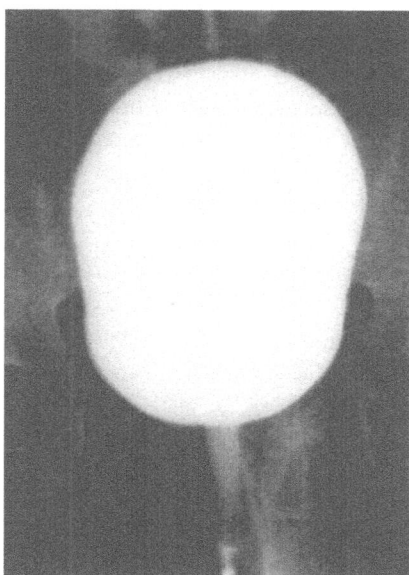

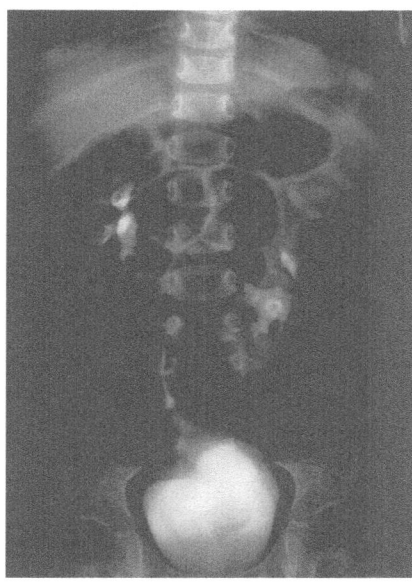

Fig. 5.2. No VUR is present during voiding cysto-urethro-graphy

Fig. 5.3. On the intravenous pyelogram a bilateral 90° rotation of the pelvicalyceal systems can be seen. The left kidney can be recognized in the pelvis. No signs of hydronephrosis are present

CASE 6 ▶ *Horseshoe Kidney with a Megaureter on the Right Side*

Clinical Course: This boy developed recurrent umbilical colics when he was 6 weeks old. Initial sonography revealed hydronephrosis on the right side (Fig. 6.1). A ^{99m}Tc-MAG$_3$ scan was suggestive of horseshoe kidney (Fig. 6.2). The split function of both kidneys was within the normal range. The decline of the time–activity curve of the left kidney following the injection of furosemide excluded obstruction. On the contralateral side, an indeterminate response curve with a 42% decrease of the time–activity curve within 10 min was seen.

The intravenous pyelogram confirmed the diagnosis of a horseshoe kidney (Fig. 6.3). The typical bilateral 90° rotation of the drainage system on both sides was noted. On the right side a megaureter and a clumsy appearance of the calyces was present. We performed a voiding cysto-urethrography, which subsequently excluded refluxing megaureter (Fig. 6.4).

On the assumption of a horseshoe kidney with a nonobstructed and nonrefluxing megaureter we started antibiotic prophylaxis, which was continued until the child was 2 years old. On a repeat ^{99m}Tc-MAG$_3$ scan performed at this time no signs of obstruction were present (Fig. 6.5).

The further clinical course was without any complications. When the boy was 4 years old, sonography demonstrated persistent dilatation of the drainage system on the right side (Fig. 6.6). On this sonogram, paravertebral parenchymal bridging was clearly demonstrated for the first time (Fig. 6.7).

Comment: In optimally prepared children a horseshoe kidney may be diagnosed by sonography alone. In our case, scintigraphic and radiological techniques were necessary to enable a proper diagnosis.

If an additional megaureter is present, further investigations are necessary to evaluate whether obstruction or reflux is present. If not, a wait-and-see strategy will be appropriate.

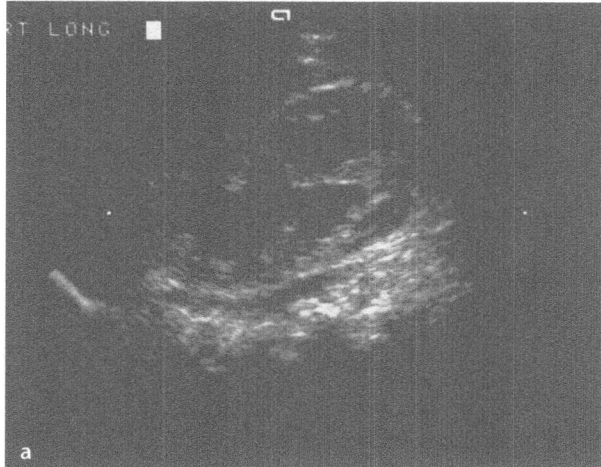

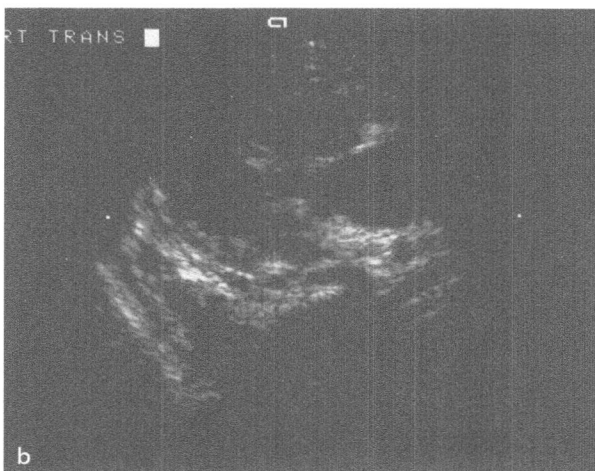

Fig. 6.1 a, b. Initial sonography demonstrates a dilatation of the drainage system on the right side

Fig. 6.2 a, b see p. 138

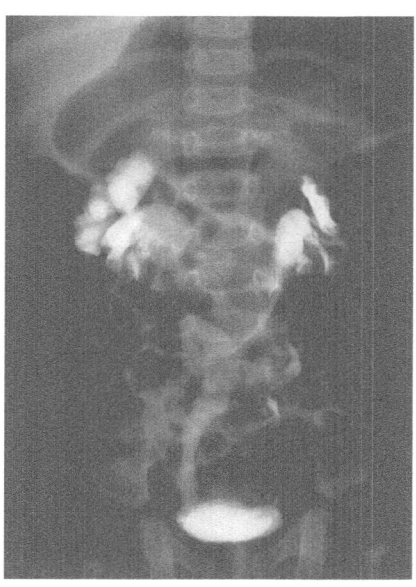

Fig. 6.3. The intravenous pyelogram confirms the diagnosis of a horseshoe kidney. The typical bilateral 90° rotation of the drainage system and the medially orientated location of the lower poles can be noted. On the right side a megaureter is present. The calyces on the right side look clumsy

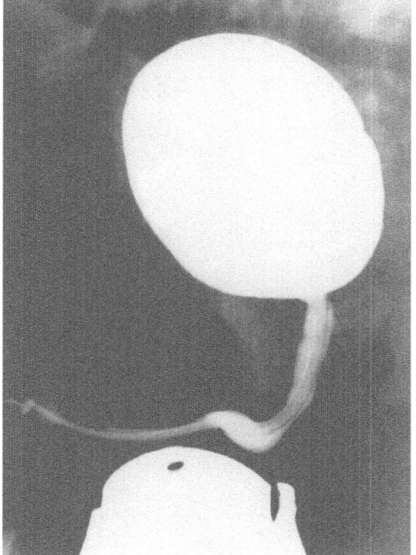

Fig. 6.4. Voiding cysto-urethrography makes it possible to exclude a refluxing megaureter. The bladder wall and the urethra look normal

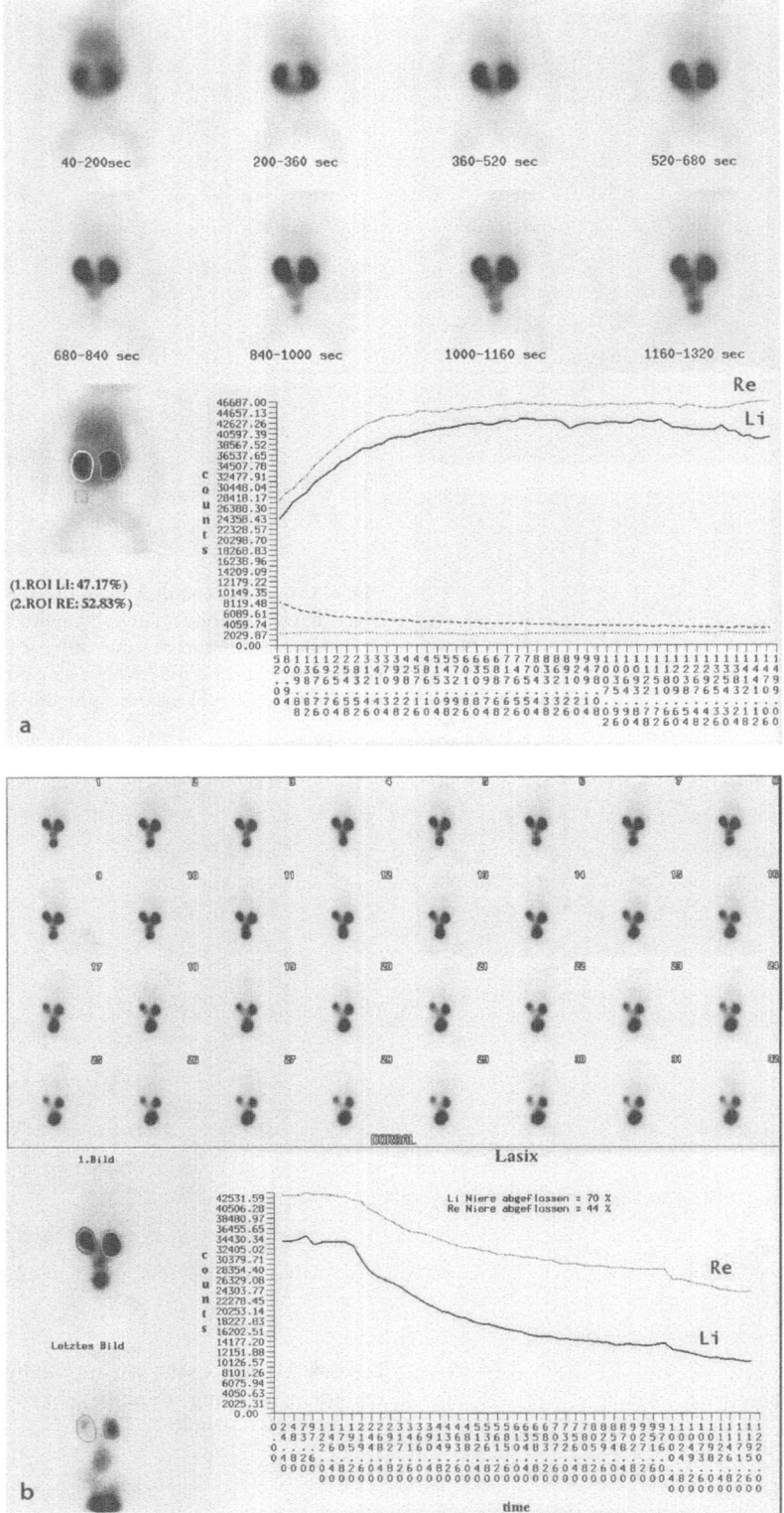

Fig. 6.2. a The ^{99m}Tc-MAG$_3$ scan during the parenchymal phase is suggestive for horseshoe kidney because the lower poles are medially orientated with evidence for parenchymal bridging. The parenchymal transit of the tracer is somewhat delayed, probably due to the child's immature tubular func-tion. The split function of both kidneys is within the normal range. **b** No signs of obstruction are present on the left side following the injection of furosemide. On the right side, an indeterminate response curve with a 42% decrease of the activity over 10 min is seen

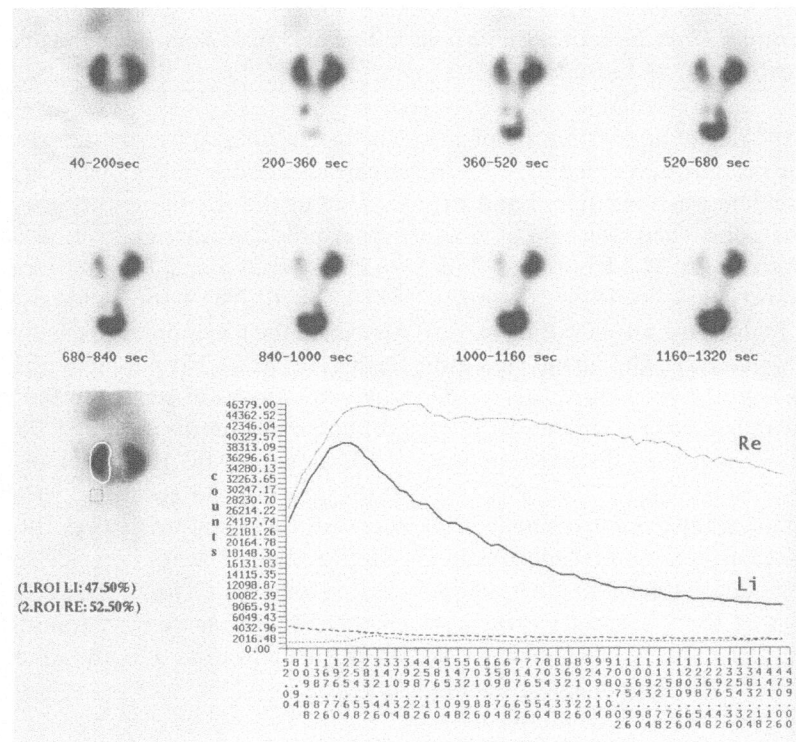

46379.00
44362.52
42346.04
40329.57
38313.09
36296.61
34280.13
c 32263.65
o 30247.17
u 28230.70
n 26214.22
t 24197.74
s 22181.26
20164.78
18148.30
16131.83
14115.35
12098.87
10082.39
8065.91
6049.43
4032.96
2016.48
0.00

Re

Li

(1.ROI LI: 47.50%)
(2.ROI RE: 52.50%)

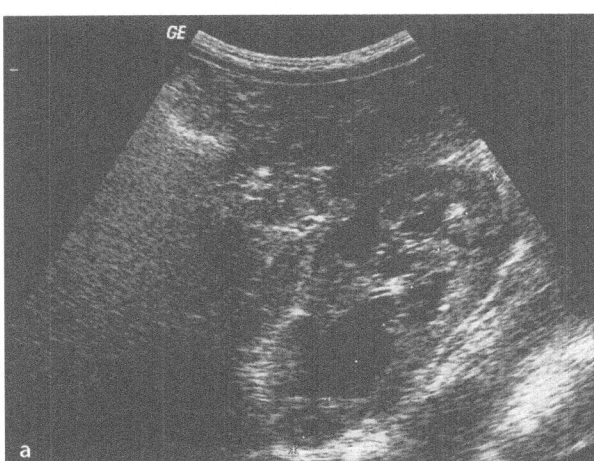

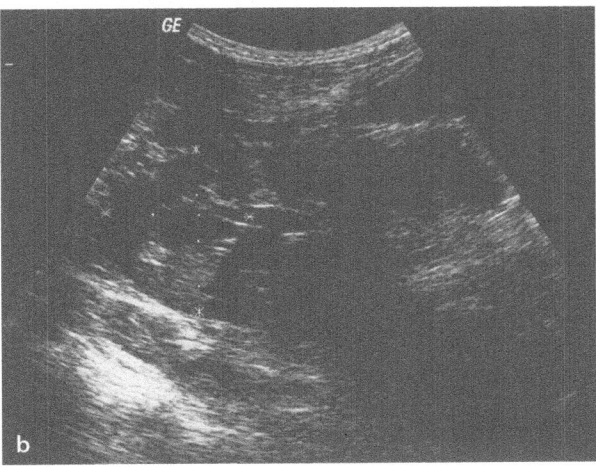

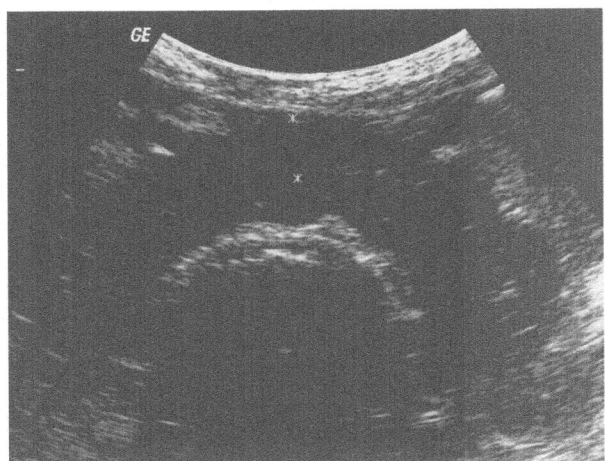

Fig. 6.5 (*above*). On the ^{99m}Tc-MAG$_3$ scan during follow-up no signs of obstruction are present. Note parenchymal bridging during the early parenchymal phase and the visualization of both ureters

Fig. 6.6 a, b (*left*). Persistence of the right-sided dilation of the drainage system during follow-up

Fig. 6.7 (*below*). Sonographic confirmation of parenchymal bridging between the kidneys

CASE 7 ▶ *Upper Urinary Tract Infection Combined with Reversible Renal Lesions Seen on* ^{99m}*Tc-DMSA Scan and Ectopic Positon of One Kidney*

Clinical Course: On the day of admission to our institution the 2 1/2-year-old girl developed high fever, vomiting and malaise. She was dehydrated and her general condition was poor. There were no obvious clinical signs of a septic focus. The laboratory findings consisted in massive leucocytosis (27,000/mm³), a CRP level of 34,5 mg/dl and an elevation of the serum creatinine (0.7 mg/dl). The urine analysis revealed pyuria (2,000/μl), leucocyte casts and proteinuria. Significant bacteriuria and growth of *Escherichia coli* were subsequently demonstrated in the urinary culture.

We immediately started antibiotic treatment with cefotaxime (100 mg/kg) and parenteral rehydration of the child. The fever persisted for a further 3 days, but the normalization of the CRP and pyuria was delayed for weeks.

Early sonography showed enlargement of the left kidney, with a significant increase of the echogenicity in the middle and upper part (Fig. 7.1). The pelvicalyceal system was only slightly dilated and not suggestive of hydronephrosis. The right kidney was recognized as being in an ectopic supravesical position (Fig. 7.2). The echogenicity and the enlargement of the left kidney began to normalize within the first week of antibiotic treatment, while a slight dilatation of the calyces was still present (Fig. 7.3).

The intravenous pyelogram during the child's first week (Fig. 7.4) showed an ectopic right kidney and clumsy calyces on both sides. We performed renal cortical scintigraphy on the 7th day of antibiotic treatment and found globally reduced ^{99m}Tc-DMSA uptake of the left kidney with a focal defect on the upper pole. An ectopic position on the right kidney (66% of split renal function) could be confirmed (Fig. 7.5a, b). The ectopic kidney exhibited a cortical defect on the lower pole, especially on the SPECT-Images (Fig. 7.6b). No parenchymal bridging between the two kidneys was seen on the SPECT images. On voiding cysto-urethrography VUR was excluded.

After successful treatment of the acute urinary tract infection no antibiotic prophylaxis was given because hydronephrosis or VUR had been excluded. No further urinary tract infections occurred during follow-up. The ^{99m}Tc-DMSA scan was repeated 1 1/2 years after acute infection and revealed a complete normalization of both kidneys without signs of scarring.

Comment: This case demonstrates that pyelonephritis may occur even in the absence of hydronephrosis or reflux. During acute upper urinary tract infection the ^{99m}Tc-DMSA scan revealed a focally reduced uptake on both kidneys in a 2 1/2-year-old girl, indicative of pyelonephritis. The scan was repeated 1 1/2 year later, and the uptake had completely normalized with no signs of renal scarring. Acute infection and ectopic positon of the right kidney was also clearly be demonstrated by ultrasound.

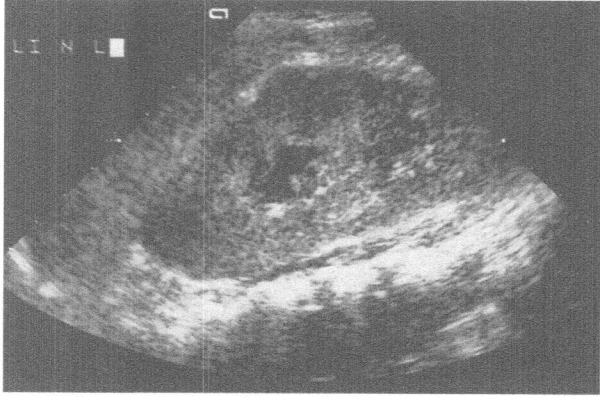

Fig. 7.1. Initial sonography of the left kidney (longitudinal section): enlargement and enhancement of the echogenicity in the middle and upper part

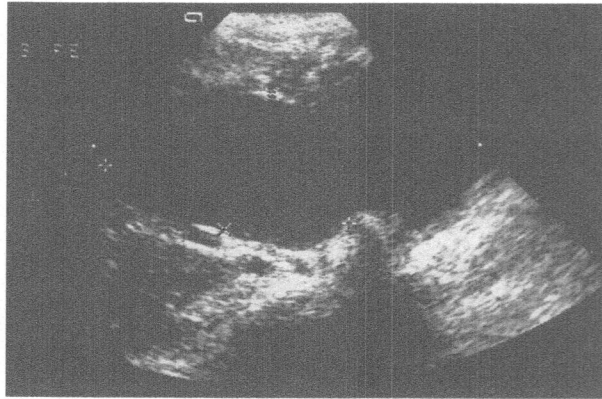

Fig. 7.2. The right kidney (longitudinal section) is seen on ultrasound to be in an ectopic supravesical position

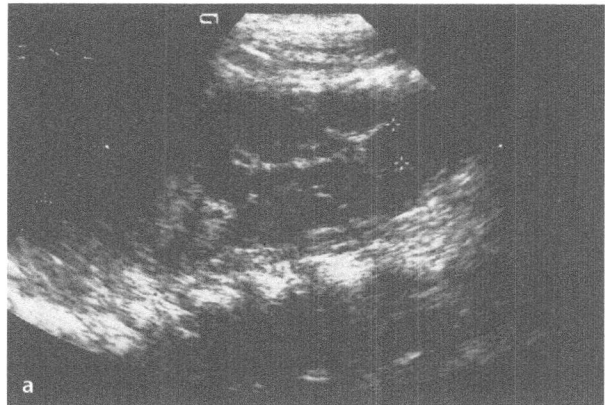

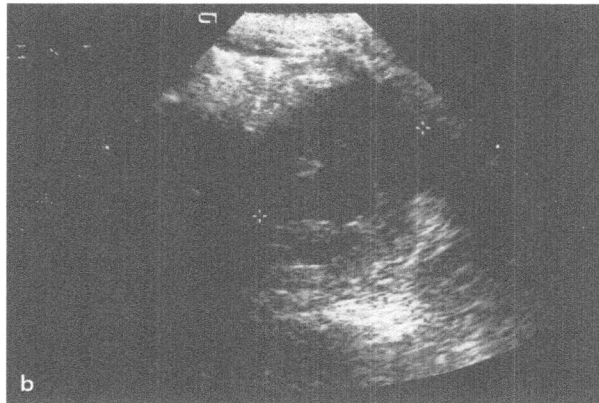

Fig. 7.3 a, b. Within the first week of antibiotic treatment the echongenicity and the enlargement of the left kidney begin to normalize, while a slight dilatation of the calyces was still present (**a** longitudinal, **b** transverse sections)

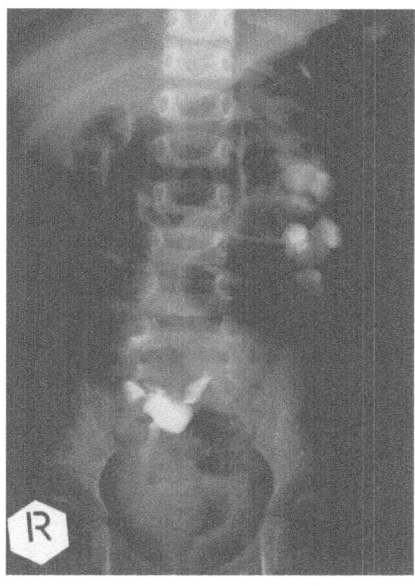

Fig. 7.4. The intravenous pyelogram shows an ectopic right kidney and no signs of renal parenchymal bridging

Fig. 7.5 a, b. ^{99m}Tc-DMSA scan. **a** On the planar scans there is a cortical defect on the upper pole of the left kidney. The right kidney is in an ectopic position in the pelvis. **b** On the SPECT images (3-D reconstruction), parenchymal bridging between the kidneys can be excluded, the defect on the upper pole of the left kidney is confirmed and an additional defect is seen at the lower pole of the ectopic kidney (*arrows*)

▼

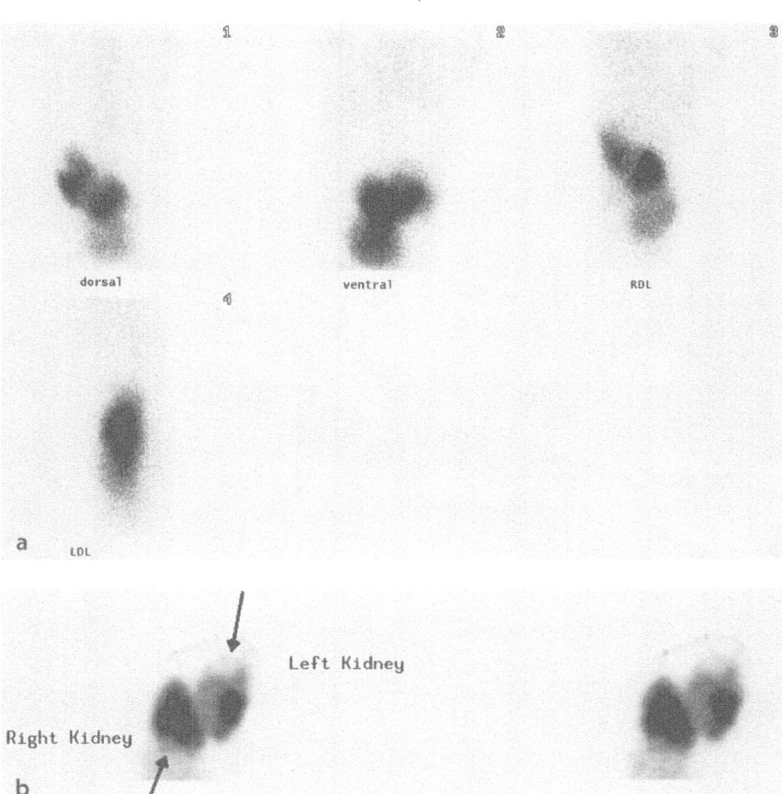

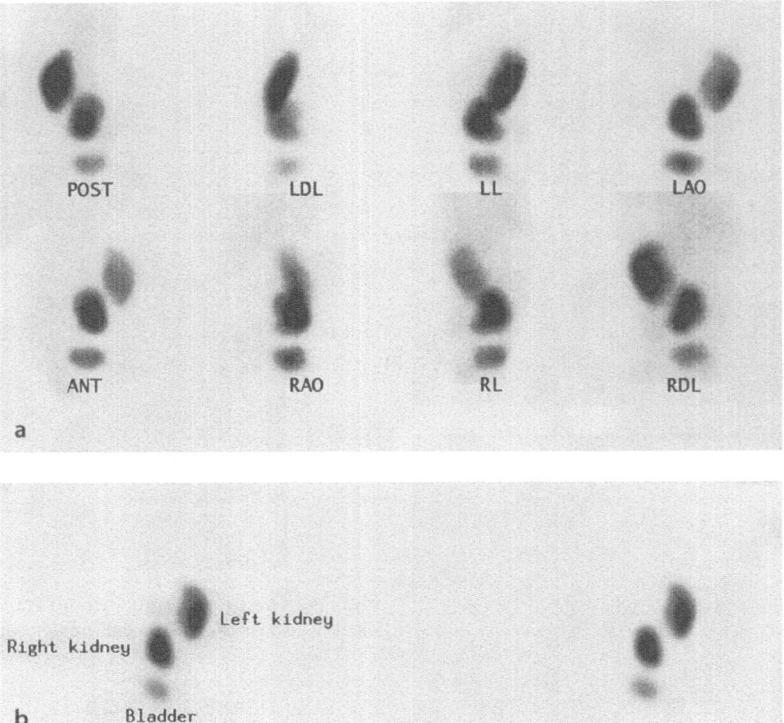

Fig. 7.6a, b. ^{99m}Tc-DMSA scan. Normalization of **a** the planar scan and **b** the SPECT images (3-D reconstruction) during follow-up

CASE 8 ▶ *Renal Damage Following Multifocal Pyelonephritis*

Clinical Course: Antibiotic treatment of otitis media was performed in this boy when he was 3 years old. Two weeks after the start of this treatment acute pyelonephritis with *Streptococcus faecalis* developed. The CRP levels (27 mg/dl) and the ESR (113 mm within the first hour) were markedly increased. Although antibiotic treatment with amoxicilline and ceftacidine was immediately started, the fever persisted for 9 days and the relief of clinical symptoms was delayed.

On the initial sonography both kidneys were found to be enlarged and both ureters were dilated in their distal parts with a diameter up to 9.5 mm (Figs. 8.1, 8.2). During further sonographic evaluations a progressive reduction in the size of the right kidney was noted, with persistent dilatation of the ureter on the same side (Figs. 8.3, 8.4). No VUR was demonstrated by voiding cysto-urethrography. The ^{99m}Tc-DMSA scan was performed 5 weeks later. The uptake of the left kidney was normal, while the right kidney exhibited multifocal areas of reduced uptake (split function: 31%; Fig. 8.5). Figure 8.6 gives an impression of the intravenous pyelogram. The pyelogram shows a right-sided dysplastic upper pole and a megaureter. On the ^{99m}Tc-MAG$_3$ scintigraphie performed 6 months later, the split function of the right kidney was impaired and there were indirect signs of a megaureter, but no signs of obstruction were present (Fig. 8.7).

Comment: During an acute upper urinary tract infection involvement of both kidneys was proven by sonography. Five weeks later the left kidney looked normal on the ^{99m}Tc-DMSA scan, but the right kidney showed multifocal defects, suggestive of renal scarring. This case demonstrates, again, that pyelonephritis can occur even in the absence of VUR and that one episode of severe upper urinary tract infection can lead to irreversible renal damage.

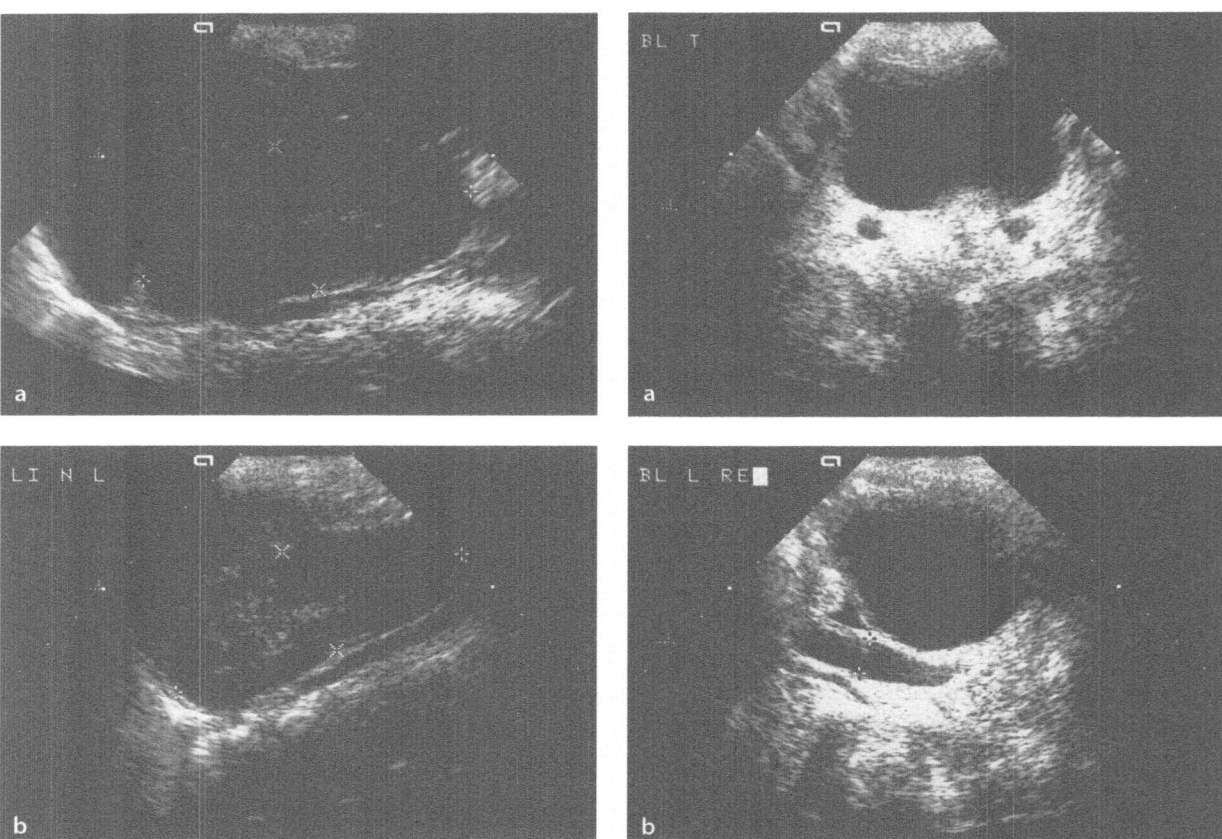

Fig. 8.1 a,b. Sonography showing acute swelling of both kidneys with poor pelvi-cortical differentiation on the initial sonography (**a** right longitudinal, **b** left longitudinal sections)

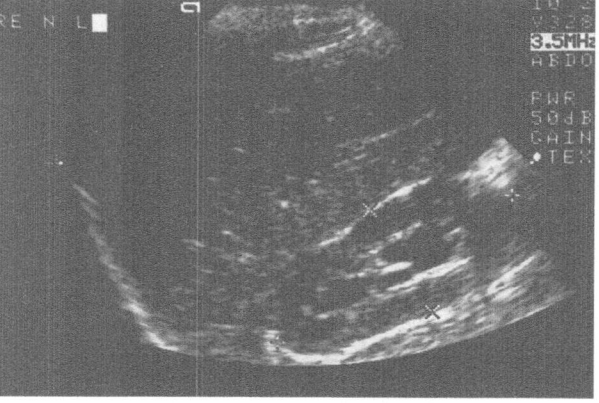

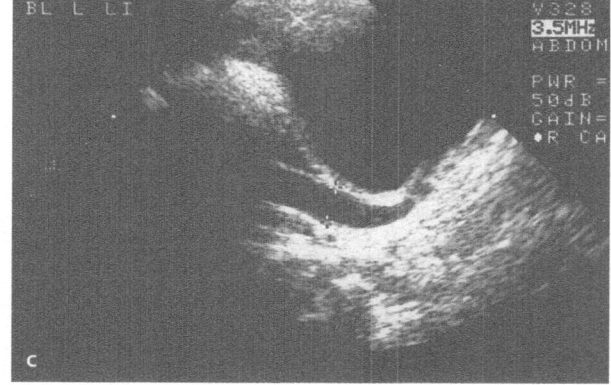

Fig. 8.2 a–c. Sonographic view of distal dilatation of both ureters (**a** transverse, **b, c** longitudinal sections)

◀

Fig. 8.3. Sonography shows reduction of the renal volume and dilatation of the renal pelvis on the right side 3 months after acute infection

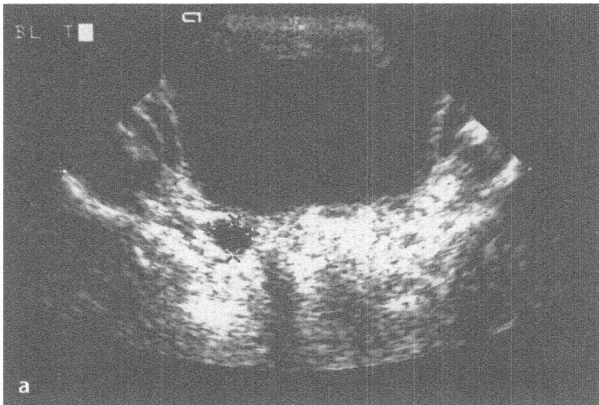

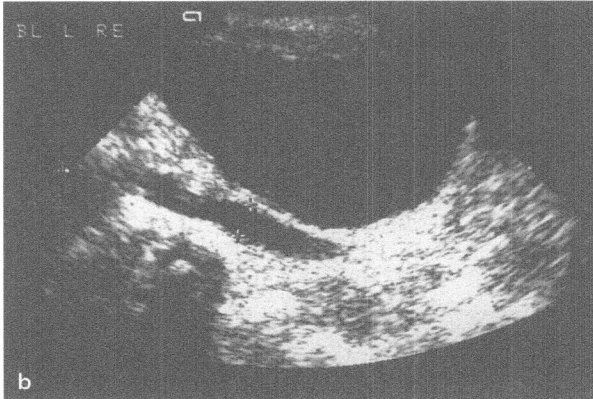

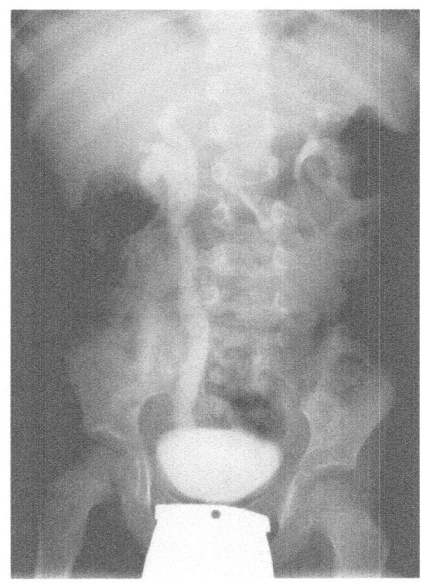

Fig. 8.6. Pyelogram showing dysplastic calyces and a mega-ureter of the right kidney

◄

Fig. 8.4 a, b. Persistent dilatation of the right ureter seen on the sonogram 3 months after acute infection (**a** transverse, **b** longitudinal sections)

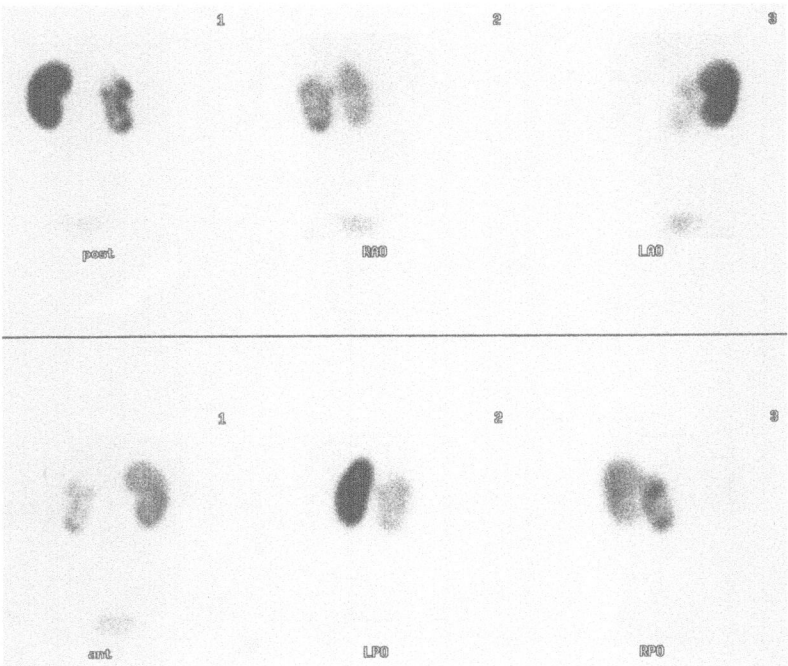

Fig. 8.5. ^{99m}Tc-DMSA scan: on the planar scan the left kidney shows a normal uptake, while the right kidney exhibits multi-focal areas of reduced uptake

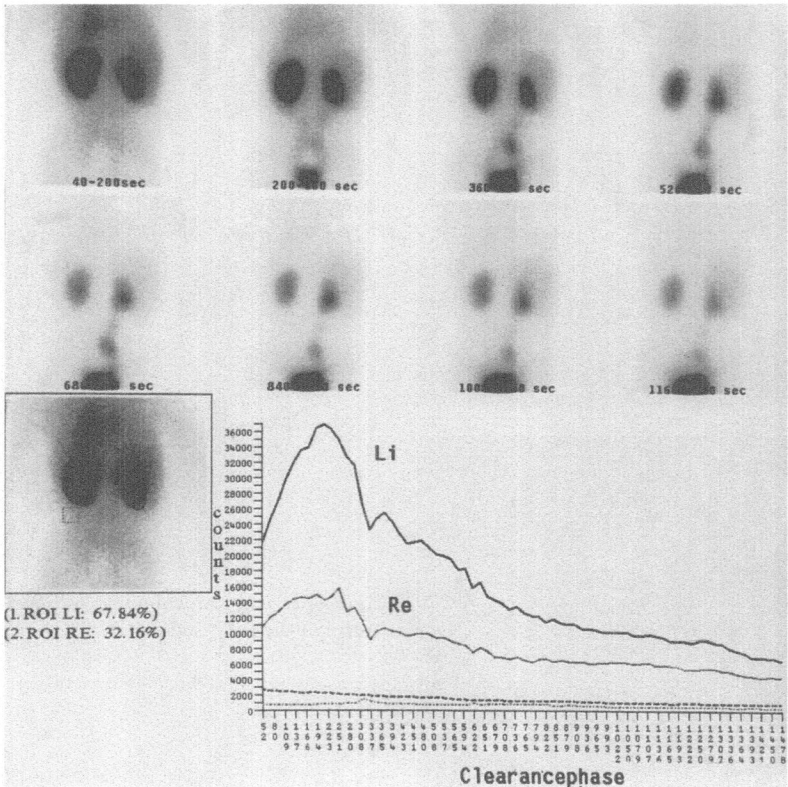

Fig. 8.7. ^{99m}Tc-MAG$_3$ scintigraphy reveals impairment of the split function of the right kidney and indirect signs of a mega-ureter can be seen during the drainage phase. No signs of obstruction are visible

CASE 9 ▶ *Subpelvic Obstruction During Early Childhood*

Clinical Course: Right hydronephrosis in this male newborn had already been diagnosed antenatally. During the neonatal period continuous sonographic monitoring revealed a progressive dilatation of the right renal pelvis. (Figs. 9.1, 9.2). When the boy was 4 weeks old we performed a ^{99m}Tc-MAG$_3$ scan. During this examination the split function of the right kidney was normal, but the furosemide study showed an impaired response of the time-activity curve to the diuretic (Fig. 9.3). Owing to the well-preserved function of the right kidney we first adopted a "wait-and-see" strategy. During subsequent weeks we found there was progressive dilatation of the right drainage system and finally decided on surgical treatment.

Preoperatively VUR was excluded by voiding cysto-urethrography (Fig. 9.4). The intravenous pyelogram showed a delayed excretion on the right side. On the 30-min images the X-ray contrast medium was seen only in the calyces, while the renal pelvis was not visualized. In contrast to these findings, the contralateral kidney looked normal (Fig. 9.5).

Surgical correction of a subpelvic obstruction was performed without any complications at 10 weeks of age. A sonographic control, performed 6 weeks later, showed regressed dilatation of the right renal pelvis and maturation of the right renal parenchyma (Fig. 9.6). Repeat ^{99m}Tc-MAG$_3$ scintigraphy demonstrated the absence of obstruction (Fig. 9.7). Sonography performed at the age of 4 years revealed parenchymal maturation of both kidneys with only residual dilatation of the drainage system on the right side (Fig. 9.8).

Comment: It is crucial to wait for a decline of the split renal function as definitive proof of obstruction. Although the function of the right kidney in this boy was well preserved, progressive dilatation of the renal pelvis and a poor diuretic response on the ^{99m}Tc-MAG$_3$ scintigraphy led to early surgical correction of a subpelvic obstruction.

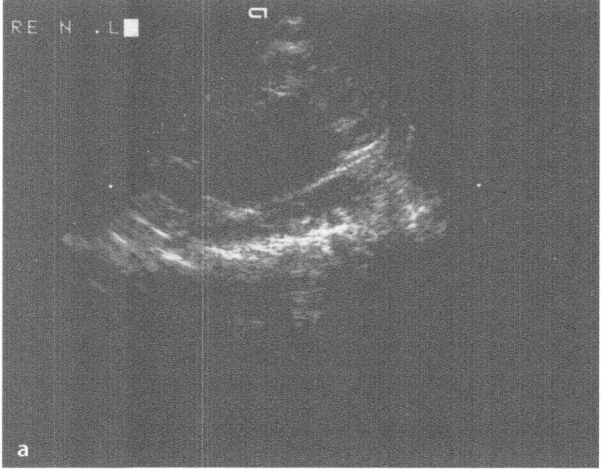

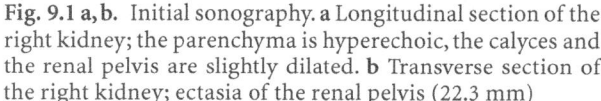

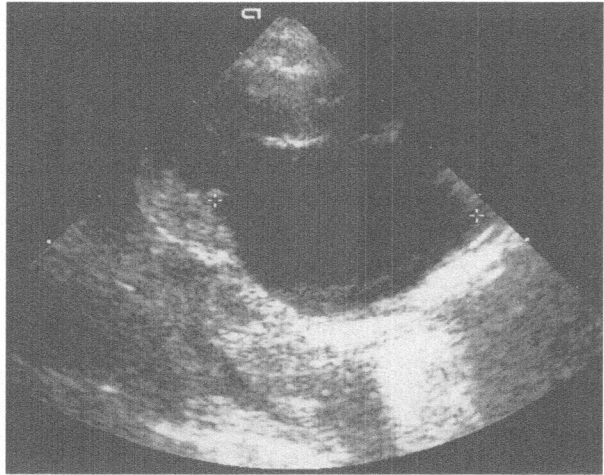

Fig. 9.2. Sonography during follow-up: progressive dilatation of the drainage system on the right side

Fig. 9.3 a, b see p. 149

Fig. 9.1 a, b. Initial sonography. **a** Longitudinal section of the right kidney; the parenchyma is hyperechoic, the calyces and the renal pelvis are slightly dilated. **b** Transverse section of the right kidney; ectasia of the renal pelvis (22.3 mm)

Fig. 9.4. VUR is excluded by voiding cysto-urethrography. ▶ The urethra and the contour of the urinary bladder look normal

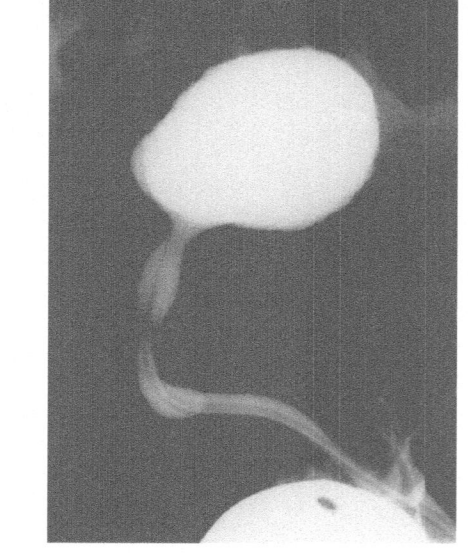

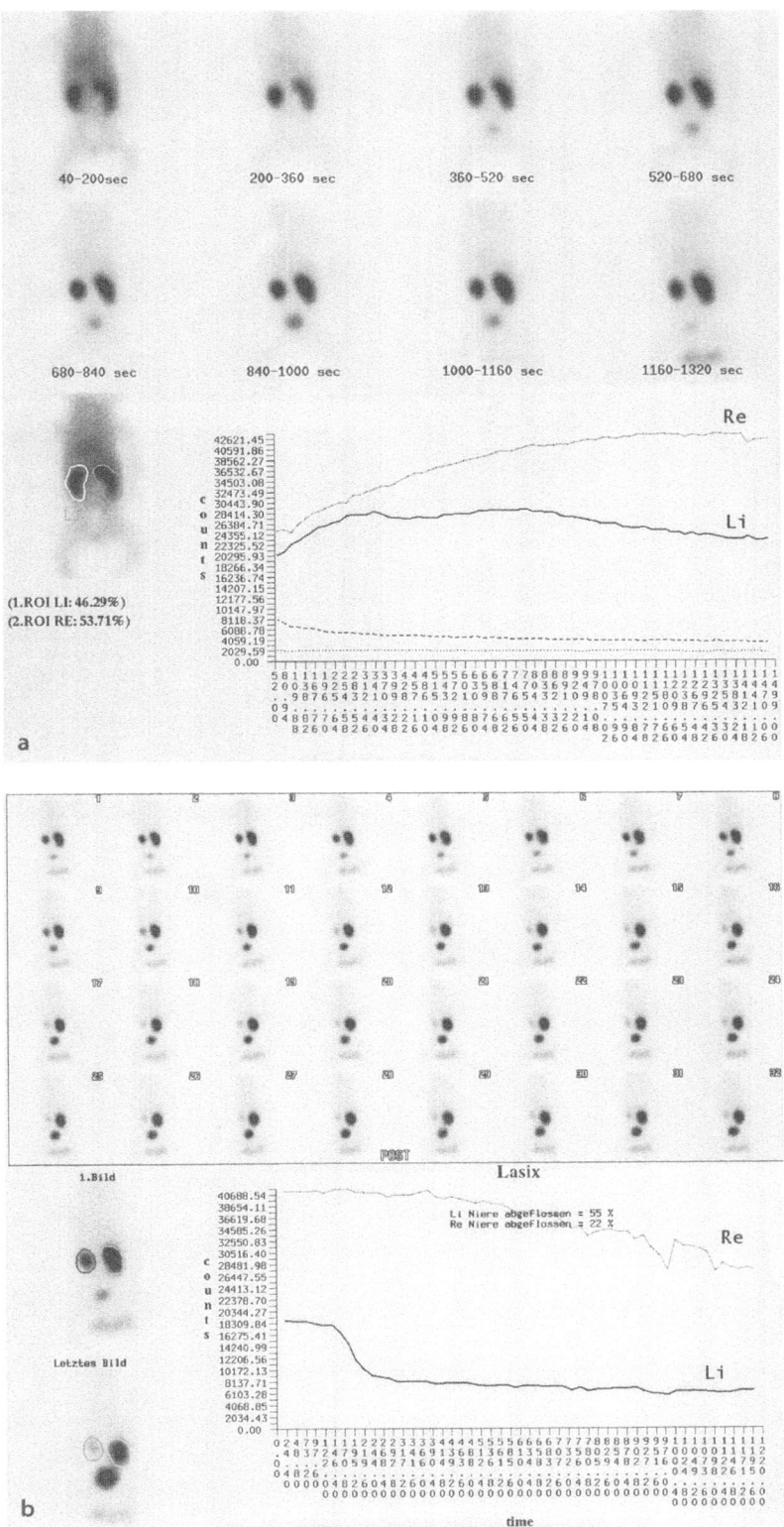

Fig. 9.3. a The ⁹⁹ᵐTc-MAG₃ scan during the parenchymal phase is suggestive of obstruction. The split function of the right kidney (53%) is well preserved. **b** On the right side there is a progressive accumulation of the tracer in the renal pelvis and only a poor response to frusemide (22% decline of the time-activity curve within 20 min)

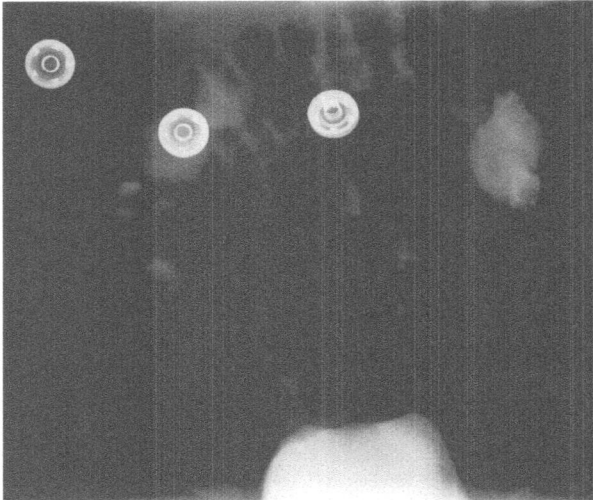

Fig. 9.5. The intravenous pyelogram shows a delayed excretion on the right side. On the 30-min images the X-ray contrast medium is seen only in the calyces, while the renal pelvis is not visualized. In contrast to these findings, the contralateral kidney looked normal

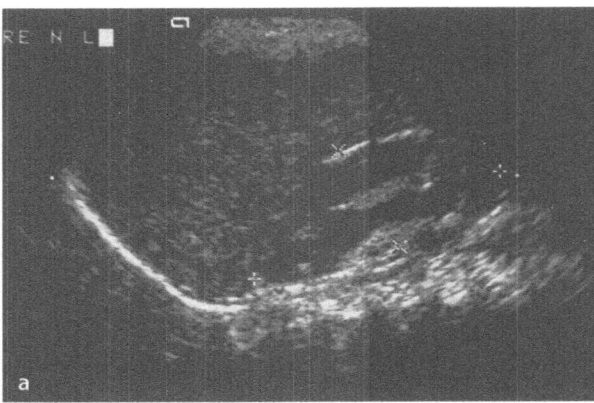

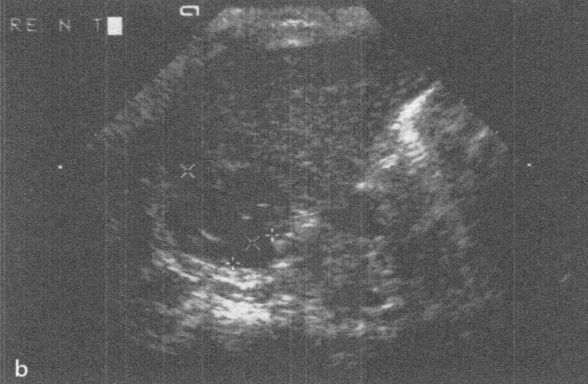

Fig. 9.6 a, b. Sonography 6 weeks postoperatively shows regressed dilatation of the right renal pelvis

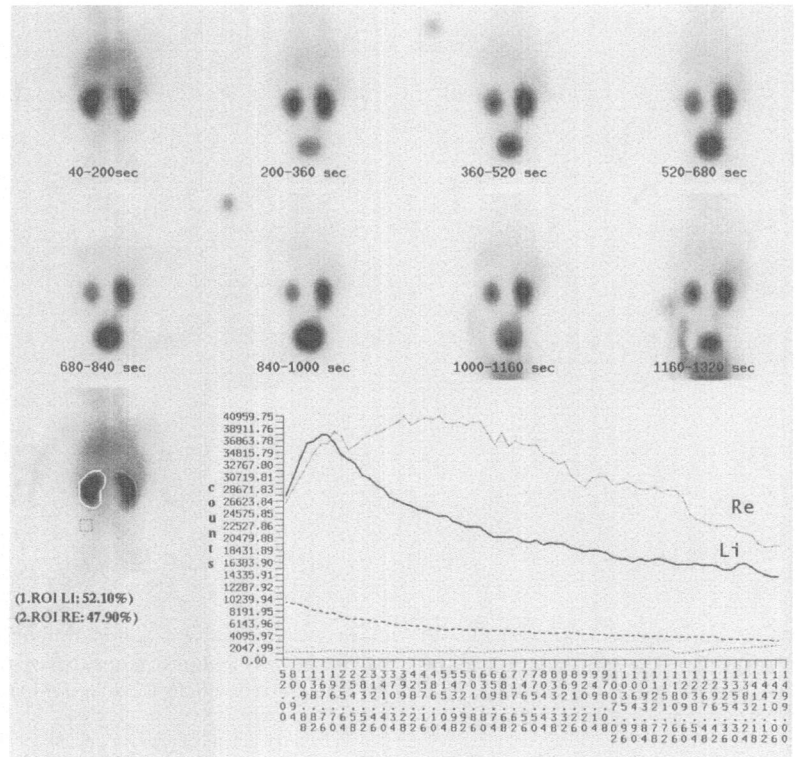

Fig. 9.7. The ^{99m}Tc-MAG$_3$ scan demonstrates the absence of obstruction

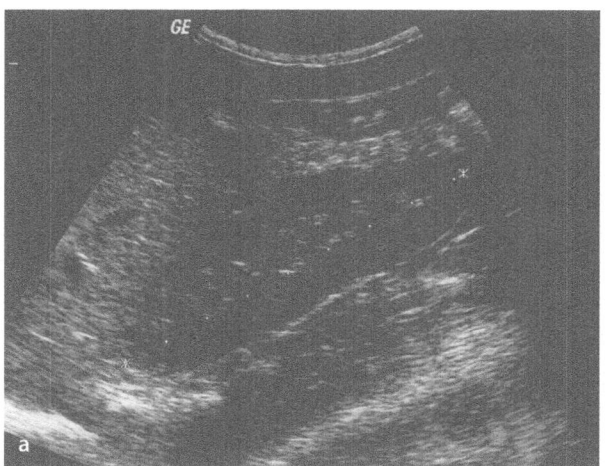

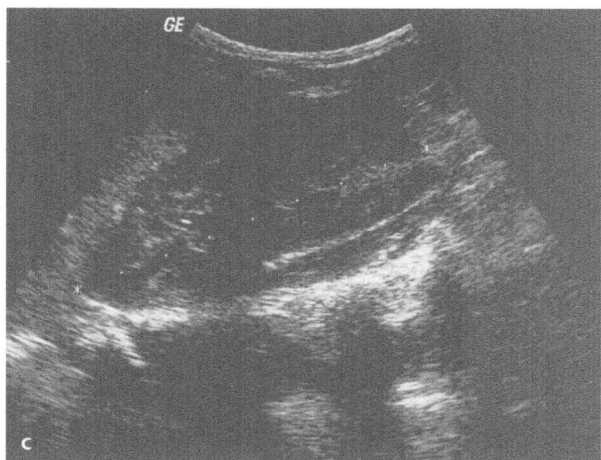

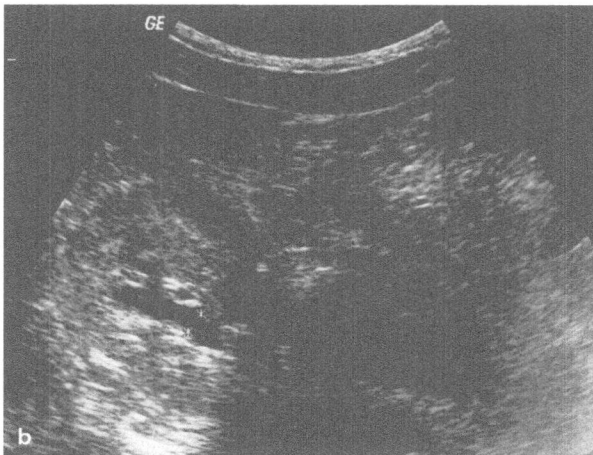

Fig. 9.8 a–c. Sonography at the age of 4. a Longitudinal section of the right kidney, showing adequate maturation of the right renal parenchyma. b Transverse section of the right kidny: the intrarenal renal pelvis is only slightly dilated, and the extrarenal pelvis looks normal. c Longitudinal section of the left kidney: normal appearance

CASE 10 ► *Recurrent Renal Colics Caused by an Extrinsic Subpelvic Stenosis*

Clinical Course: This 13-year-old child had recurrent renal colics on the left side. Hydronephrosis of the left kidney had been already diagnosed by sonography and on a pyelogram by an outdoor urologist. The patient reported that these symptoms occurred especially after drinking fairly large quantities.

On our first sonography (Fig. 10.1 a, b), which was performed when our patient felt well, we found no abnormalities on the right kidney and only slight ectasia of the renal pelvis on the left side (Fig. 10.1 c, d). We repeated the sonography when the girl was symptomatic, and at the time we found a massive dilatation of the left drainage system (Fig. 10.2).

The ^{99m}Tc-MAG$_3$ scintigraphy performed when the patient was disease free showed a normal split function of the left kidney and an accumulation of the tracer in the renal pelvis, which was suggestive of obstruction (Fig. 10.3 a). The diuretic study gave an indeterminate result (Fig. 10.3 b).

The intravenous pyelogram gave definitive evidence of an extrinsic subpelvic stenosis (Fig. 10.4), and following this procedure surgery was performed. Intraoperatively we found that the intermittent hydronephrosis was due to an aberrant vessel. Following the surgical correction, which was performed according to the Anderson-Hynes method, the patient became symptom free. Sonographic re-evaluation 2 years after surgery showed complete normalization (Fig. 10.5).

Comment: While subpelvic obstruction in siblings is usually asymptomatic, intermittent renal colics together with a massive dilatation of the pelvicalyceal system may occur during later childhood, as demonstrated in this case. As a rule, diagnosis is not possible except in the symptomatic patient.

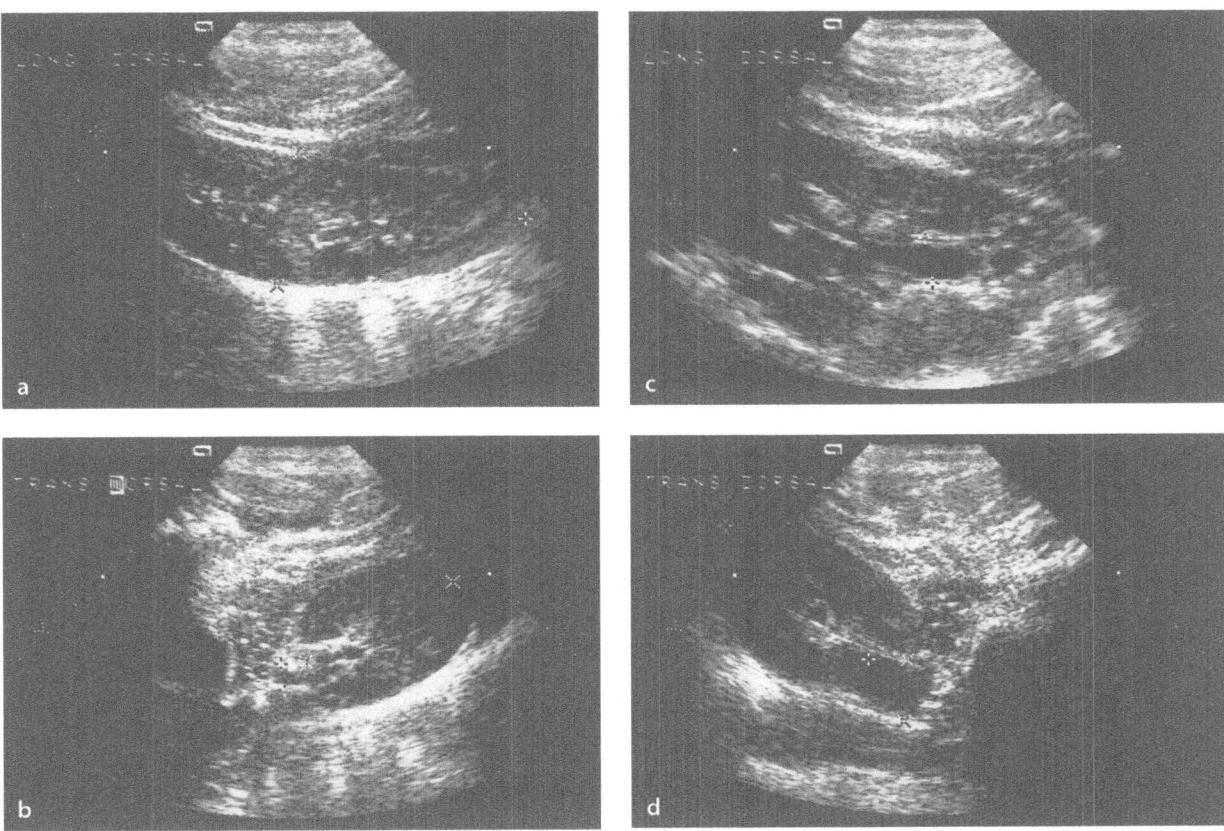

Fig. 10.1 a–d. Sonography during a symptom-free interval. **a, b** Right kidney (**a** transverse, **b** longitudinal sections). **c, d** Left kidney (**c** transverse, **d** longitudinal sections). Slight dilatation of the renal pelvis (indicative of hydronephrosis grade I) can be seen

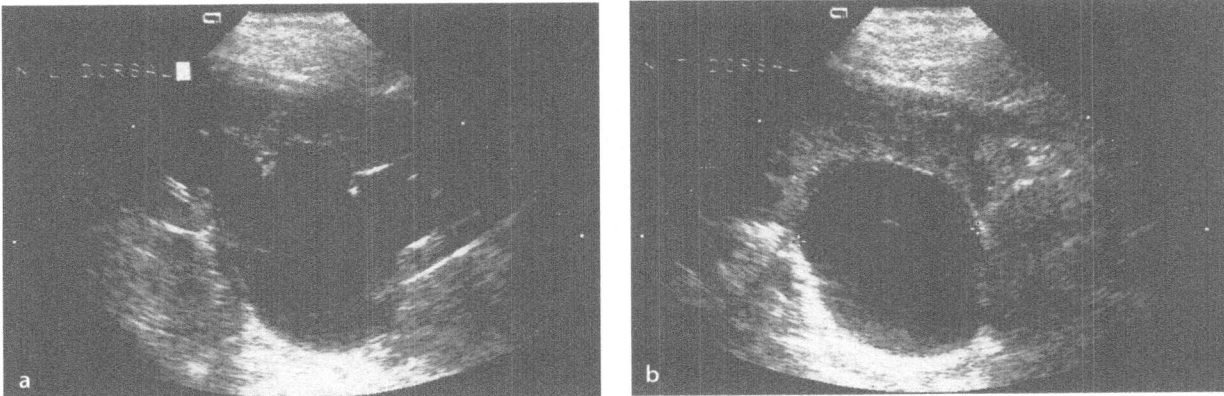

Fig. 10.2 a, b. Massive dilatation of the left drainage system can be noted during a colic

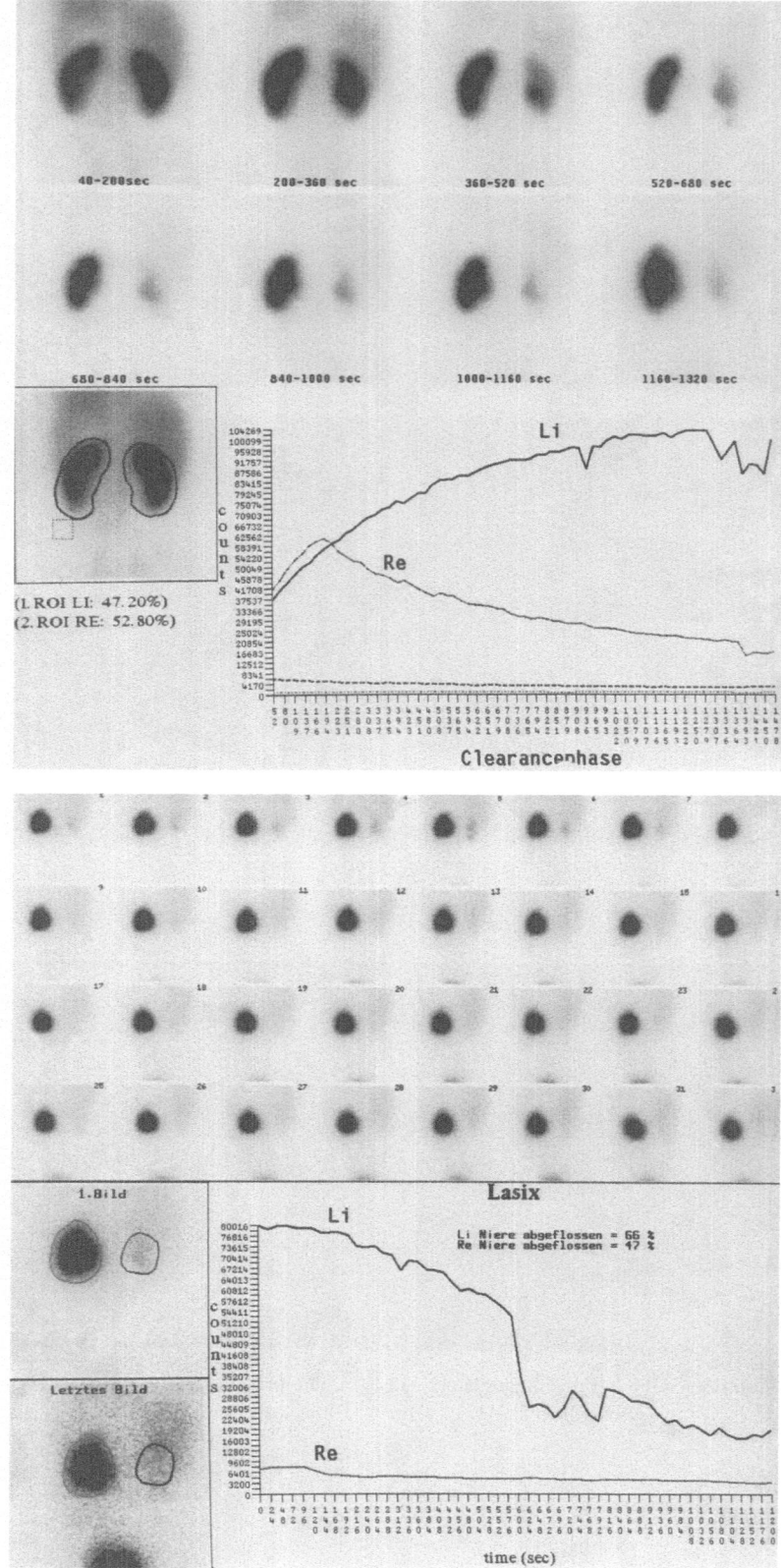

Fig. 10.3a, b. A ^{99m}Tc-MAG$_3$ scan performed when the patient was free of symptoms. **a** The left kidney showed a normal split function with an accumulation of the tracer in the renal pelvis suggestive of obstruction. **b** The diuretic study was nondiagnostic

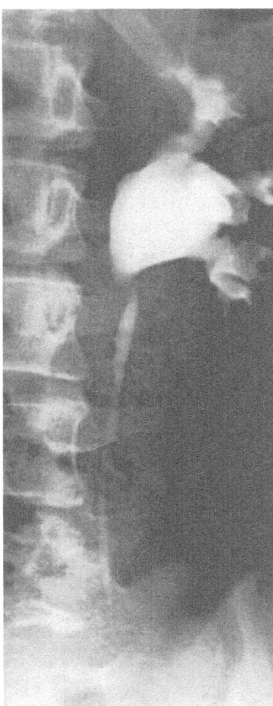

Fig. 10.4. On the pyelogram the renal pelvis of the left kidney is filled with the X-ray contrast medium. A clear interruption of the contrast column at the pelvi-ureteral junction due to an aberrant vessel can be noted

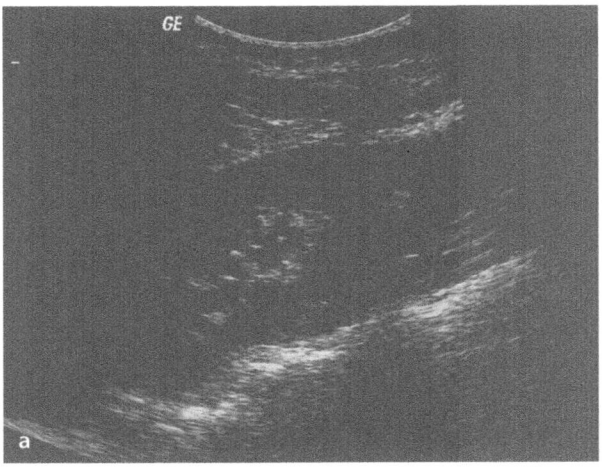

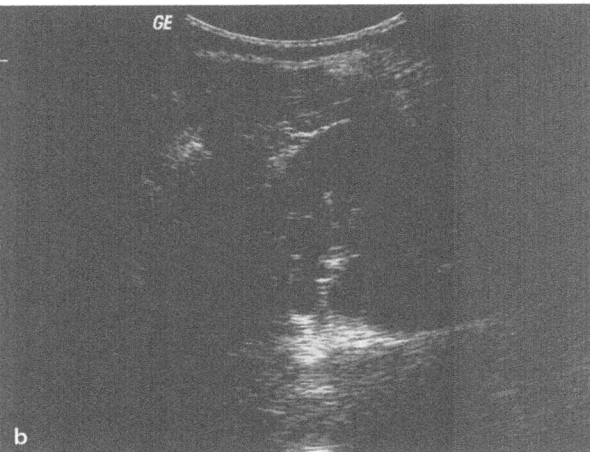

Fig. 10.5 a, b. Sonographic follow-up of the left kidney 2 years postoperatively. Longitudinal sections of the left kidney. **a** Normal parenchyma, no dilatation of the renal pelvis or calyces. **b** Only a minimal dilatation of the renal pelvis is seen

CASE 11 ▶ *Dilatation of the Renal Pelvis Without Obstruction*

Clinical Course: A dilatation of the left renal pelvis was seen on the ultrasound when the girl was examined for premature thelarche at the age of 4 years. We found significant ectasia of the calyces and the intra- and extrarenal pelvis on the left side (hydronephrosis grade III). The parenchyma looked normal. The contralateral kidney and drainage system showed no abnormalities (Fig. 11.1).

A ^{99m}Tc-MAG$_3$ scan was performed, on which a normal split function of the left kidney (53%) was found. During the parenchymal phase, the tracer accumulated in the renal pelvis. The time–activity curve after furosemide showed a decline of the activity by more than 50% within 10 min, indicative of a nonobstructed drainage system (Fig. 11.2).

During follow-up the dilatation of the left renal pelvis persisted but did not increase. When the girl was 7 years old, we repeated the sonogram and found the dilatation had remained unchanged (Fig. 11.3). The ^{99m}Tc-MAG$_3$ scan at this time showed a significant improvement of the drainage on the left side (Fig. 11.4). The split function of this kidney was well preserved.

Comment: Dilatation of a drainage system even for years can occur without significant obstruction and renal damage, as demonstrated in this case. Diuretic scintigraphy is reliable in most cases to exclude obstruction.

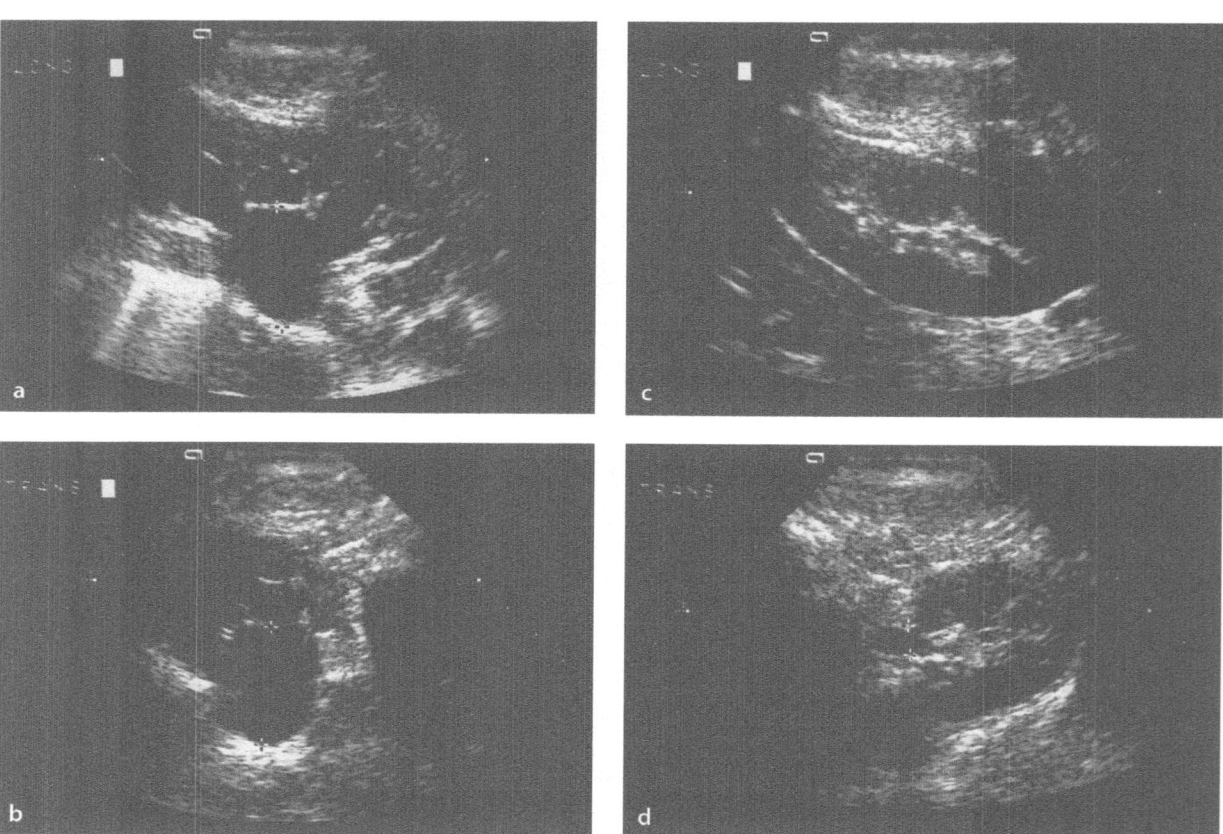

Fig. 11.1 a–d. Initial sonography. **a, b** Left kidney: a longitudinal section; dilatation of the calyces and the renal pelvis. **b** Transverse section: significant dilatation of the drainage system. **c, d** Right kidney (**c** longitudinal, **d** transverse section: no abnormalities are noted)

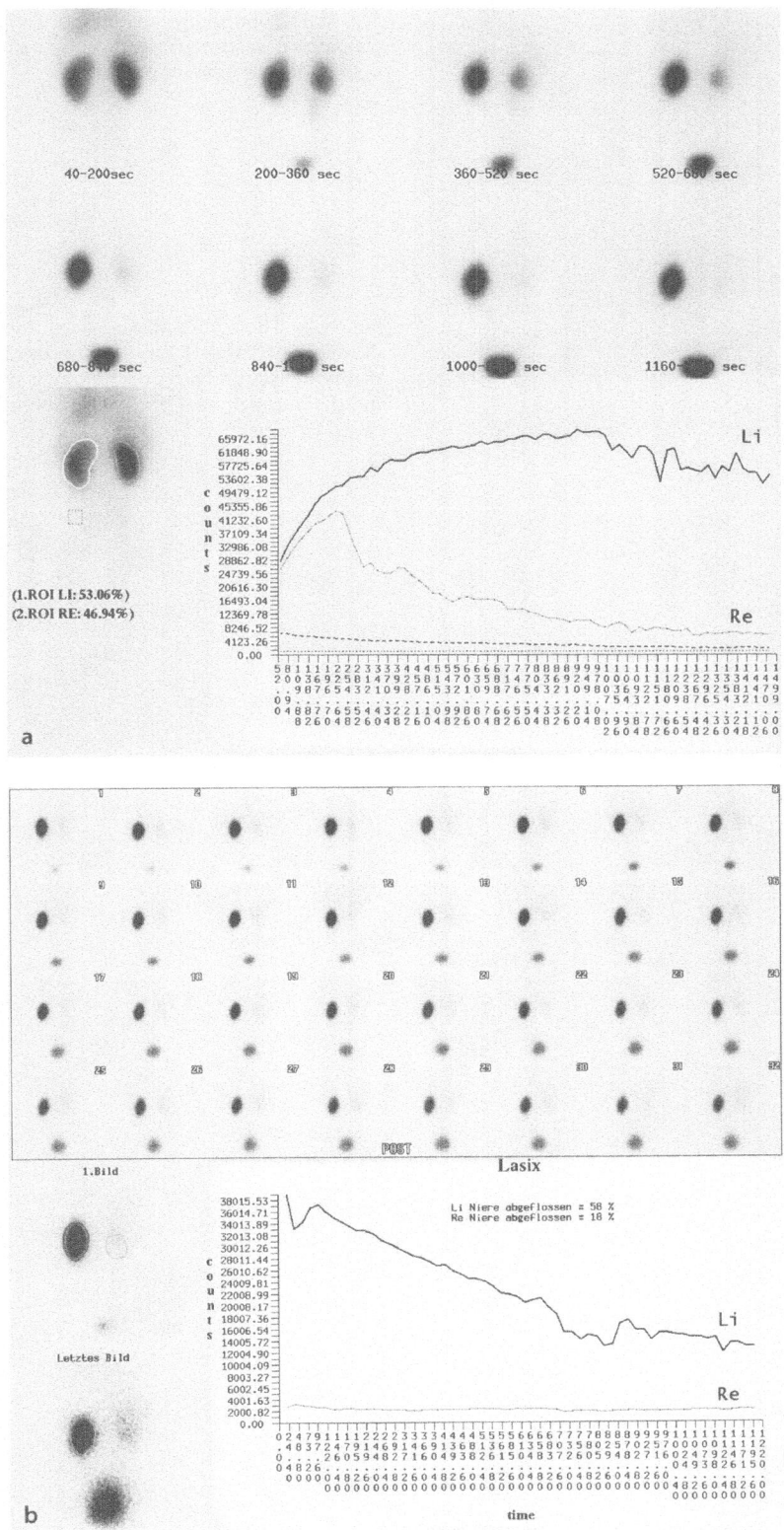

Fig. 11.2. a The initial ^{99m}Tc-MAG$_3$ scan shows an accumulation of the tracer in the renal pelvis on the left side during the parenchymal phase. **b** The time–activity curve after furosemide shows a decline of the activity by more than 50% within 10 min, indicating that no obstruction is present

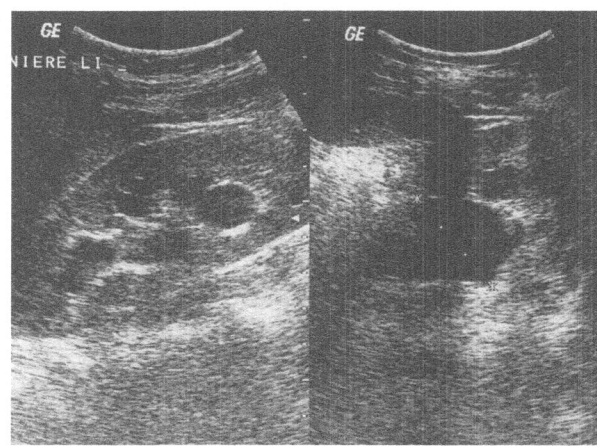

Fig. 11.3. Sonography of the left kidney (longitudinal and transversal sections): persistent dilatation of the drainage system during follow-up

◀

Fig. 11.4. The ^{99m}Tc-MAG$_3$ scan during follow-up. The drainage of the left kidney improved spontaneously, with transient accumulation of the tracer in the renal pelvis during the parenchymal phase and spontaneous decline of the time–activity curve

▼

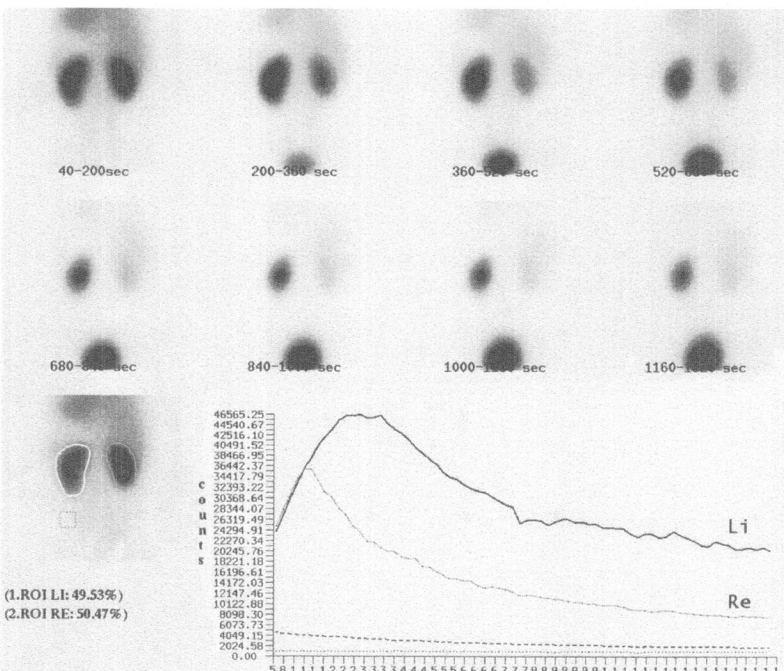

CASE 12 ► *Prenatally Diagnosed Unilateral Dilation of the Renal Pelvis*

Clinical Course: During the fetal period unilateral right hydronephrosis had been recognized in this child. These findings were confirmed postnatally during the boy's first days of life (Fig. 12.1) Sonography revealed high-grade hydronephrosis on the right side with dilation of the renal pelvis and the calyces. We started antibiotic prohylaxis and discharged the child.

When he was 4 week old, we performed a ^{99m}Tc-MAG$_3$ scan. The split function of the affected kidney was well preserved (48%). The tracer showed accumulation in the pelvicalyceal system, but the diuretic response was normal with a decline of the time–activity curve by 50% within 10 min (Fig. 12.2). As the scintigraphic findings were more favourable we adopted a "wait-and-see" stategy.

When our patient was 9 months old we repeated sonography and found regression of the calyceal dilatation, while the dimensions of the renal pelvis seemed to be unchanged (Fig. 12.3).

Repeated ^{99m}Tc-MAG$_3$ scintigraphy confirmed the improvement. The split function was unchanged and the drainage from the right renal pelvis had now improved and was showing a spontaneous decline of the curve during the excretion phase of the scintigraphic study. The furosemide study, although not mandatory in such a situation, again excluded obstruction (Fig. 12.4).

During follow-up the boy was monitored sonographically. The last sonogram, performed at the age of 3, showed no significant dilatation of the drainage system to be present (Fig. 12.5).

Comment: Although high-grade dilation of the drainage system was present, functional imaging with ^{99m}Tc-MAG$_3$ excluded obstruction in this boy and prevented unnecessary surgery. Note the good concordance of the sonographic and scintigraphic findings.

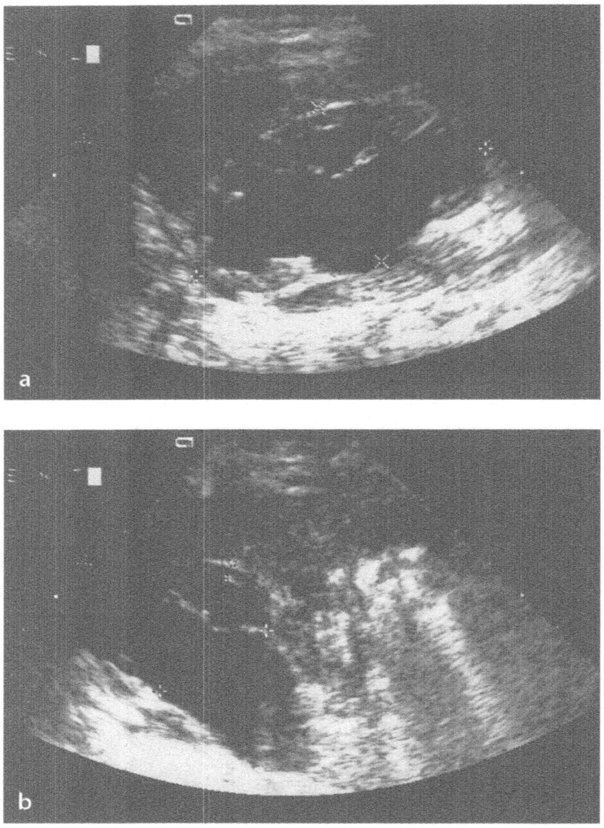

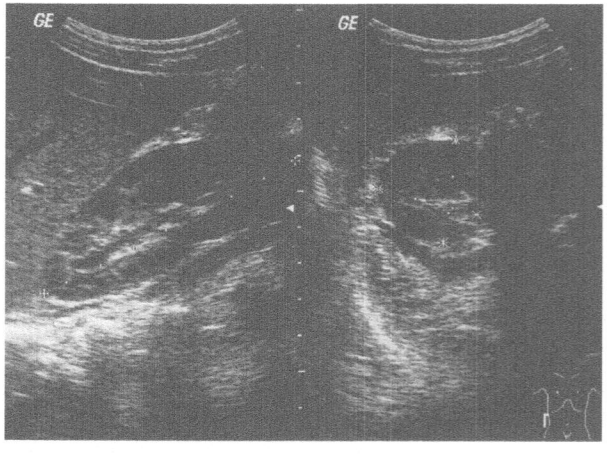

Fig. 12.1a, b. Initial sonography. **a** Longitudinal section of the right kidney: the parenchyma looks thinned. There is high-grade dilatation of the calyces and the renal pelvis. **b** Transverse section of the right kidney

Fig. 12.2a, b see p. 161

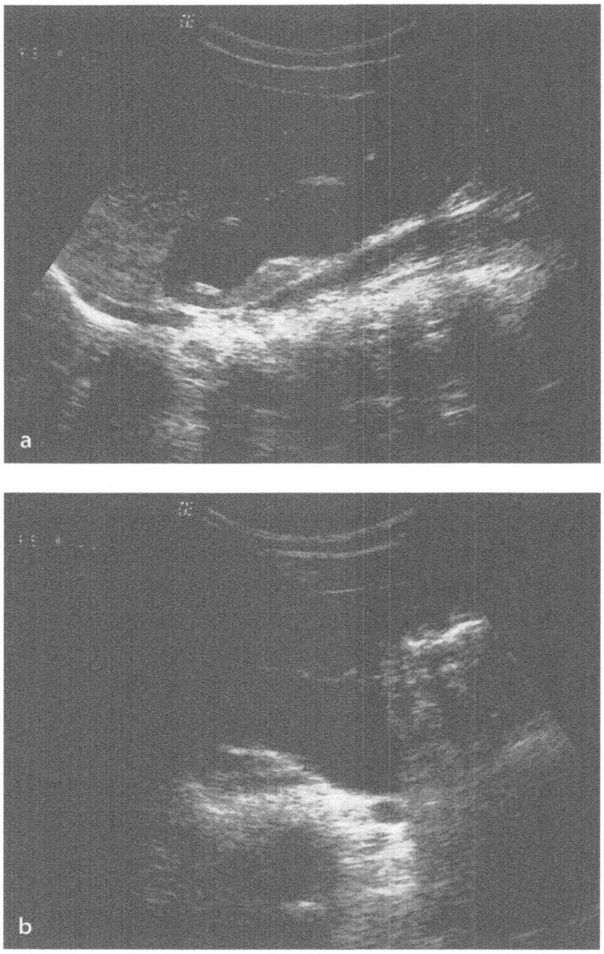

Fig. 12.3a, b. Sonography during follow-up: only slight dilatation of the calyces. No improvement of the dilatation of the right renal pelvis

Fig. 12.4a, b see p. 162

Fig. 12.5. The last sonogram, performed at the age of 3, shows a normal parenchyma of the right kidney; the kidney volume is within the normkal range, and no significant dilatation of the drainage system is present

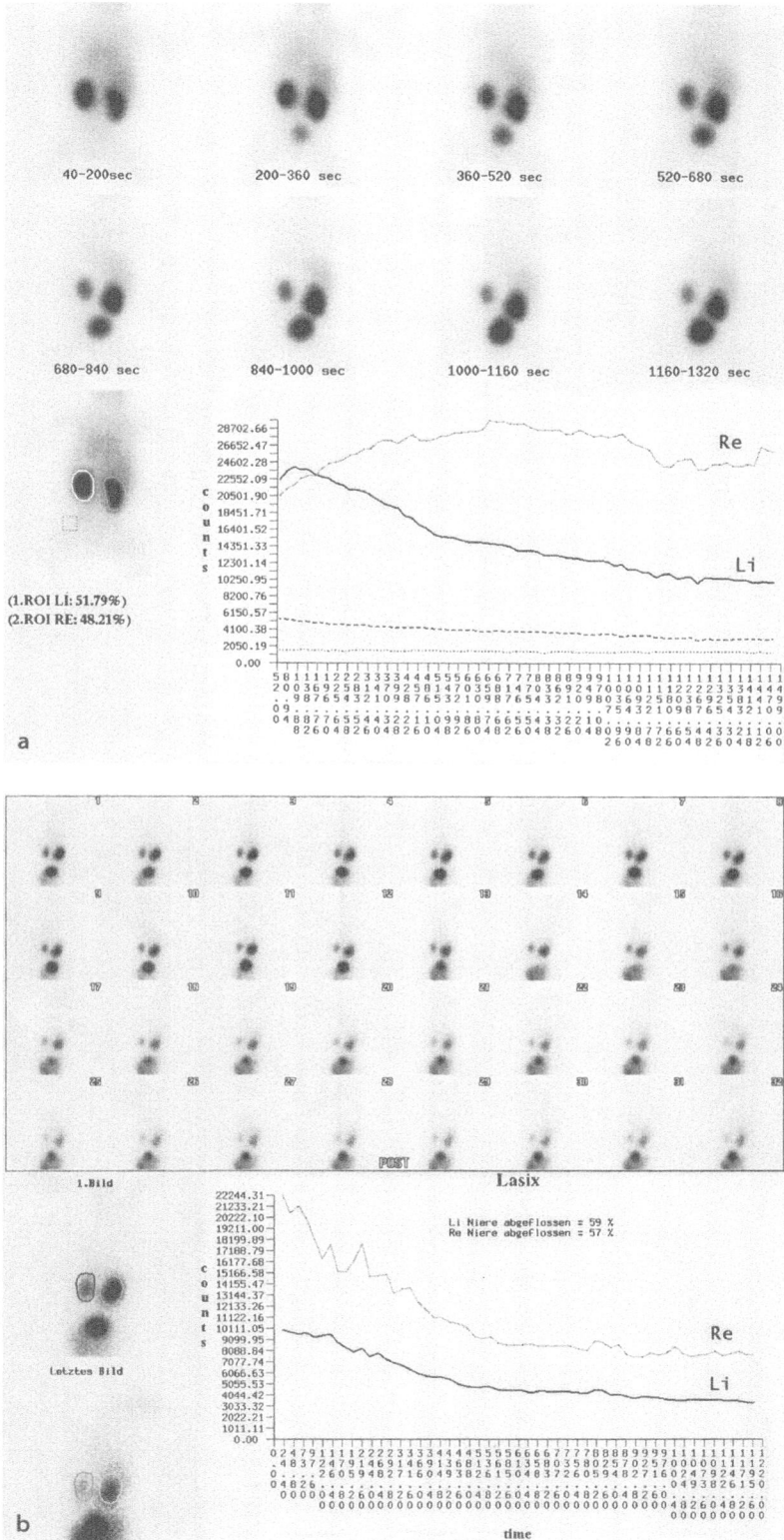

Fig. 12.2 a, b. First ^{99m}Tc-MAG$_3$ scan. **a** The split function of the affected kidney is preserved (48%). **b** The tracer is shown to have accumulated in the pelvicalyceal system, but the diuretic response is normal with decline of the time–activity curve by 50% within 10 min

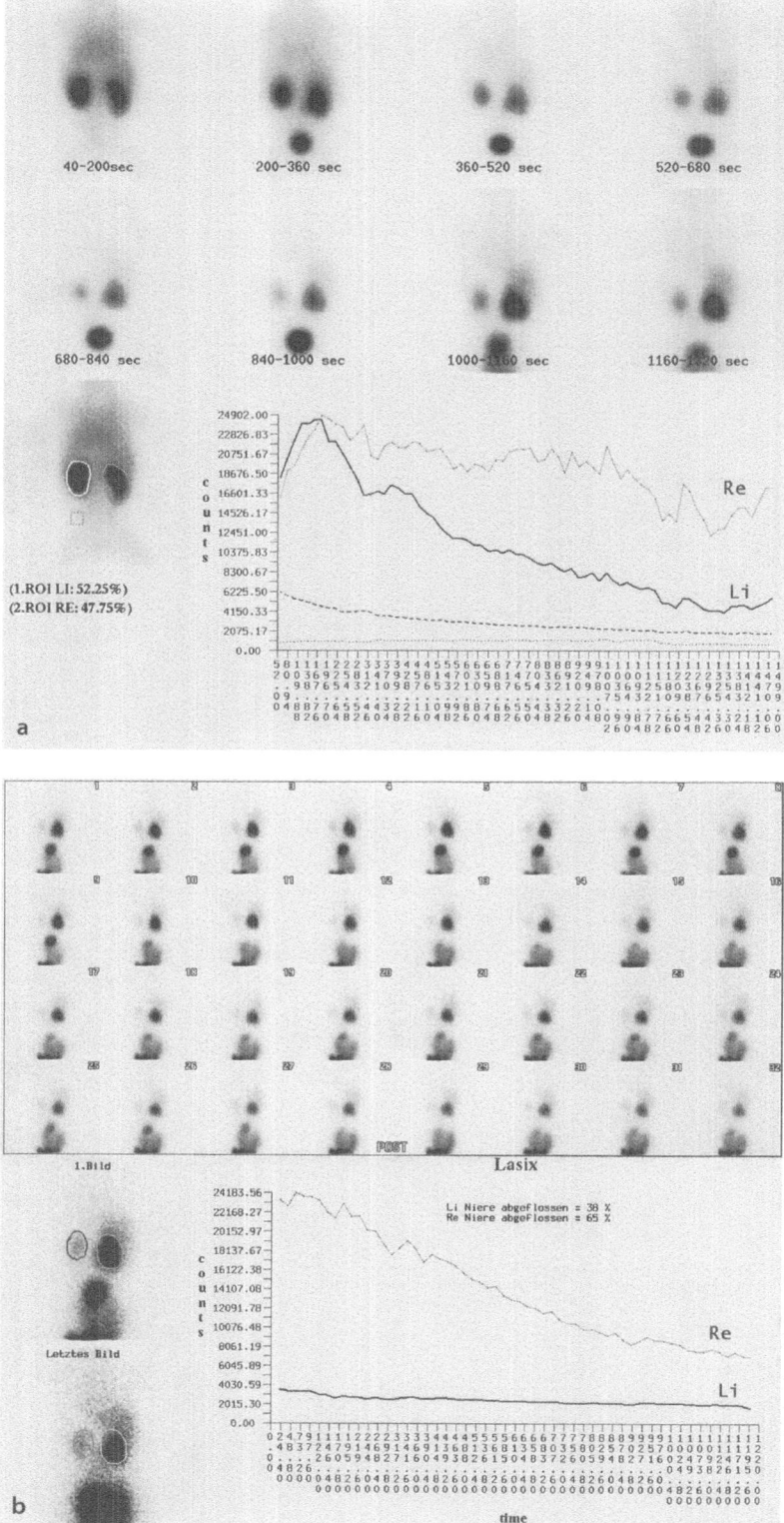

Fig. 12.4a, b. The ⁹⁹ᵐTc-MAG₃ scan during follow-up. The function of the right kidney is well preserved, with no significant change since the first scintigraphy. **a** Although there is an accumulation of the tracer in the pelvicalyceal system on the right side, the drainage during the excretion phase of the study has improved. **b** The furosemide response excludes obstruction (55% fall of the time–activity curve within 10 min)

CASE 13 ▶ *Intermittent Colics with Macrohaematuria Due to Extrinsic Subpelvic Stenosis*

Clinical Course: Surgical correction of hypospadias had been peformed in this boy during early childhood. When he was 16 years old painless haematuria developed, followed by a renal colic.

Nephroliths and glomerulonephritis were subsequently excluded. On sonography we found ectasia of the extra- and intrarenal drainage system on the right side (Fig. 13.1). The renal parenchyma was well preserved.

Besides slight impression of the proximal right ureter, the intravenous pyelogram exhibited no major pathologic findings (Fig. 13.2). The ^{99m}Tc-MAG$_3$ scintigraphy and the furosemide study (Fig. 13.3) revealed an indeterminate pattern. The split function of the right kidney was preserved. The ^{99m}Tc-MAG$_3$ scan was repeated 9 months later because renal colics persisted. We found no change in the partial function, and the furosemide-study did not confirm any relevant obstruction (Fig. 13.4).

The MRI urography confirmed dilatation of the right renal pelvis (Fig. 13.5). No abnormalities were seen in the renal parenchyma. MR angiography with gadopentetate dimeglumine showed normal renal arteries and a right polar artery, atypically situated behind the caval vein and the renal pelvis leading to the lower right pole (Fig. 13.6). An extrinsic subpelvic narrowing was also seen on the retrograde pyelogram (Fig. 13.7).

Comment: In this case an extrinsic subpelvic stenosis due to an aberrant vessel was the most probable diagnosis to explain the child's intermittent colics. MR angiography is the procedure of choice for the diagnosis if a vascular malformation is suggested as a cause hydronephrosis.

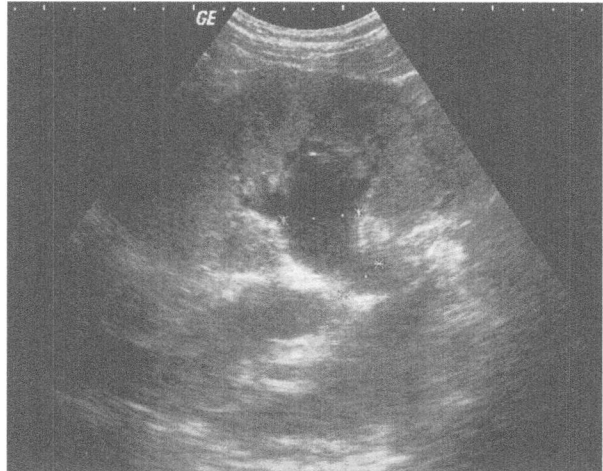

Fig. 13.1. The initial sonography (longitudinal section) of the right kidney demonstrates significant hydonephrosis

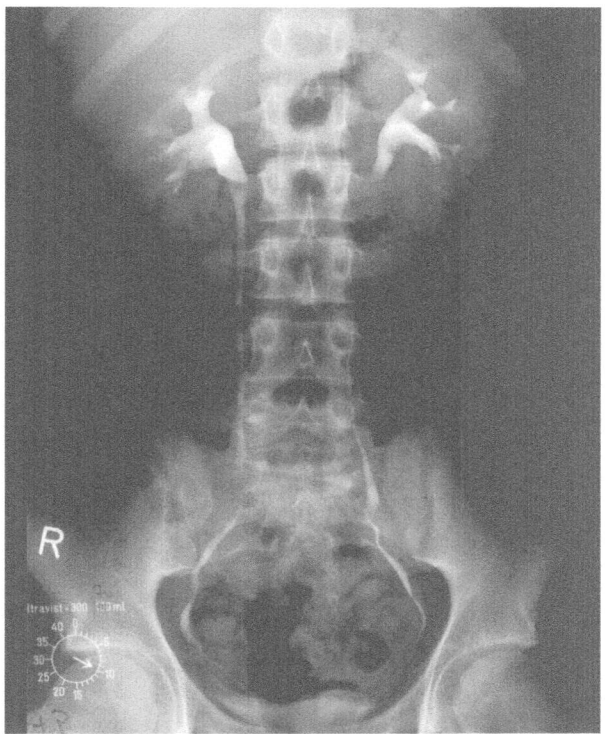

Fig. 13.2. The pyelogram shows a subpelvic impression of the ureter suggestive of an extrinsic narrowing by an aberrant vessel

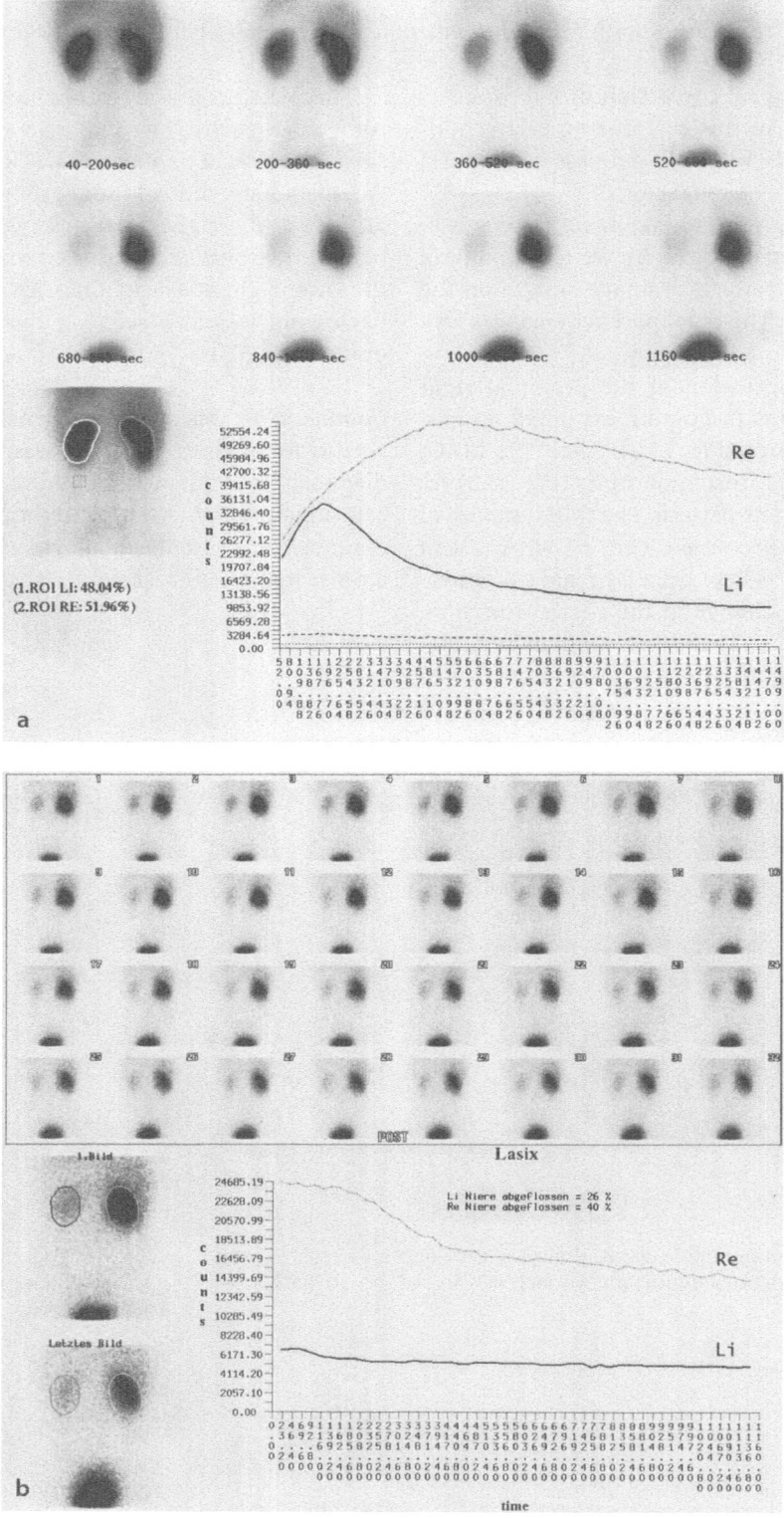

Fig. 13.3. a ^{99m}Tc-MAG$_3$ scan shows a normal split function of the right kidney, with an accumulation of tracer but a spontaneous fall of the time–activity curve during the first 20 min. **b** This pattern is not suggestive of obstruction, although the furosemide study gives an indeterminate result

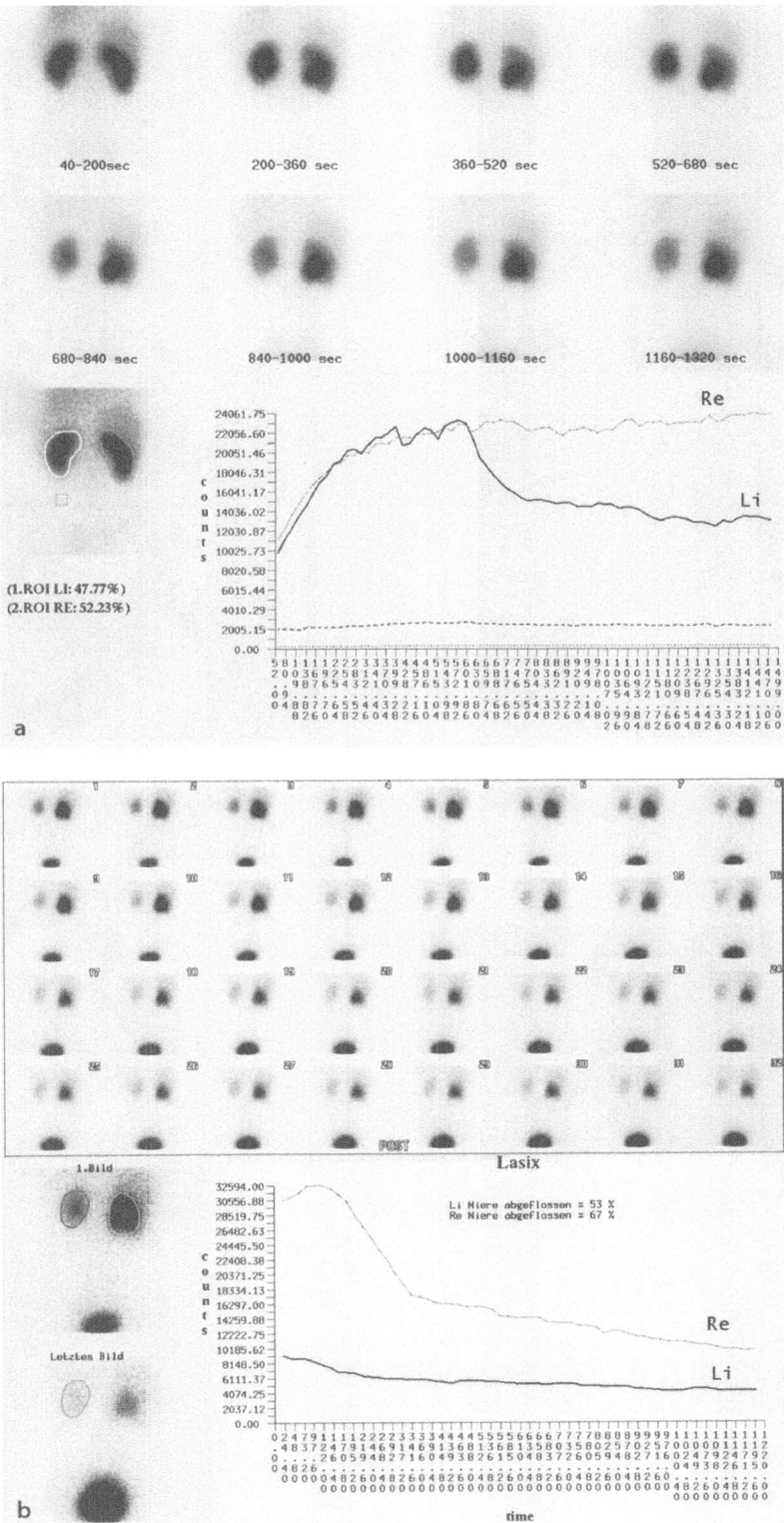

Fig. 13.4. a On the repeat ^{99m}Tc-MAG$_3$ scan 9 months later than that of Fig. 13.3, no change in the partial function can be found. **b** The furosemide study did not show an obstructive pattern

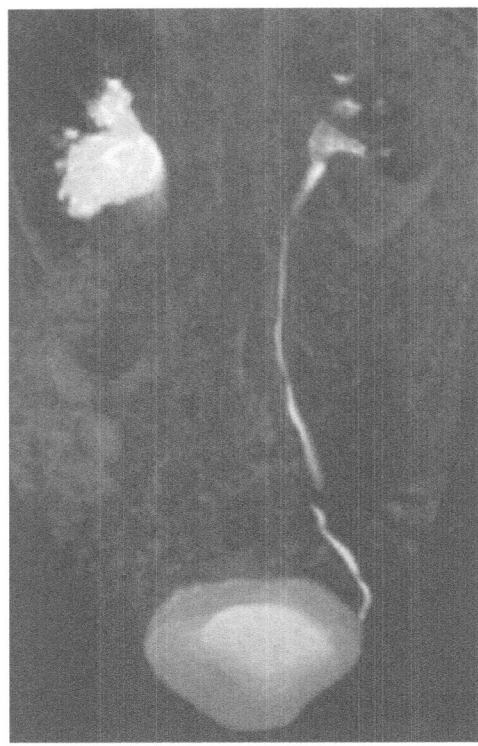

Fig. 13.5. MR urography reveals hydronephrosis of the intra- and extrarenal pelvis

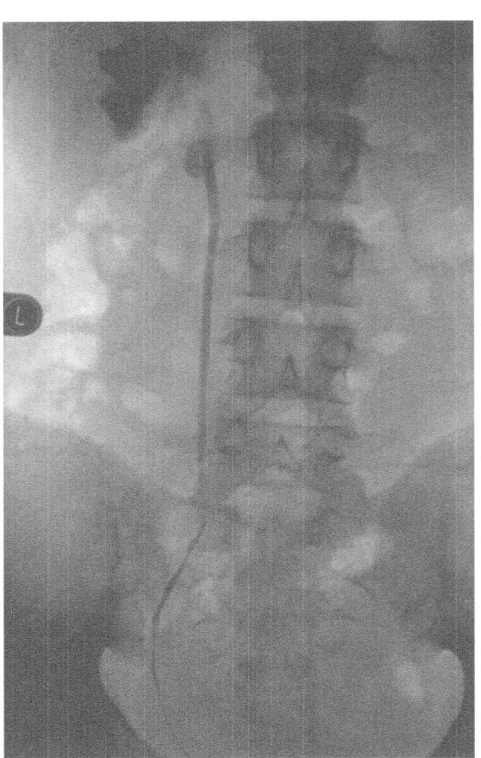

Fig. 13.7. On the retrograde pyelogram the ureter looks normal below the pyelo-ureteral junction but shows an extrinsic subpelvic narrowing due to the vascular malformation confirmed by MR angiography

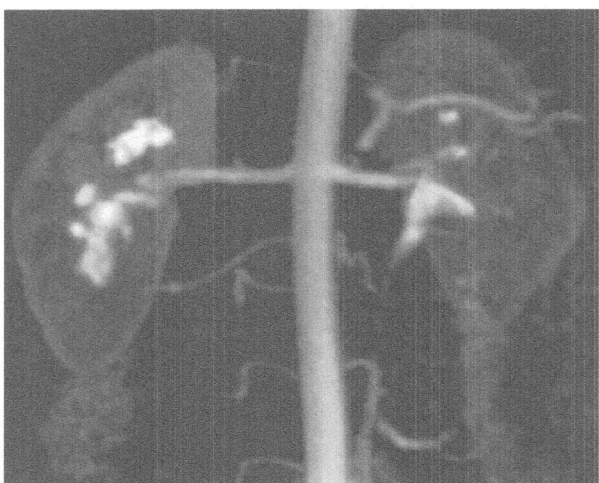

Fig. 13.6. MR angiography shows normal renal arteries and a right polar artery atypically situated behind the vena cava and the renal pelvis leading to the right lower pole

CASE 14 ▶ *Prune Belly Syndrome (Unilateral Manifestation)*

Clinical Course: In this boy a dilatation of the right urinary tract had already noted on the prenatal sonography (Fig. 14.1). The child was born by a caesarian section during the 36th week of gestation and was immediately transferred to the paediatric department. The child's right abdominal wall was flabby without a palpable tumour. In addition we noted bilateral cryptorchidism.

An unusually large urinary bladder was seen on the first postnatal sonography. A slight thickening of the bladder wall was present. The left kidney looked normal, while the right kidney exhibited a dilatation of the drainage system combined with a thin parenchyma. The combination of abdominal muscle deficiency, cryptorchidism and hydroureter/hydronephrosis was in keeping with prune belly syndrome (Fig. 14.2).

On the 5th day we performed intravenous pyelography (Fig. 14.3), which demonstrated an extremely dilated right drainage system. Besides a dilated distal ureter no urological abnormalities were recognized on the contralateral side. The bladder has also a pathologic configuration.

We started antibiotic prophylaxis. When the child was 6 months old we performed a ^{99m}Tc-MAG$_3$ scan, which exhibited normal split function without evidence of obstruction. During his further clinical course the boy developed well and no urinary tract infection occurred. Physiotherapy led to a maturation of the hypoplastic abdominal wall. When he was $2^1/_2$ years old the cryptorchidism was surgically corrected by autotransplantation of the testicles, which were found near the iliac vessels.

In subsequent years the boy developed a steadily increasing bladder capacity and residual urine. We performed voiding cysto-urethrography and found an large bladder with irregular margins, which raised the suspicion of an apical diverticulum. No spontaneous micturition was possible during the procedure, so that the urethra could not be investigated (Fig. 14.4). Following the catheterization the boy developed his first urinary tract infection. We started micturition training together with medical therapy, but it did not prove possible to achieve reduction of the residual urine. In addition, progressive dilatation of the right drainage system was noted (Fig. 14.5). Beginning at the age of 12 intermittent catheterization of the urinary bladder became necessary, which was successful as sonographic monitoring showed a decrease in the right-sided hydronephrosis (Fig. 14.6). The ^{99m}Tc-MAG$_3$ scan at this time showed no deterioration of the right kidney function (Fig. 14.7 a). The response of the time–activity curve to furosemide was pathologic, probably due to a full bladder at the beginning of diuretic scintigraphy (Fig. 14.7 b). During puberty the boy developed normally.

Comment: This is an unusual case of unilateral prunc belly syndrome. Intermittent catheterization is necessary to prevent complications due to megacystis. The kidney function was preserved during the years, and following autotransplantation of the testicles normal genital maturation has taken place.

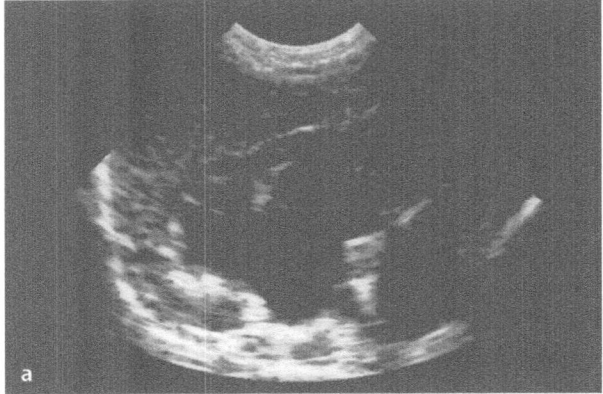

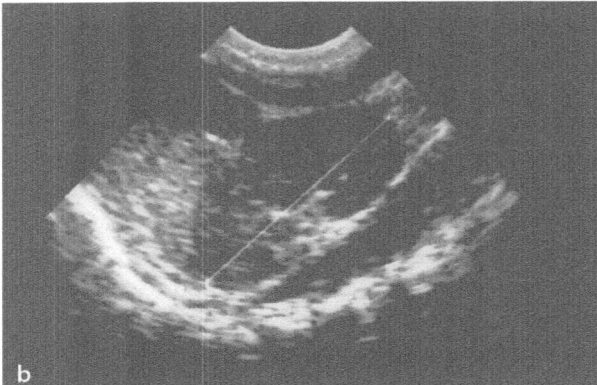

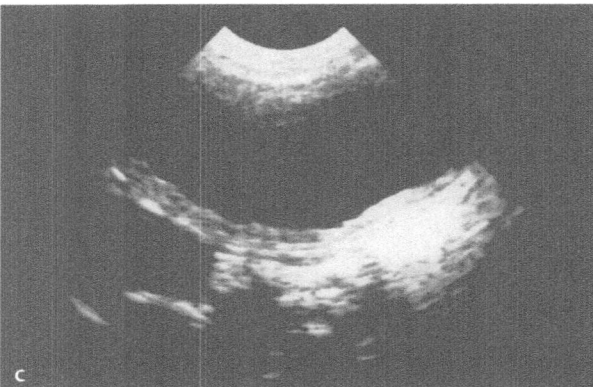

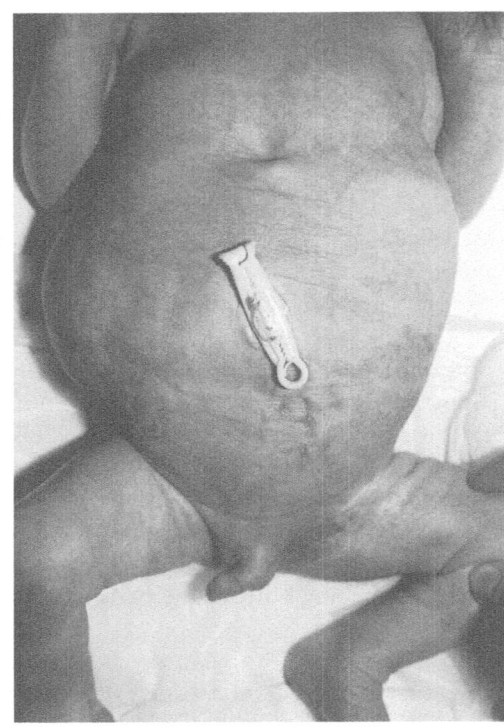

Fig. 14.2. Extensive distension of the abdominal wall and bilateral cryptorchidism are typical of prune belly syndrome

Fig. 14.1 a–c. Sonographic examinations during the first days of the boy's life. **a** Right kidney (longitudinal section): dilatation of the renal pelvis and thinning of the parenchyma. **b** The left kidney looks normal. **c** Transverse section of the urinary bladder, showing thickening of the bladder wall. A dilated distal ureter can be noted paravesically on the right side

▶

Fig. 14.3. Intravenous pyelography: the pyelogram shows extreme dilatation of the right drainage system. A dilatation of the distal ureter on the contralateral side is present. The urinary bladder is suggestive of a diverticulum of the bladder dome

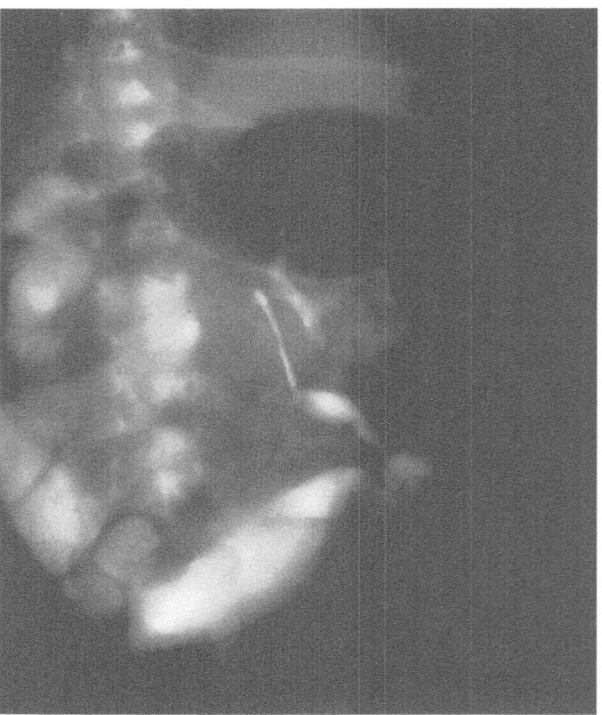

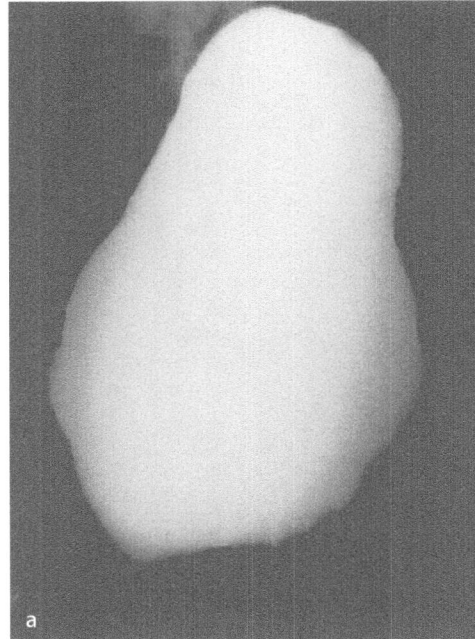

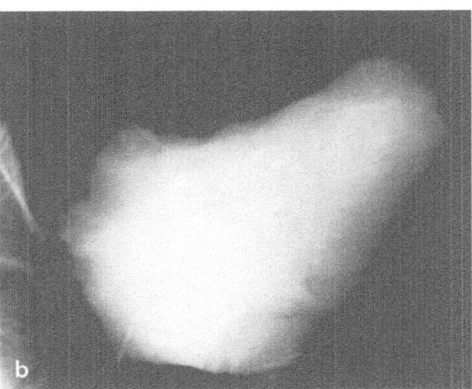

Fig. 14.4 a, b. Voiding cysto-urethrography performed at the age of 6. The bladder is enlarged and shows irregular margins

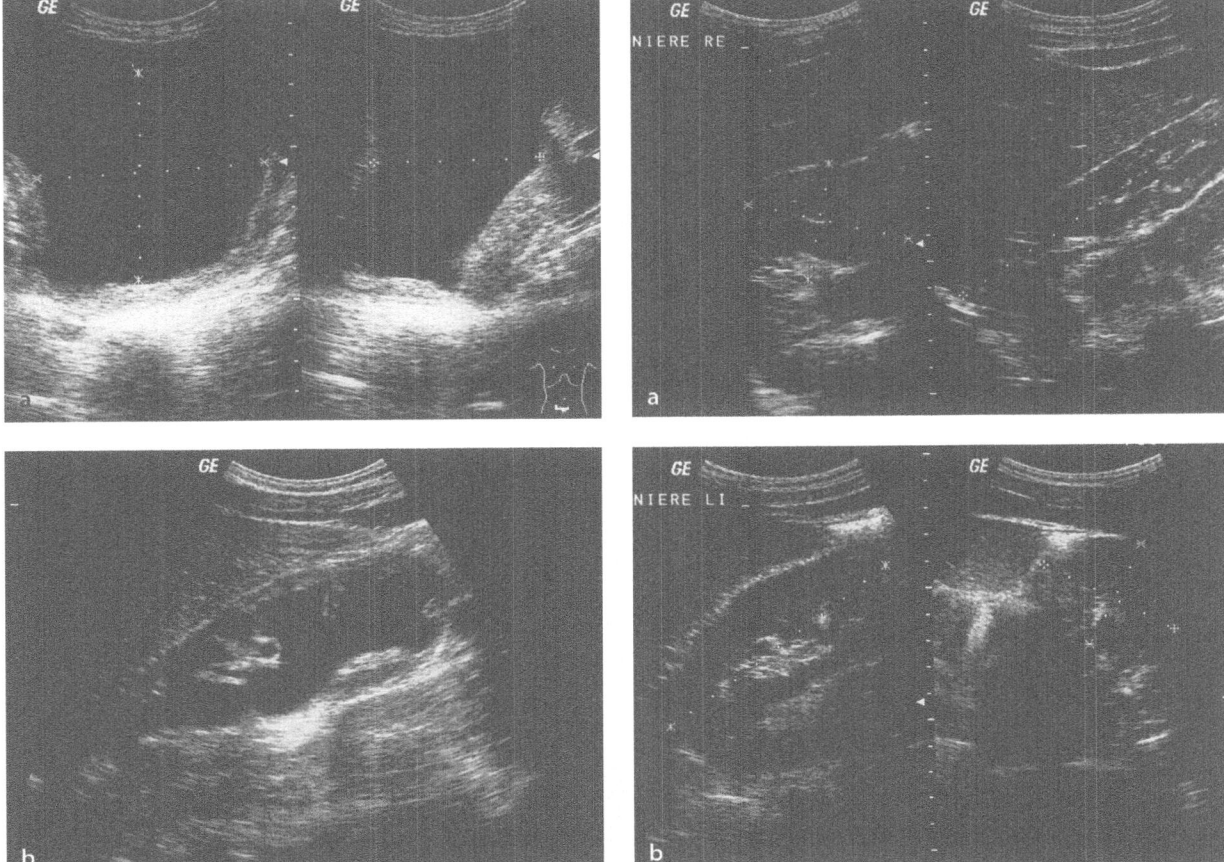

Fig. 14.5. a Large quantities of residual urine (124 ml) are present in the urinary bladder after micturition. **b** The right-sided drainage system is dilated

Fig. 14.6. a Following intermittent catherization, the dilatation of the right renal pelvis clearly decreases. **b** Sonography at the age of 11: normal appearance of the left kidney

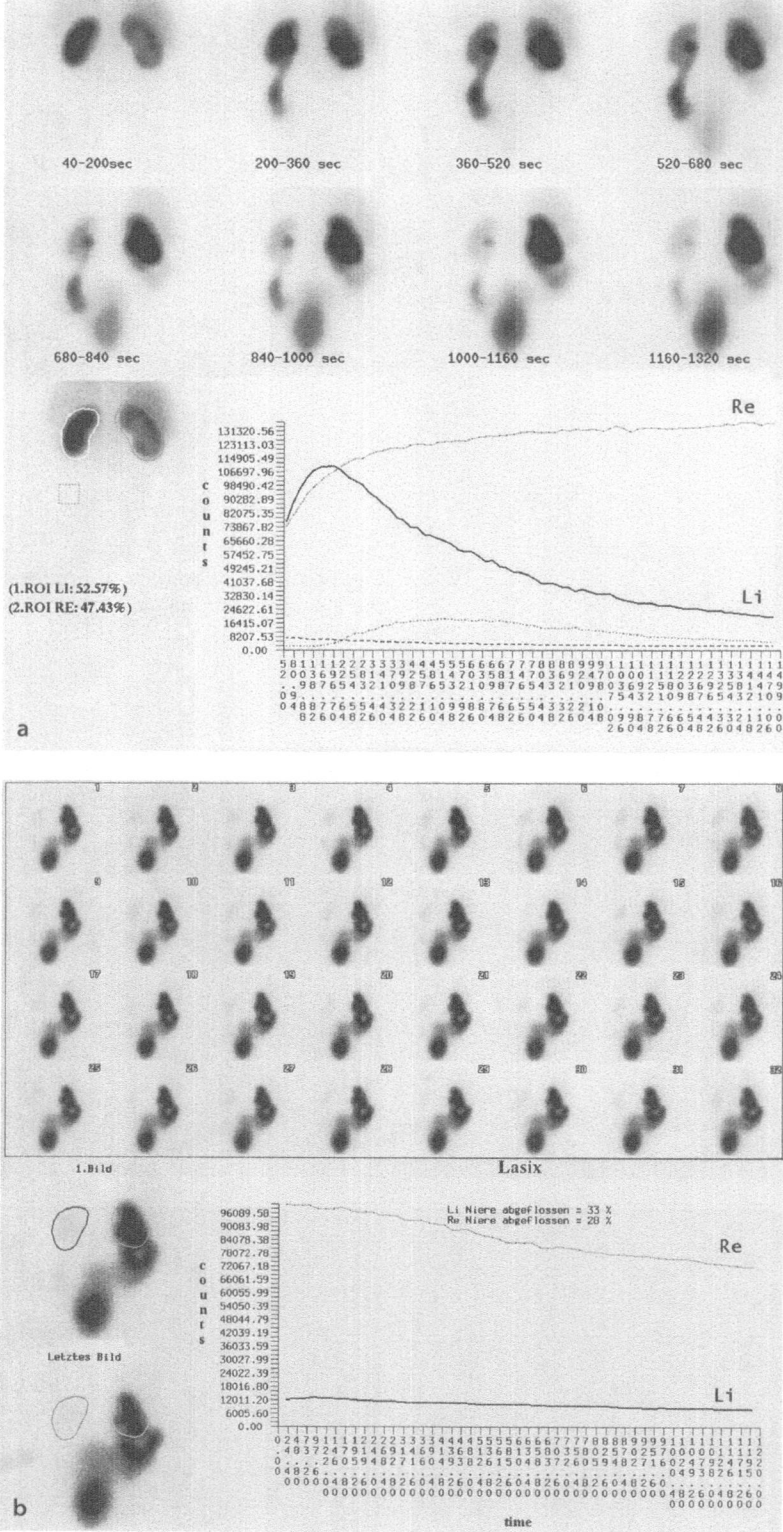

Fig. 14.7a, b. ^{99m}Tc-MAG$_3$ scan. **a** The function of both kidneys is well preserved. The split function is normal. **b** False-positive diuretic scintgraphy, probably due to a full bladder during the study

CASE 15 ▶ *Obstructive Megaureter*

Clinical Course: Hydronephrosis on the left side had already been diagnosed prenatally by US. Amniorrhexis of the mother led to the child's birth during the 37th week. The newborn was hospitalized in the paediatric department with a suspected neonatal infection. We found bacterial colonization of the skin with group B β-haemolytic streptococci and no bacterial growth on blood or urine cultures.

The first US was performed on the first postnatal day. The distal left ureter was extensively dilated (Fig. 15.1a, b). A normal right kidney (Fig. 15.1c) was present. The whole left upper urinary tract was dilated and thinning of the left kidney parenchyma could be noted (Fig. 15.1d–f). Repeated sonography (Fig. 15.2) gave similar results. We performed voiding cysto-urethrography on the 14th postnatal day. No abnormalities of the urethra were seen. The contrast media refluxed in a large dilated left ureter, while no reflux was found on the contralateral side. Additionally a Hutches' diverticulum was seen (Fig. 15.3).

Following this procedure it was decided to wait, on the assumption of a refluxing megaureter. During follow-up, after 4 weeks persistent dilatation of the whole left drainage system was noted (Fig. 15.2).

^{99m}Tc-MAG$_3$-scintigraphy was performed in the boy's first week of life. While the perfusion and function of the right kidney were normal, the function of the left kidney was heavily impaired (Fig. 15.4). A ^{99m}Tc-MAG$_3$ scan was performed 4 weeks postnatally to determine the split function of the left dysplastic kidney, which was found to be only 14%.

When the boy was 6 weeks old, antegrade pyelography via a percutaneous drainage of the left renal pelvis was performed (Fig. 15.5). A filamentous constriction of the left sided megaureter was diagnosed and therefore gave evidence for primary obstruction of the drainage system. The drainage had to be removed subsequently owing to a dislocation 4 weeks later. Although antibiotic prophylaxis was continued, an upper urinary tract infection later occurred.

Although severe dysplasia of the left kidney with a poor residual function was present, it was decided to perform reimplantation of the left ureter, to prevent further urinary tract infections and to preserve the function of the left kidney. Surgery according to Politano-Leadbetter combined with modelling of the left ureter was performed when the boy was 3 months old.

Following surgical correction, MAG$_3$ scintigraphy was repeated and showed that the function of the left kidney had not deteriorated further (Fig. 15.6). On ultrasound the calyceal system of the left kidney was only slightly dilated at this time.

Comment: Reflux of a megaureter does not exclude additional obstruction Fig. 15.7. Early surgical correction in this boy helped to prevent further urinary tract infections and to preserve the kidney's residual function.

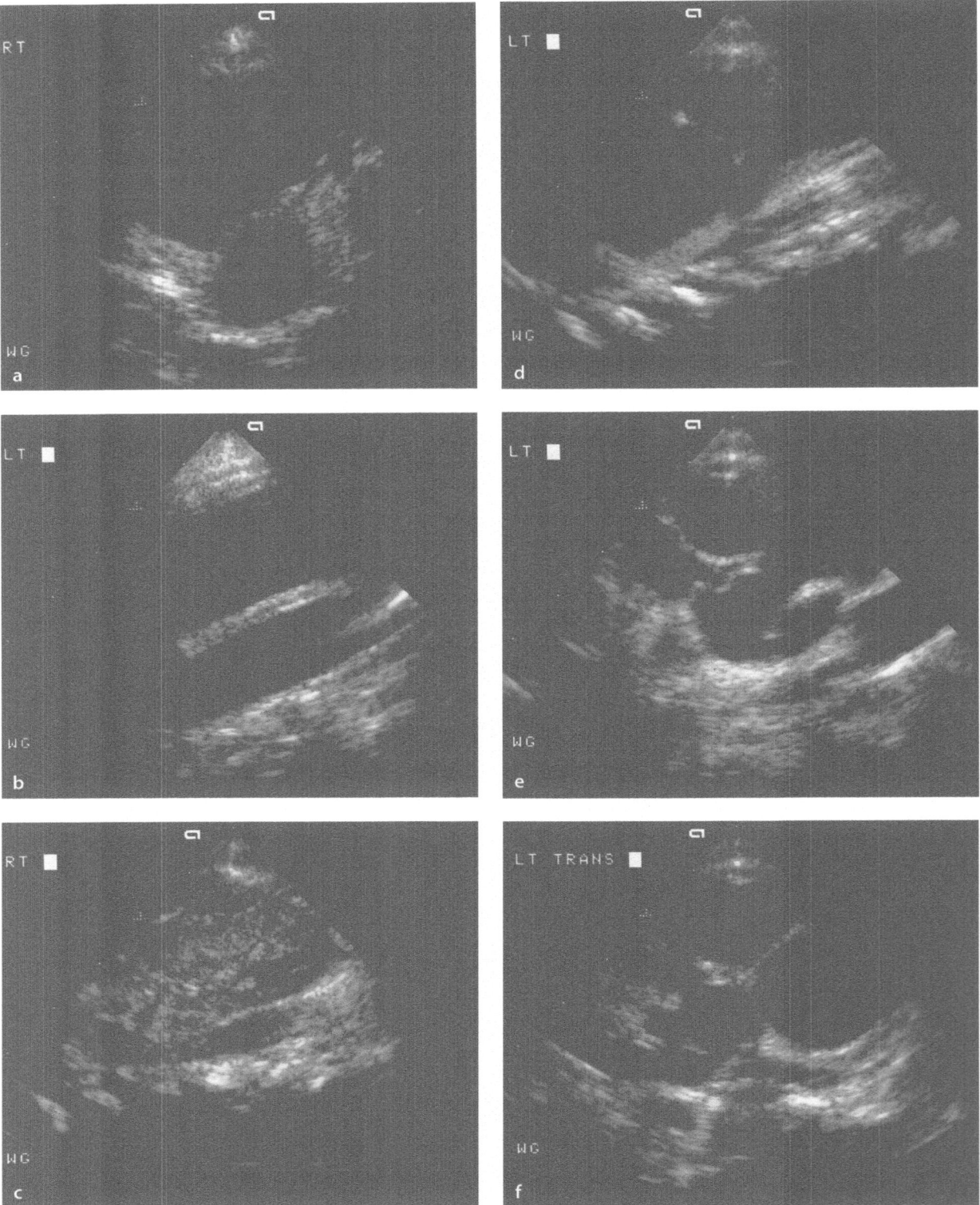

Fig. 15.1 a–f. Sonography during the boy's first day. **a, b** The distal left ureter is extensively dilated (**a** transverse section, **b** longitudinal section). **c** A normal right kidney (longitudinal section) is present. **d–f** Dilatation of the whole left upper urinary tract and thinning of parenchyma of left kidney

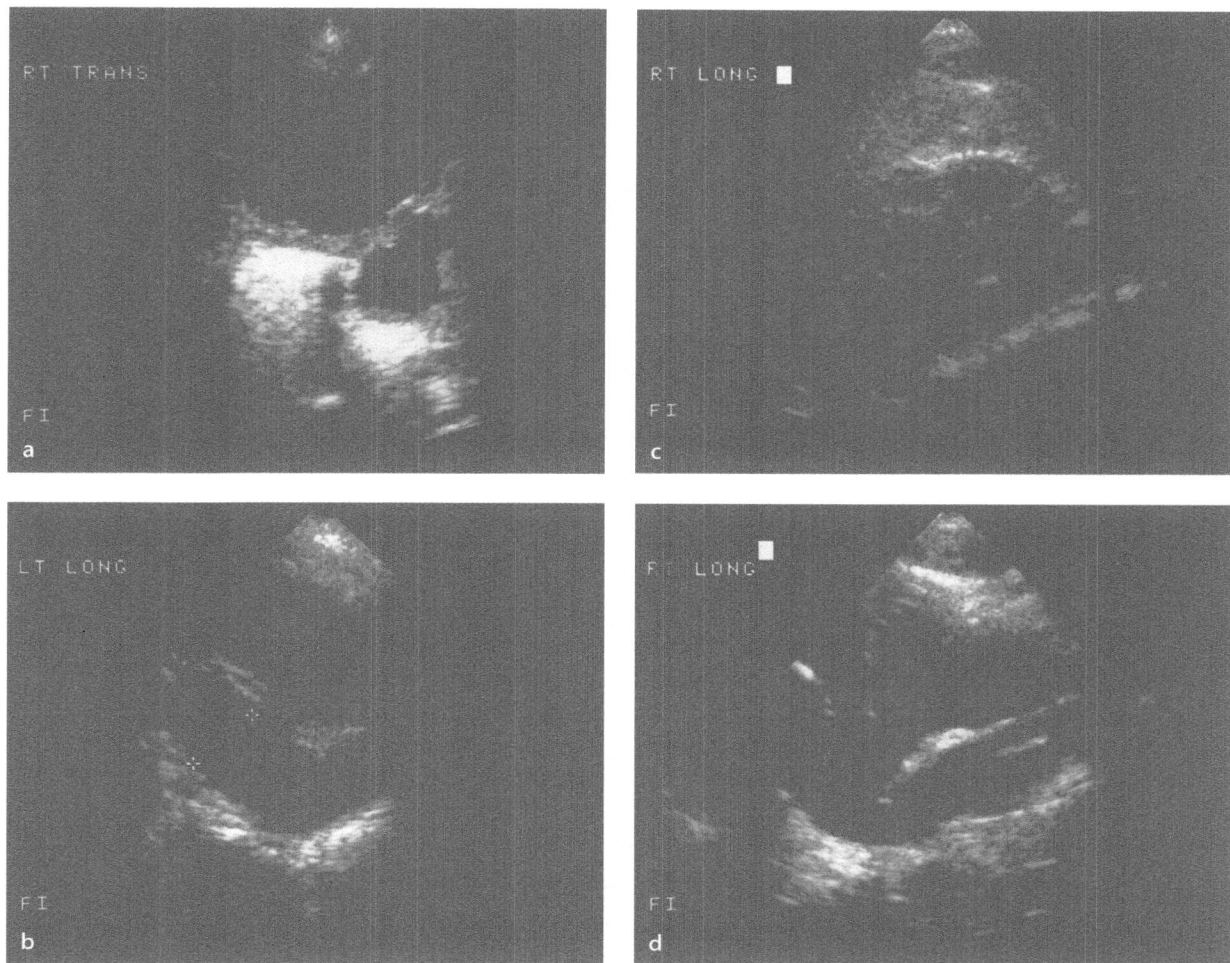

Fig. 15.2 a–d. Sonography 4 weeks later. **a, b** Persistent massive dilatation of the left ureter is seen paravesically. **c** The right kidney appears normal. **d** The left kidney exhibits marked dilatation of the calyces

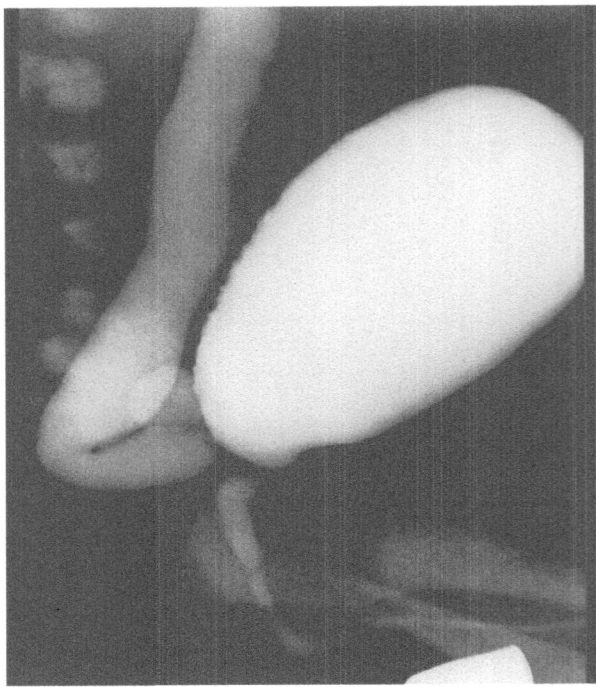

Fig. 15.3. Reflux into the left megaureter demonstrated on the voiding cysto-urethrogram. The presence of a Hutches' diverticulum can be noted in a paravesical position

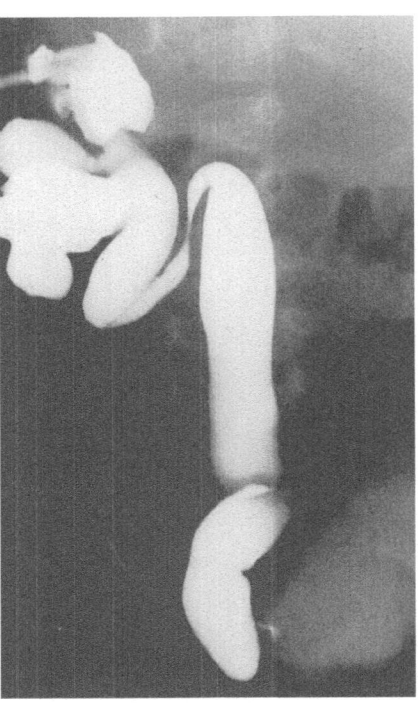

Fig. 15.5. Antegrade pyelography via percutaneous drainage of the left renal pelvis. A filamentous constriction of the megaureter was diagnosed, giving evidence of primary obstruction of the drainage system

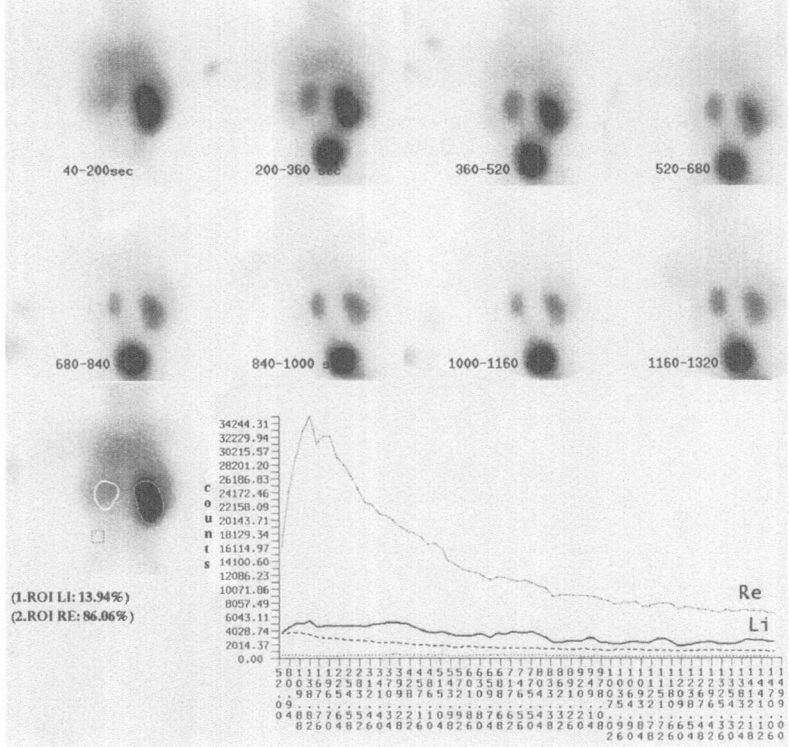

Fig. 15.4. The split renal function of the left kidney on ^{99m}Tc-MAG$_3$ scintigraphy during the first examination was only 14%. The right kidney appeared hypertrophic on the scan

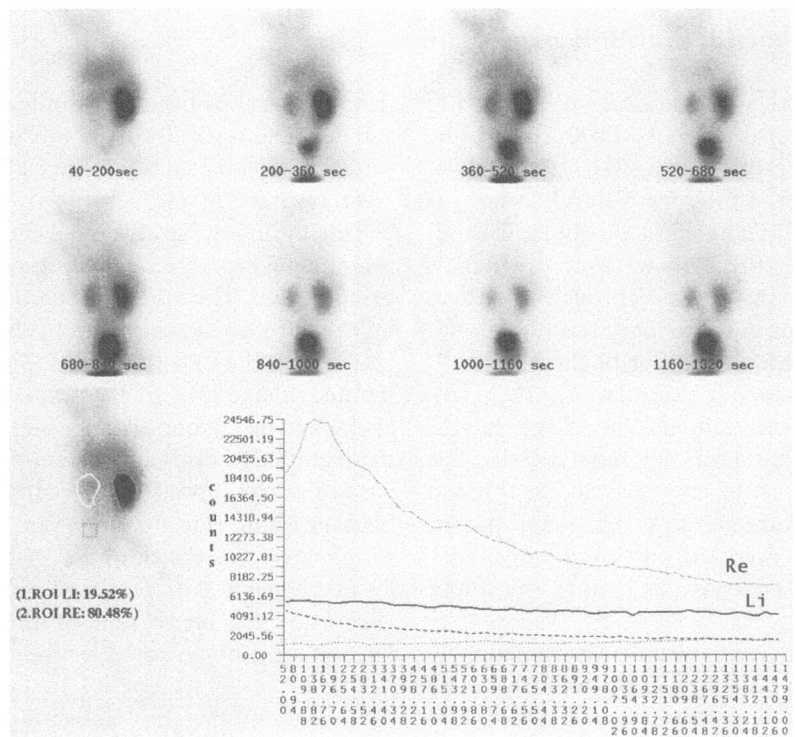

40–200sec

200–360 sec

360–520 sec

520–680 sec

680–840 sec

840–1000 sec

1000–1160 sec

1160–1320 sec

(1.ROI LI: 19.52%)
(2.ROI RE: 80.48%)

▲
Fig. 15.6. The split renal function of the left kidney on ^{99m}Tc-MAG$_3$ scintigraphy during postsurgical examination was 19% and thus had not deteriorated further

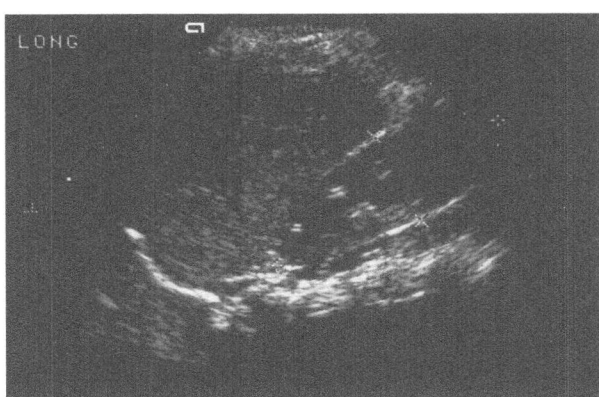

◄
Fig. 15.7. Sonography following surgical correction (longitudinal section): the calyceal system of the left kidney is only moderately dilated

CASE 16 ▶ *Congenital Bilateral Megaureter*

Clinical Course: In this boy, dilatation of the left ureter and the left renal pelvis had been prenatally diagnosed by sonography during the 31st week of pregnancy. Dilatation of the contralateral ureter was recognized antenatally. The child was born without complications during the 39th week of pregnancy. Two other children in the family were healthy with no known malformations of the urinary tract.

The first sonography 24 h after birth showed dilatation of both ureters (Fig. 16.1 a–c). The right kidney exhibited massive dilatation of the calyces and moderate dilatation of the renal pelvis. The parenchyma on this side appeared to be thinned (Fig. 16.1 d, e). Contralaterally, the renal parenchyma was well preserved and only moderate dilatation of the extrarenal pelvis (11.3 mm) was found (Fig. 16.1 f).

Postnatal antibiotic prophylaxis was immediately started. We performed voiding cysto-urethrography on the 7th postnatal day. Subvesical obstruction, a urethral value, and VUR were subsequently ruled out by this procedure (Fig. 16.2). ^{99m}Tc-MAG$_3$ scintigraphy was performed when the boy was 1 month old. The split function of the kidneys was within the normal range. Although serum creatinine levels were normal, renoparenchymal transit of the tracer was delayed, perhaps because of immaturity of the renal tubules. The renal drainage was well preserved with no signs of obstruction, especially during diuretic scintigraphy (Fig. 16.3 a, b).

During follow-up the renal retention parameters remained within the normal range and the child developed well. The width of the pelvicalyceal system on the left side decreased and subsequently normalized within the first 10 months. The distal ureters remained dilated (Fig. 16.4). On sonography performed at the age of 13 months only moderate dilatation of the right-sided drainage system was noted. The paravesical ureters could not be visualized owing to poor bladder filling (Fig. 16.4). At this time the antibiotic prophylaxis was discontinued. A mild hydronephrosis on the right side persisted on repeat sonograms (Fig. 16.5). The boy is now 19 months old and there have so far been no complications.

Comment: In this boy congenital bilaterial megaureter was present. Because this condition had been diagnosed prenatally, early postnatal diagnostic tests could be performed, and these excluded reflux and obstruction. Urinary tract infection could be successfully prevented by antibiotic prophylaxis.

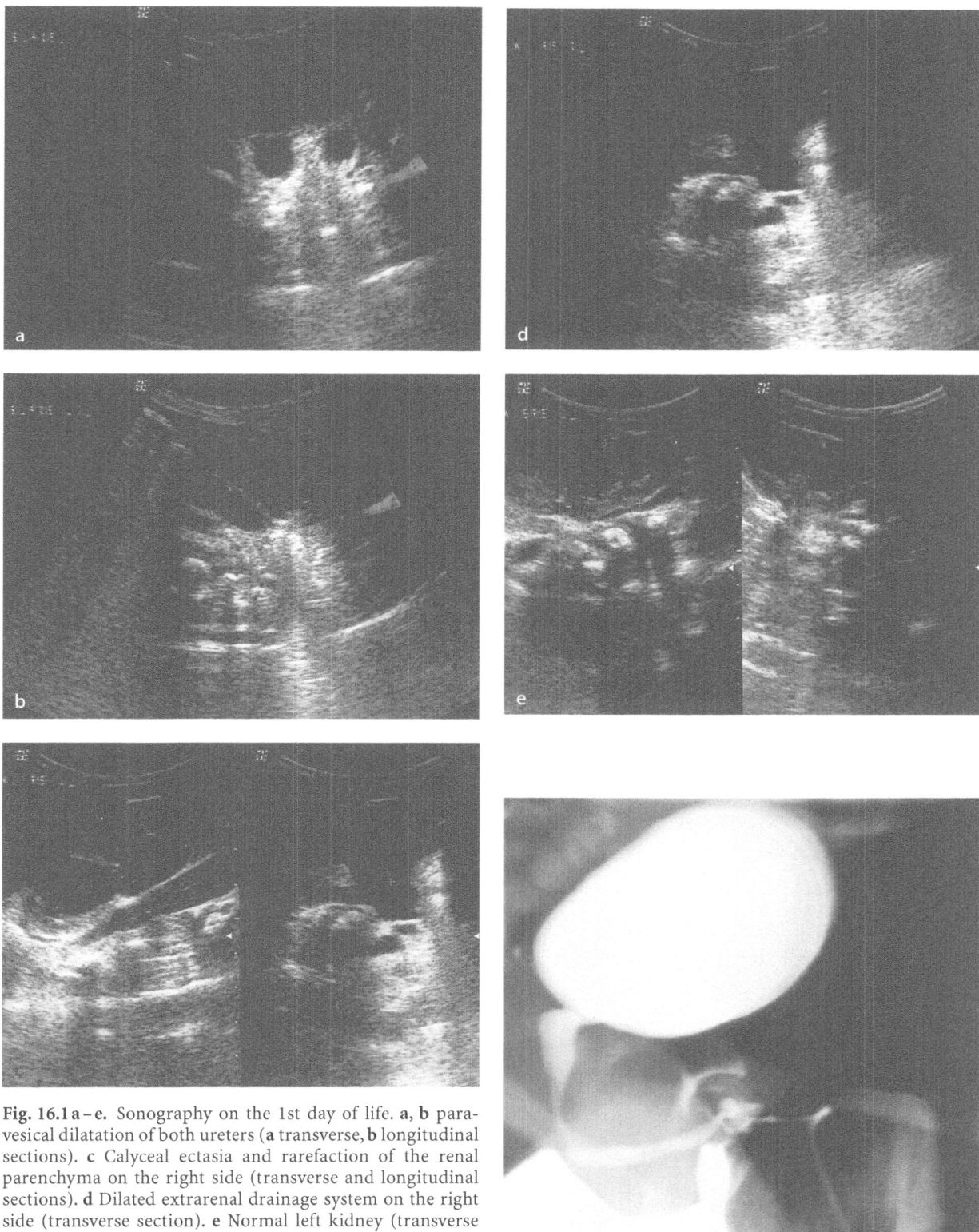

Fig. 16.1 a – e. Sonography on the 1st day of life. **a, b** paravesical dilatation of both ureters (**a** transverse, **b** longitudinal sections). **c** Calyceal ectasia and rarefaction of the renal parenchyma on the right side (transverse and longitudinal sections). **d** Dilated extrarenal drainage system on the right side (transverse section). **e** Normal left kidney (transverse and longitudinal sections)

Fig. 16.2. No reflux can be demonstrated on the voiding cysto-urothrogram. The wall of the bladder looks normal. A urethral valve can be excluded

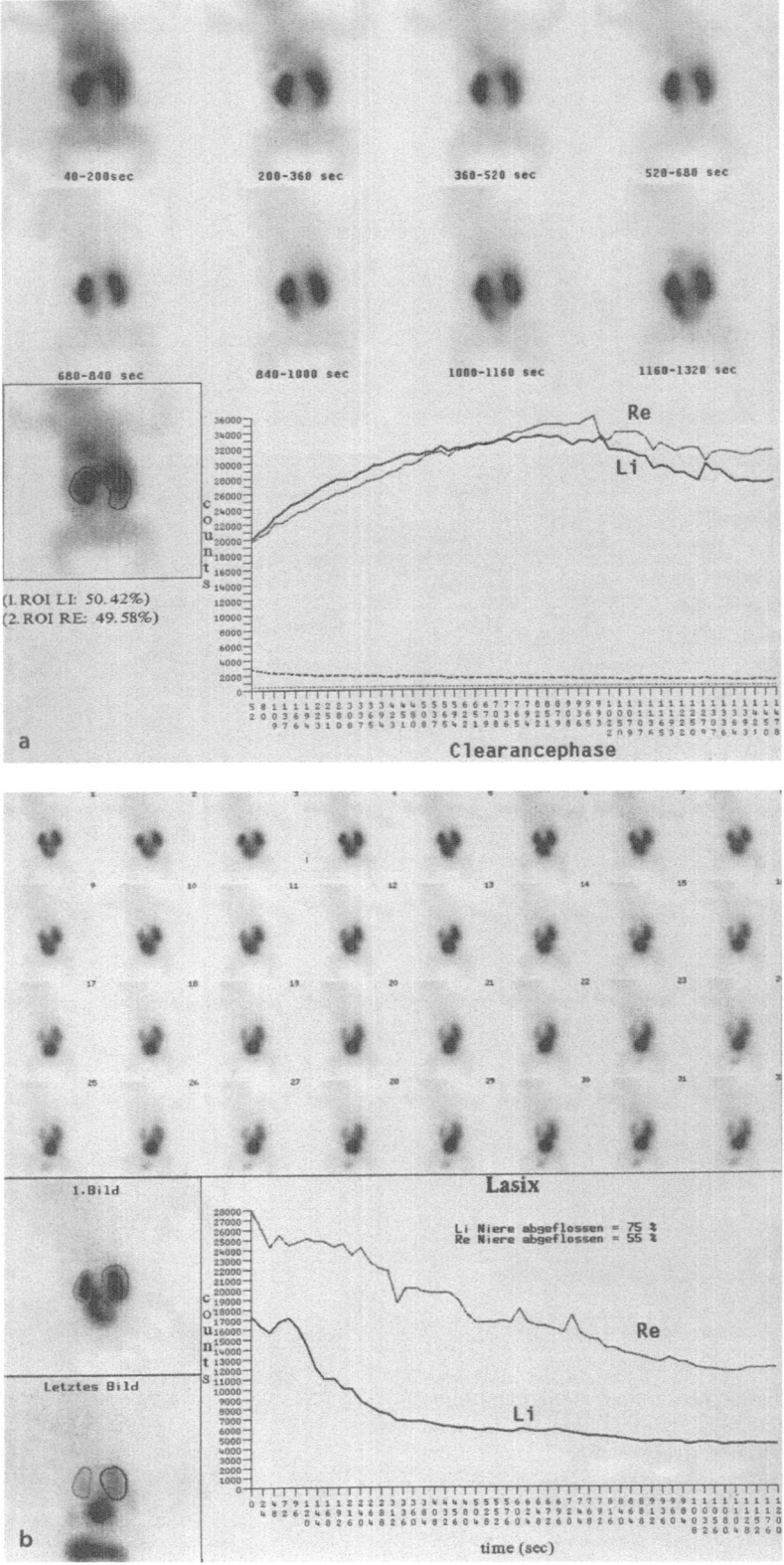

Fig. 16.3 a, b. ^{99m}Tc-MAG$_3$ scintigraphy at the age of 4 weeks: the renoparenchymal transit of the tracer is delayed, perhaps because the renal tubules are immature. The renal drainage is well preserved with no signs of obstruction. During the scintigraphic study, including diuretic scintigraphy, transient retention of ^{99m}Tc-MAG$_3$ was noted in the drainage system on both sides

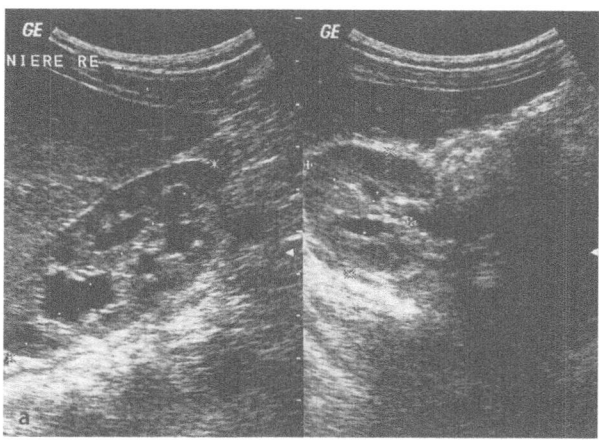

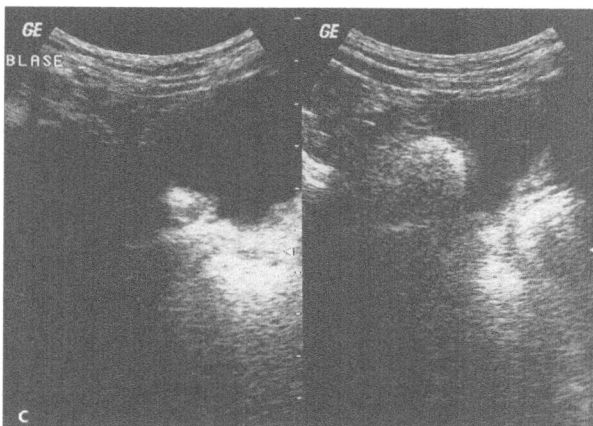

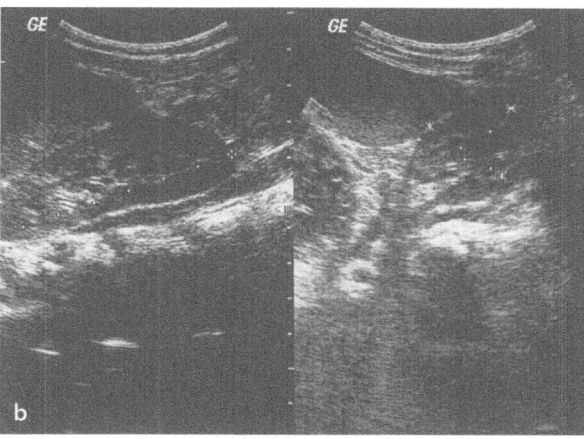

Fig. 16.4a–c. Sonography at the age of 13 months. **a** Hydronephrosis grade III on the right. **b** Normal drainage system on the left side. **c** Poor urinary bladder filling: the ureters are not visible

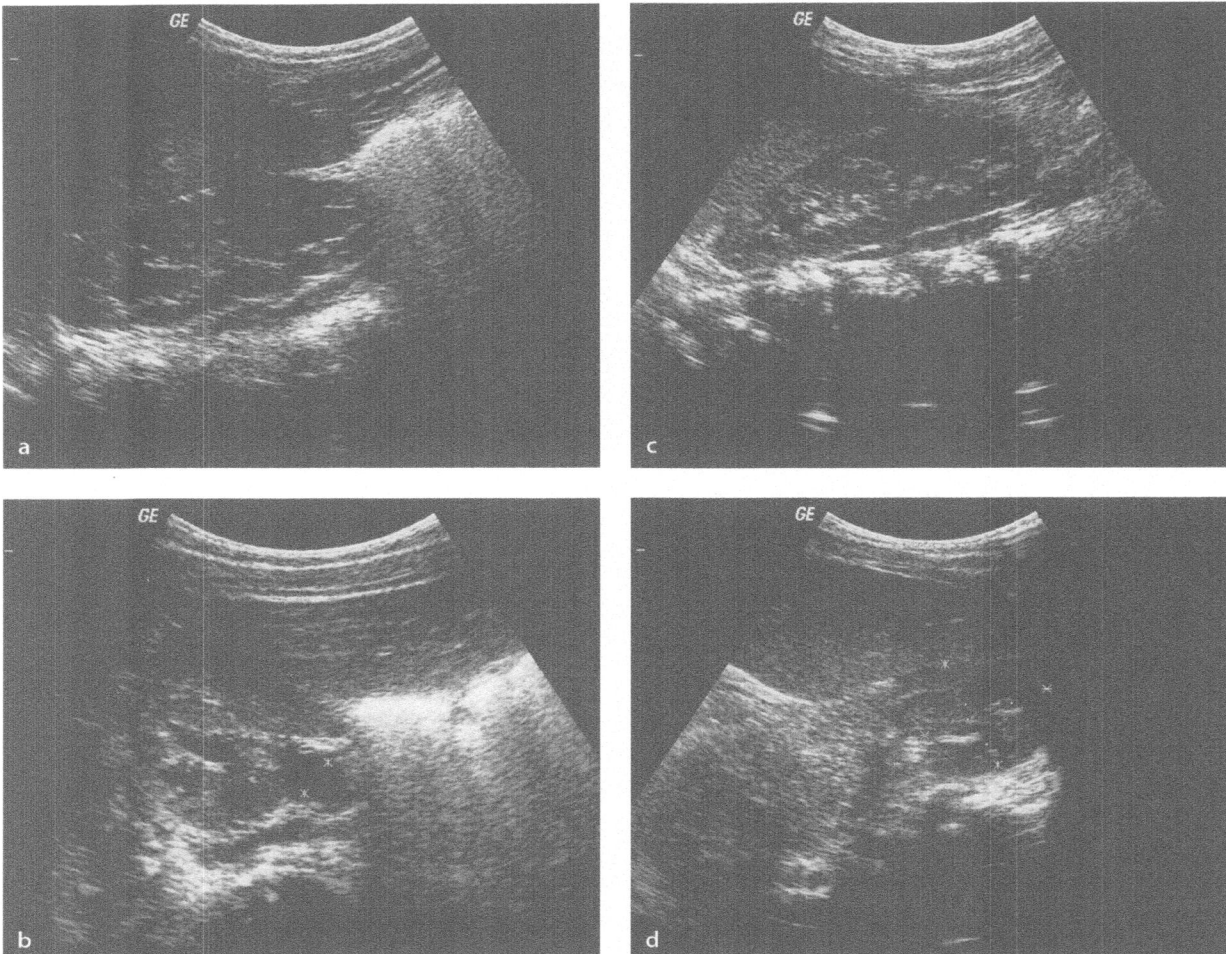

Fig. 16.5a–d. Sonography at the age of 19 months. **a, b** Hydronephrosis grade III on the right. **c, d** Normal left kidney

CASE 17 ▶ *Incontinence Caused by an Ectopic Ureter*

Clinical Course: A girl now 6 years old was admitted to our department with incontinence characterized by continously dribbling of urine. Because of this urological problem, which became evident at the age of 2 years, she had been in medical care since she was 3 years old. At that time a VUR was found by voiding cysto-urethrography. At the same time a left sided renal duplication was recognized on the intravenous pyelogram (Fig. 17.1). Following subureteric collagen injection on the right side, the VUR persisted. The mother of the child reported continous leakage of urine, although a transurethral catheter was left in place after surgery, but this information did not receive any attention.

At the age of 5 years the girl underwent a urodynamic examination, and sphincter-detrusor dyssynergia was diagnosed. A neurogenic bladder, which had been suggested, was subsequently ruled out by MRI. Bladder training was initiated, but proved of no benefit.

The characteristics of this incontinent girl with a suspected renal duplication were highly suggestive for an ectopic ureter as the most likely reason for her incontinence. On ultrasound we found a liquid lesion on the upper pole of the left kidney, most probably reflecting dysplasia (Fig. 17.2). Cystoscopy revealed orthotopic single ureteral orifices on both sides. On retrograde pyelography the renal collecting systems on both sides were completely contrasted, but the additional ureter that had been diagnosed by intravenous pyelography was missed (Fig. 17.3). When the introitus vaginae was inspected, an ectopic ureteral orifice was recognized in the left vaginal wall (Fig. 17.4). Upper pole heminephrectomy was subsequently performed (Fig. 17.5), and afterwards the girl became continent.

Comment: Ectopic ureters result either from a single ureteric bud (single ectopic ureter) or, more often, from a second ureteric bud (in renal duplication). In male subjects ectopic ureters do not lead to incontinence, because the ectopic orifice is always situated cranial to the external sphincter. In girls dribbling urinary incontinence is the main symptom of ectopic ureters, because the ectopic orifices are found distal to the vesical sphincter. If these anatomic realities are not afforded due consideration, many unnecessary examinations and treatment efforts with no benefit will be performed, as in this girl.

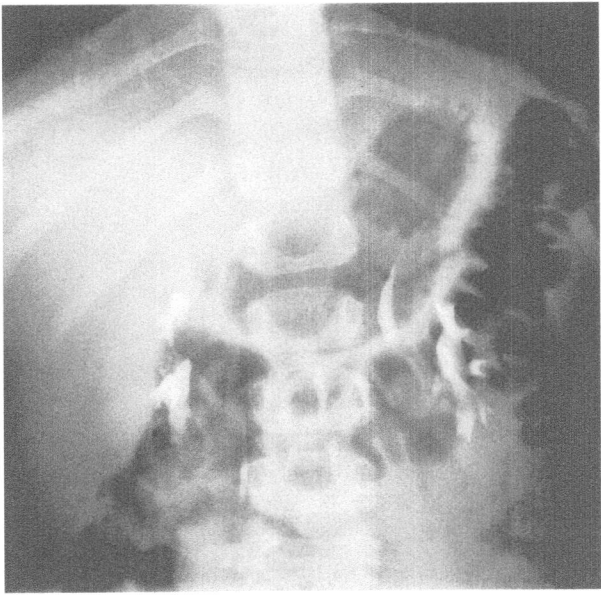

Fig. 17.1. A second ureter on the left side medial to the renal pelvis on the intravenous pyelogram, suggestive of a left sided renal duplication

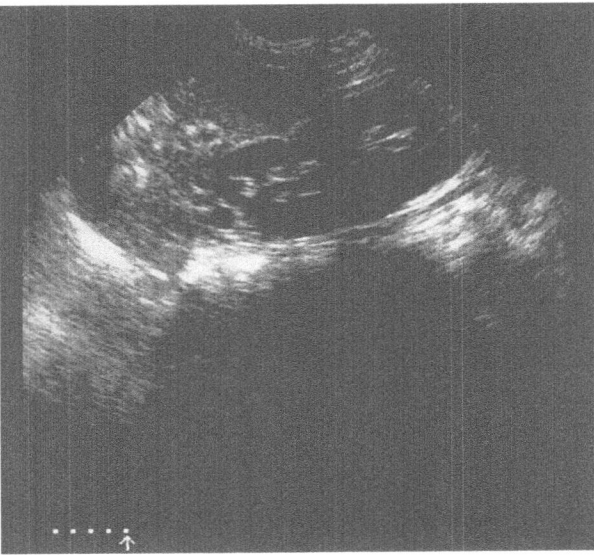

Fig. 17.2. During ultrasonography a liquid lesion is seen on the upper pole of the left kidney affected by dysplasia

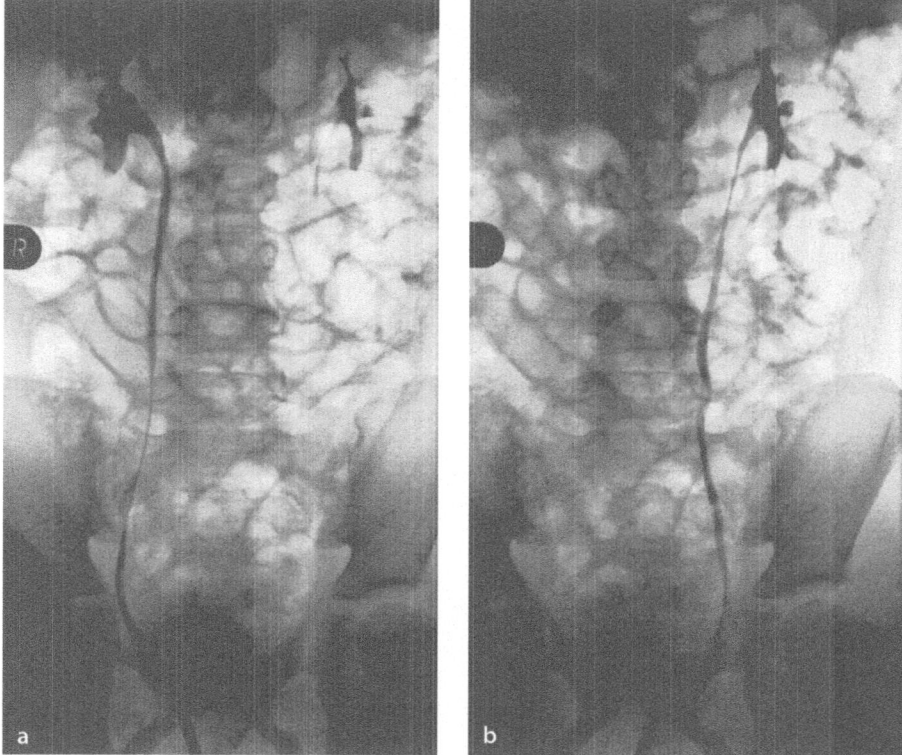

Fig. 17.3 a, b. Retrograde pyelography. Completely contrasted renal collecting system on the right side. Obviously normally contrasted renal pelvis on the left side, but no sign of the additional ureter seen on the intravenous pyelogram

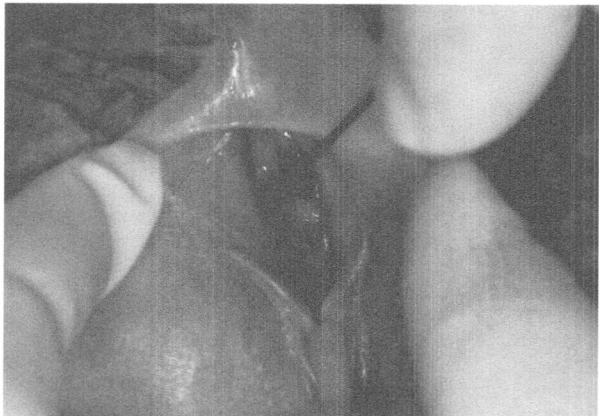

Fig. 17.4. Macroscopic view of the introitus vaginae: ectopic ureteral orifice in the left side of the vaginal wall (*arrow*)

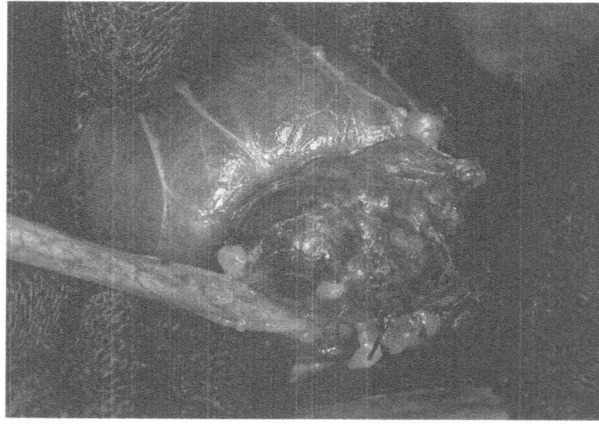

Fig. 17.5. Intraoperative view: dysplastic upper pole with enlarged and already transected ectopic ureter

CASE 18 ▶ *Bilateral Single Ectopic Ureter*

Clinical Course: This 1-year-old girl was referred to the paediatric department with a febrile urinary tract infection. During this episode, which was probably not the first one, sonography was performed as the first-line investigation. Figure 18.1 shows a smaller left kidney with dilatation of the left ureter. There were indirect signs of upper urinary tract infection, such as a poor demarcation between the parenchyma and the pelvicalyceal system.

During catheterization, in order to perform voiding cysto-urethrography the catheter was placed directly in an ectopic right ureter. The examination revealed a duplicated ureter on the right side. No vesico-ureteral reflux could be demonstrated contralaterally (Fig. 18.2). On the intravenous pyelogram the pyelon of the right kidney was dysplastic. A megaureter combined with a marked deformation of the left renal pelvis was found (Fig. 18.3).

Following this procedures and antibiotic therapy we did not have the opportunity to perform further examinations until the child was 2 years old. During this period at least seven urinary tract infections occurred. Subsequently the split function of the left kidney was diminished to 28% on ^{99m}Tc-MAG$_3$ scintigraphy (Fig. 18.4). On the radionuclide scan wie found tracer retention in the distal left-sided megaureter, with no signs of obstruction. On cystoscopy

bilateral ectopic ureter was diagnosed subsequently. Crosstrigonal reimplantation of the ectopic ureters combined with modelling of the megaureter was performed 6 months later.

Following surgery, urinary tract infections persisted and urinary incontinence became obvious. The family of the child again consulted other hospitals, but a definitive diagnosis could not be established. The girl was again referred to our department when she was 8 years old. We performed cystometry which led to a diagnosis of very low bladder capacity and loss of sphincter function (Fig. 18.5). One year later an artificial sphincter was implanted (Fig. 18.6). Following this procedure the incontinence resolved completely.

Comment: This case demonstrates the rare syndrome of bilateral ectopic ureter. Typical features of this condition are relapsing urinary tract infections and intractable urinary incontinence caused by incomplete maturation of the neck of the urinary bladder. The diagnosis can only be established by a combination of different diagnostic procedures. These children should preferably be treated with an artificial sphincter or plastic surgery of the urinary bladder neck with augmentation of bladder.

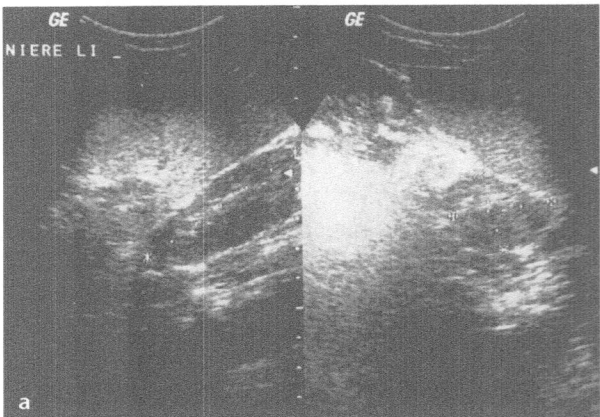

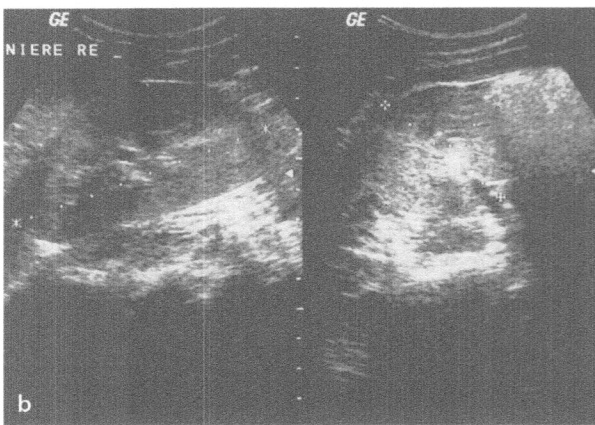

Fig. 18.1 a, b. Sonography of **a** left kidney (longitudinal and transverse sections) and **b** right kidney (longitudinal and transverse sections) shows that the left kidney is smaller and the right kidney is normally developed

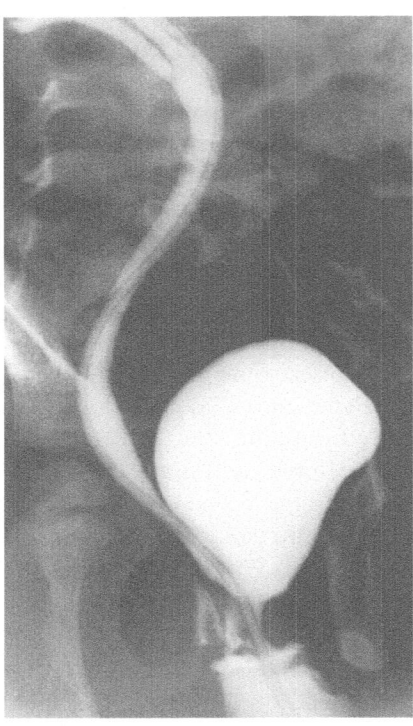

Fig. 18.2. No reflux can be demonstrated on the left sight by voiding cysto-urethrogram. The catheter is located in the ectopic right ureter

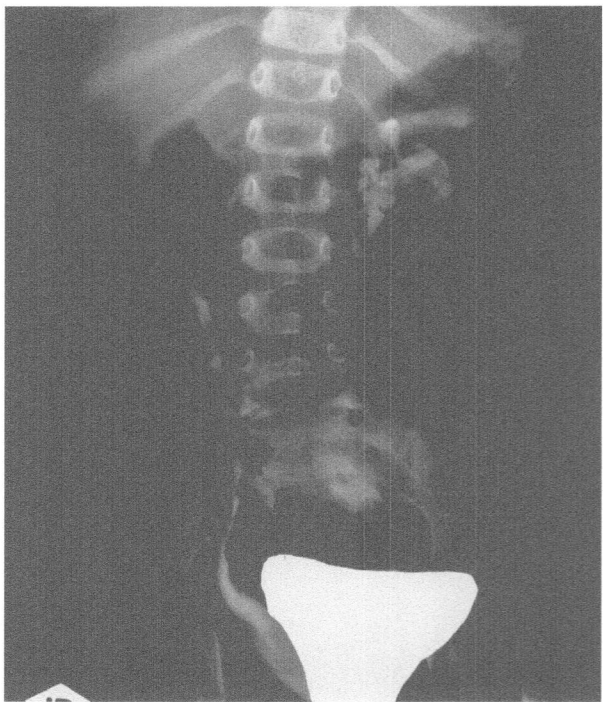

Fig. 18.3. On the intravenous pyelogram the right pyelon is dysplastic. There is marked deformation of the left pyelon combined with a megaureter

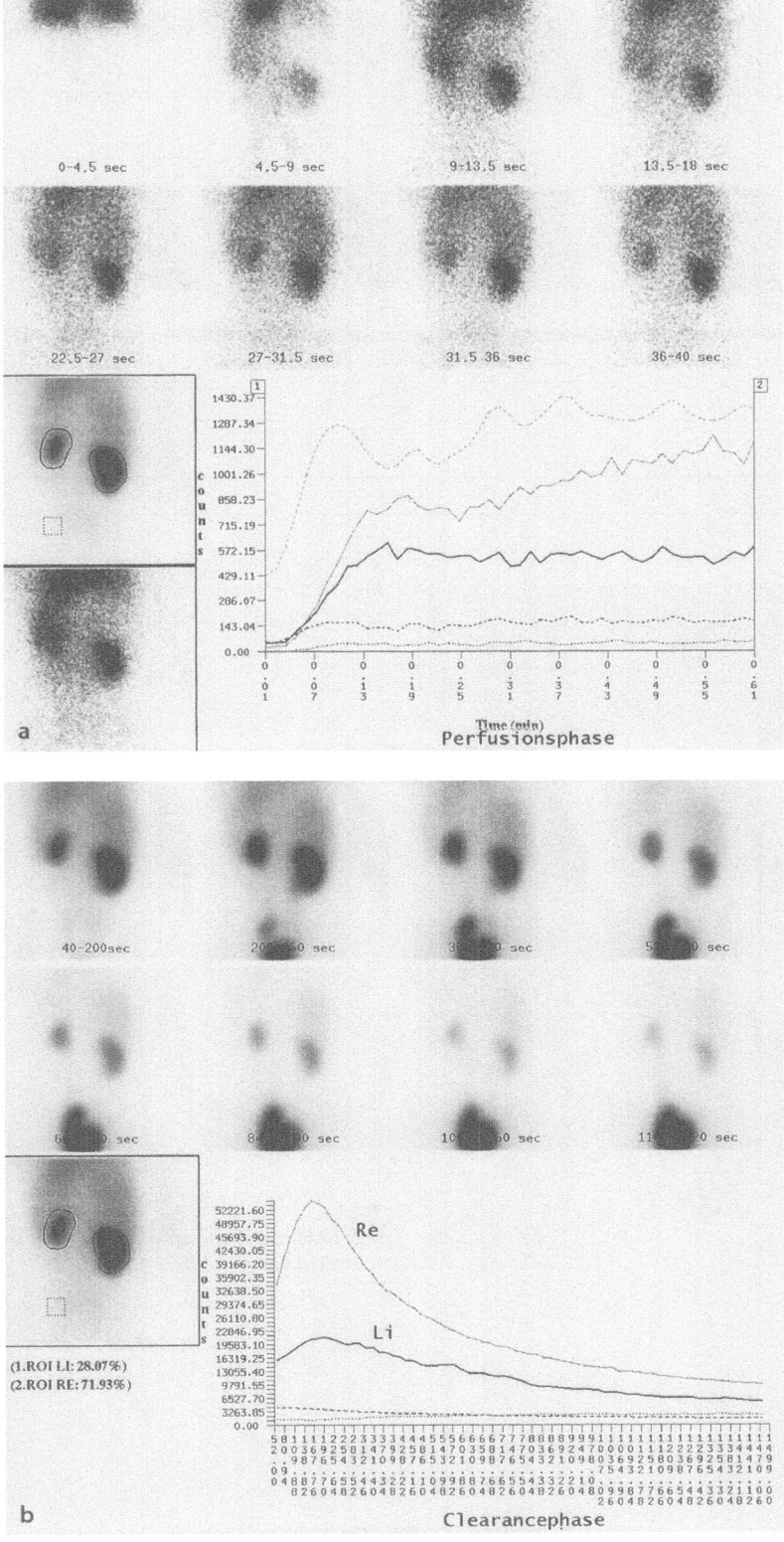

Fig. 18.4. **a** Reduced perfusion of the left kidney. **b** The split renal function of the left kidney revealed by ^{99m}Tc-MAG$_3$ scintigraphy is only 28 %; retention of the tracer can be noted in the left-sided distal megaureter with no signs of obstruction

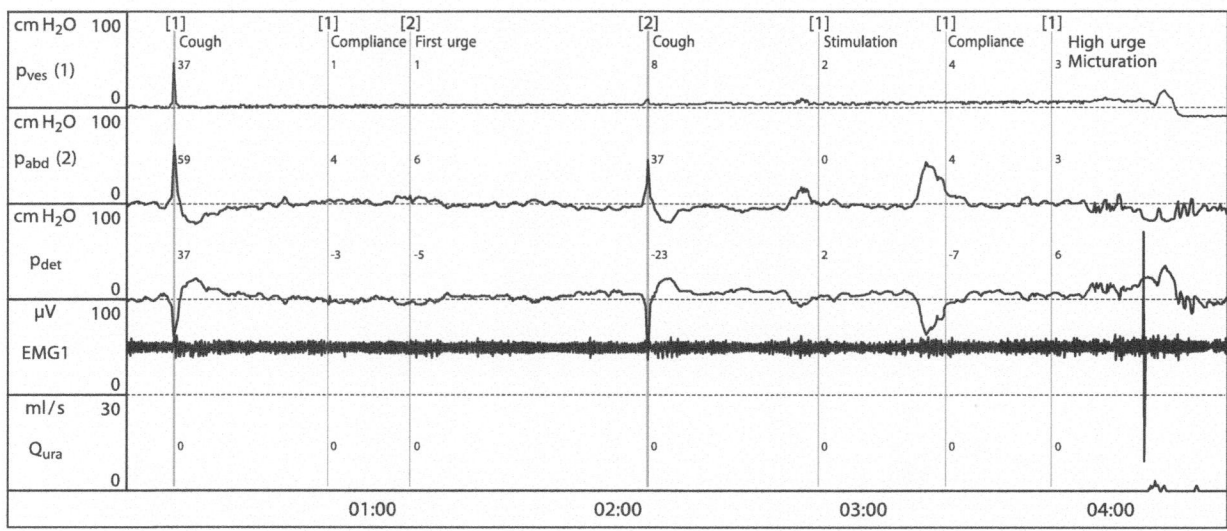

Fig. 18.5. Cystometry shows very low bladder capacity and loss of sphincter function

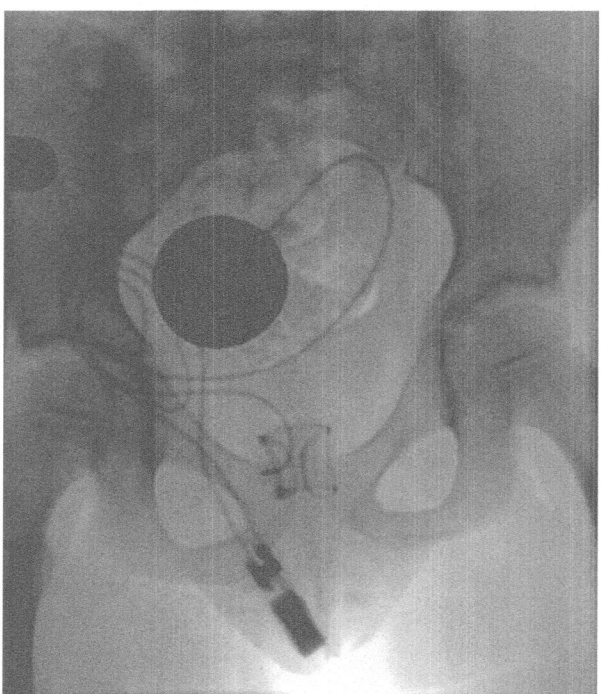

Fig. 18.6. Artificial sphincter with inflation device, cuff, and spherical reservoir

CASE 19 ▶ *Duplex System with Ectopic and Obstructive Megaureter*

Clinical Course: During sonographic screening in another hospital a massive dilatation of the left pelvicalyceal system and the left ureter was noted in a newborn girl. The child was admitted to our department with the suspicion of an obstructive megaureter.

On our first sonography advanced dilatation of the left urinary drainage system could be confirmed. While the drainage system of the lower pole of the left kidney was ectatic, a space-occupying cystic lesion was found in the upper medial pole, together with marked rarefaction of the renal parenchyma. This combination was highly suggestive of a duplex system (Fig. 19.1).

VUR was subsequently ruled out by voiding cysto-urethrography (Fig. 19.2). During catheterization of the urinary bladder the catheter was seen on ultrasonography to have moved spontaneously into the distal part of the left-sided megaureter, thus providing evidence for an ectopic ostium (Fig. 19.3). Retrograde X-ray contrast media filling of the catheter confirmed the diagnosis of an ectopic megaureter, which was draining the upper (dysplastic) pole of the left kidney (Fig. 19.4).

The ^{99m}Tc-MAG$_3$ scan showed decreased perfusion and function of the left kidney, with an inadequate response to furosemide indicating obstruction, while normal results were obtained in the contralateral kidney (Fig. 19.5).

Intravenous urography showed poor excretion of the contrast medium in a large dilated pyelon on the upper pole of the left kidney. The lower pole exhibited considerably less dilatation of the calyces. The urinary bladder was displaced, probably by the megaureter, which could not be visualized (Fig. 19.6).

Heminephrectomy and ureterectomy were performed. During the follow-up no further complications occurred.

Comment: An extopic and obstructive megaureter draining the upper part of a duplex system was diagnosed by selective catherization and from the observation of an obstructive response curve on the diuretic scintigram. Duplex systems cannot be visualized by dynamic scintigraphy because of the limited resolution of radionuclide scanning.

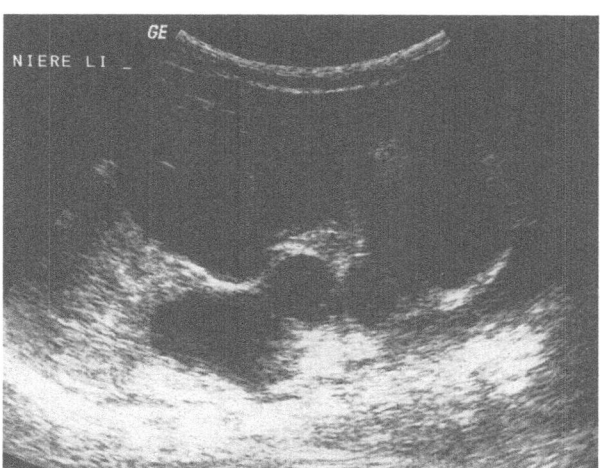
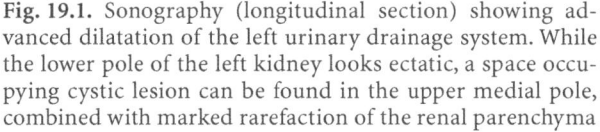

Fig. 19.1. Sonography (longitudinal section) showing advanced dilatation of the left urinary drainage system. While the lower pole of the left kidney looks ectatic, a space occupying cystic lesion can be found in the upper medial pole, combined with marked rarefaction of the renal parenchyma

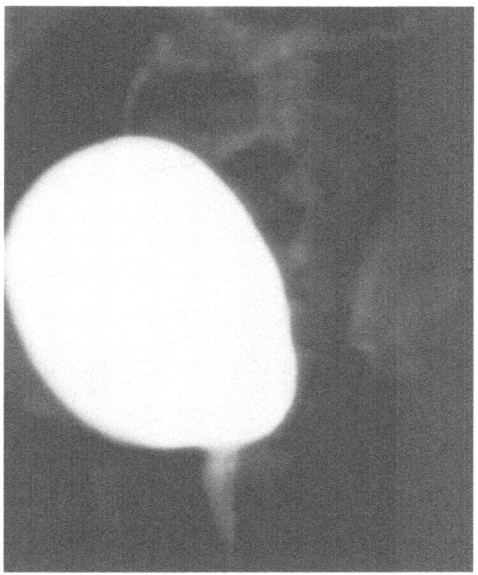

Fig. 19.2. No reflux can be demonstrated on the voiding cysto-urethrogram

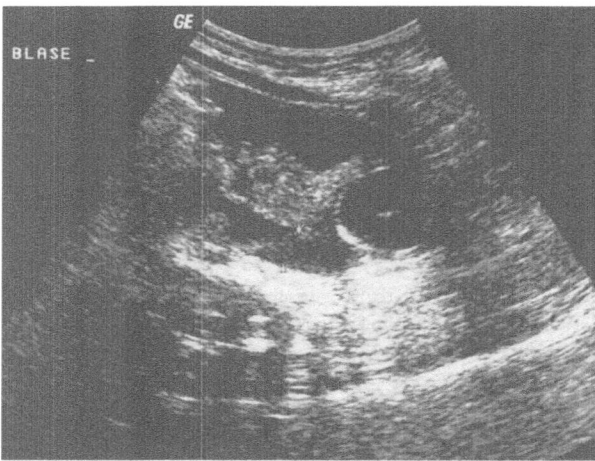

Fig. 19.3. Sonography (transverse section) shows a mega-ureter on the left side, paravescial with the catheter in the lumen

Fig. 19.5 a, b see p. 189

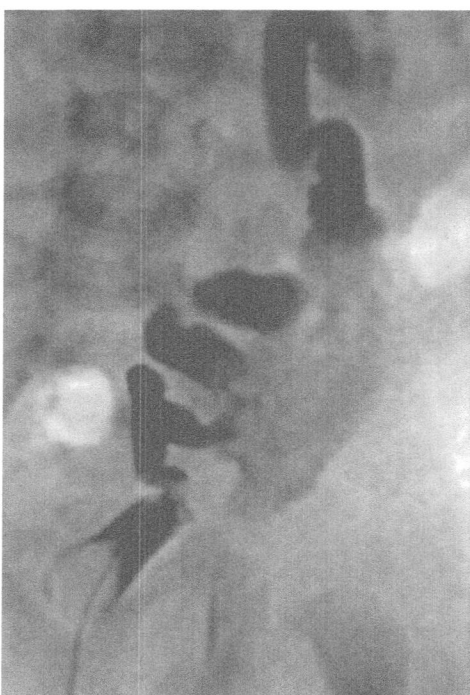

Fig. 19.4. Retrograde pyelography confirms the presence of an ectopic megaureter draining the upper pole of the left kidney

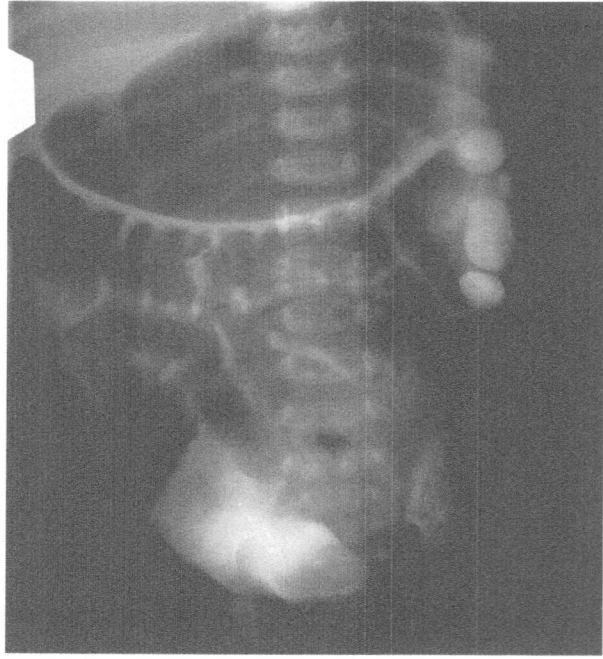

Fig. 19.6. Intravenous urography shows poor excretion of the contrast medium in a large dilated pyelon on the upper pole of the left kidney. The lower pole exhibits less pronounced dilatation of the calyces. The urinary bladder is displaced, probably by the megaureter, which cannot be visualized

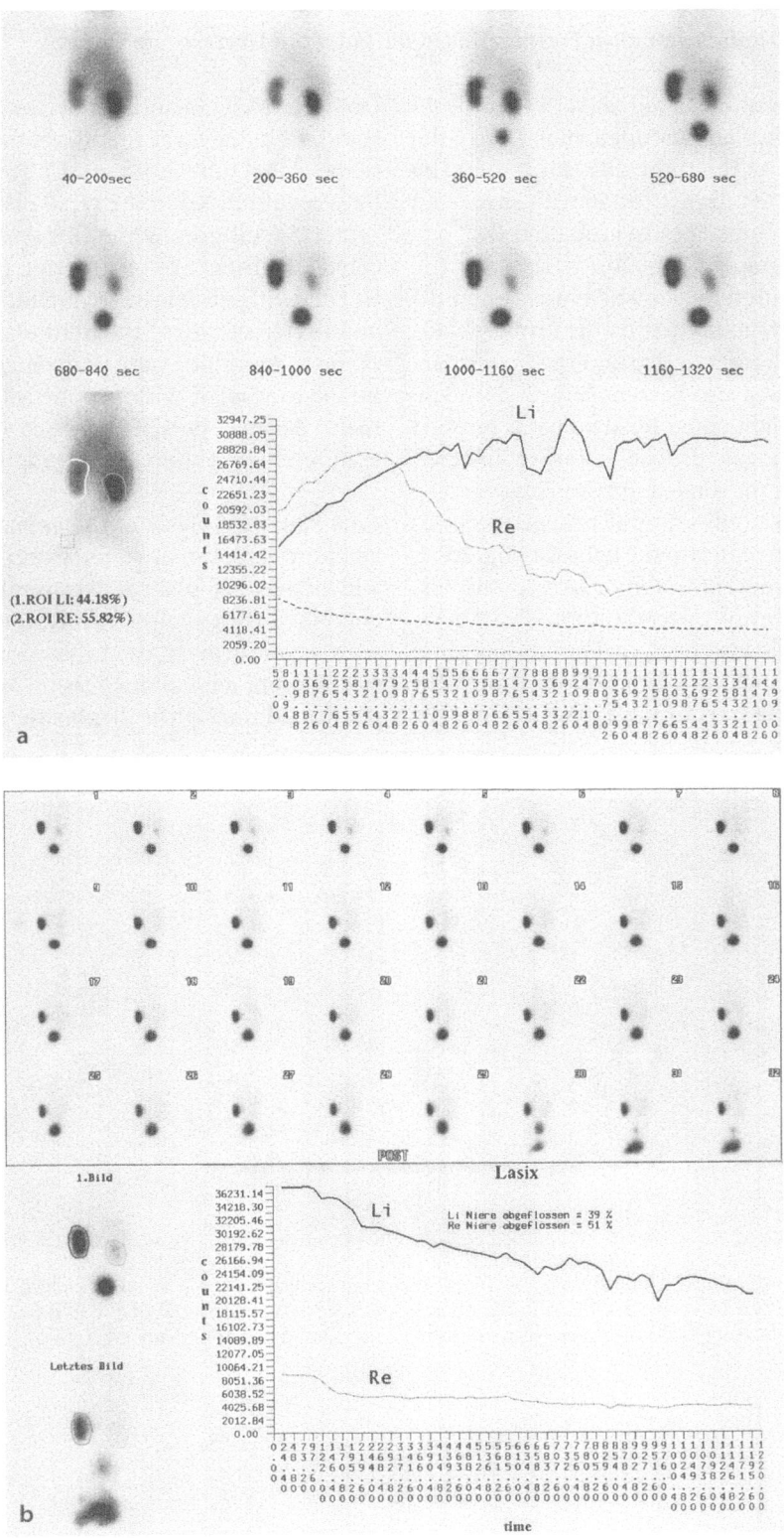

Fig. 19.5. a The ^{99m}Tc-MAG$_3$ scan shows decreased perfusion and function of the left kidney (44%) with an inadequate response to furosemide (39% decrease within 20 min) indicating obstruction, while **b** normal results were obtained for the contralateral kidney

CASE 20 ▶ *Renal Duplication with Dysplastic Upper Pole and Ureterocele*

Clinical Course: Fever occurred in a 5-month-old child, and sonography demonstrated dilatation of the upper urinary tract on the right side (Fig. 20.1). The infant was admitted to our institution with suspected pyelonephritis due to obstructive uropathy.

Our initial sonography (Fig. 20.1a) revealed the typical features of a ureterocele, which was clearly diagnosed as a cystic structure within the urinary bladder. Dilatation of the right ureter and the upper part of the right kidney was also present (Fig. 20.1b). The parenchyma of the right upper renal pole was rarefied and an echogenic mass, probably due to infected urine, was present in the dilated upper urinary tract.

The voiding cysto-urethrography revealed second-grade vesico-ureteral reflux on the left side (Fig. 20.3). The intravenous urography demonstrated the absence of upper calyces of the right kidney with normal excretion into the lower calyceal group, a finding considered to be typical for renal duplication with dysplasia of the upper part of the kidney (Fig. 20.4).

On ^{99m}Tc-MAG$_3$ scintigraphy the global function of the right kidney was found not to be impaired (46% of the global tubular function). The tracer was seen to have accumulated in the renal pelvis (Fig. 20.5a). On diuretic scintigraphy the furosemide response indicated the absence of obstruction (Fig. 20.5b).

Following antibiotic treatment, heminephrectomy and ureterectomy of the nonfunctioning upper part of the right kidney were performed. After surgery the infant continued with prophylactic antibiotic treatment, because persistent vesico-ureteral reflux was seen on direct voiding scintigraphy (Fig. 20.6).

Comment: Dysplasia of the upper part of the affected kidney is common in renal duplication. The ureter, which may be obstructive, is usually ectopic and combined with an ureterocele. Our patient presented with a first urinary tract infection and sonographic suspicion of a renal duplication and ureterocele, was confirmed during the diagnostic work-up.

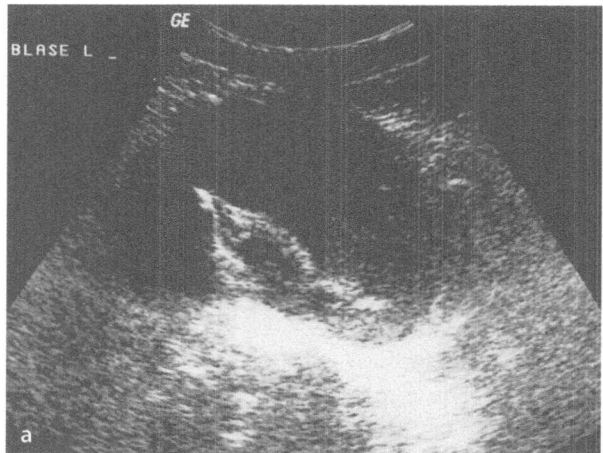 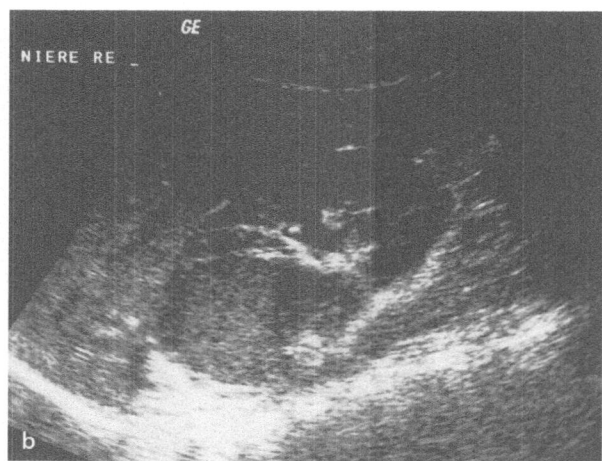

Fig. 20.1 a, b. a First sonography (longitudinal sections at bladder). A ureterocele can be recognized as a cystic structure within the urinary bladder. **b** The drainage system of the upper (dysplastic) part of the right kidney is dilated. An echogenic mass, probably due to infected urine, is present in the dilated upper urinary tract

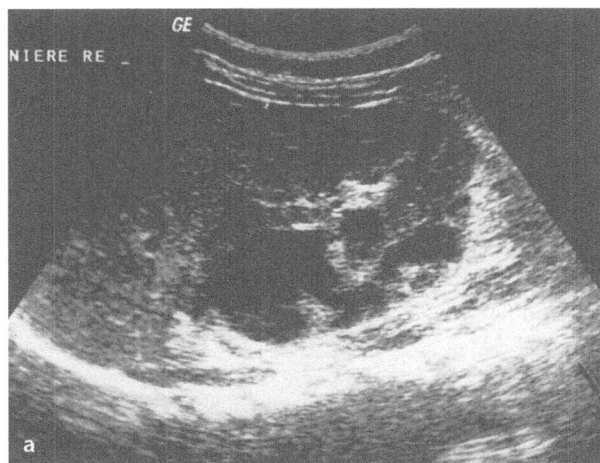

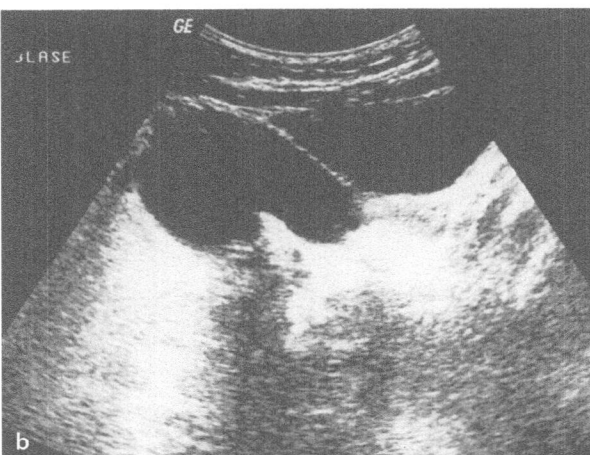

Fig. 20.2 a, b. The second sonography (longitudinal sections) shows a dilatation of the renal pelvis in the upper pole and **b** the ureter with less echogenic content corresponding to clear urine following antibiotic treatment

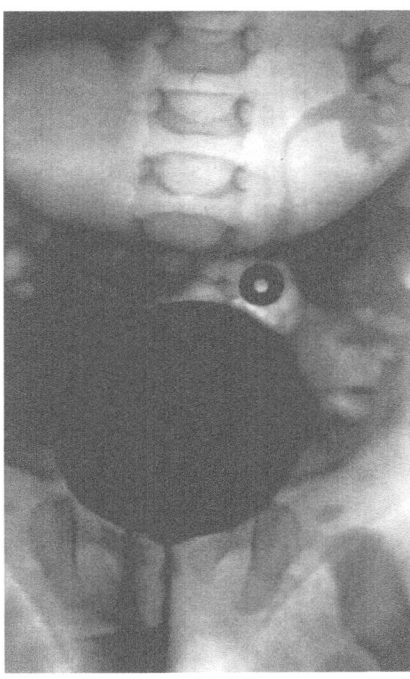

Fig. 20.3. Voiding cysto-urethrography demonstrates second-grade vesico-ureteral reflux in the left kidney

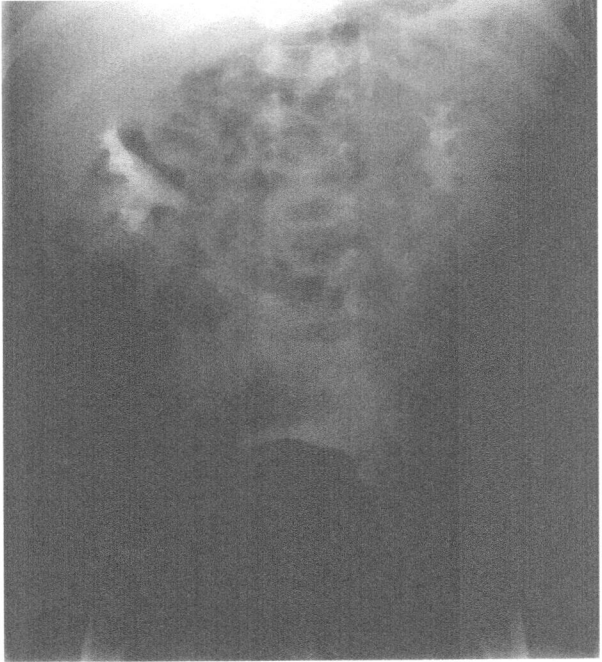

Fig. 20.4. Urography: the upper calyces of the right kidney are not seen. Normal excretion into the lower calyceal group, a finding typical for renal duplication with dysplasia of the upper pole

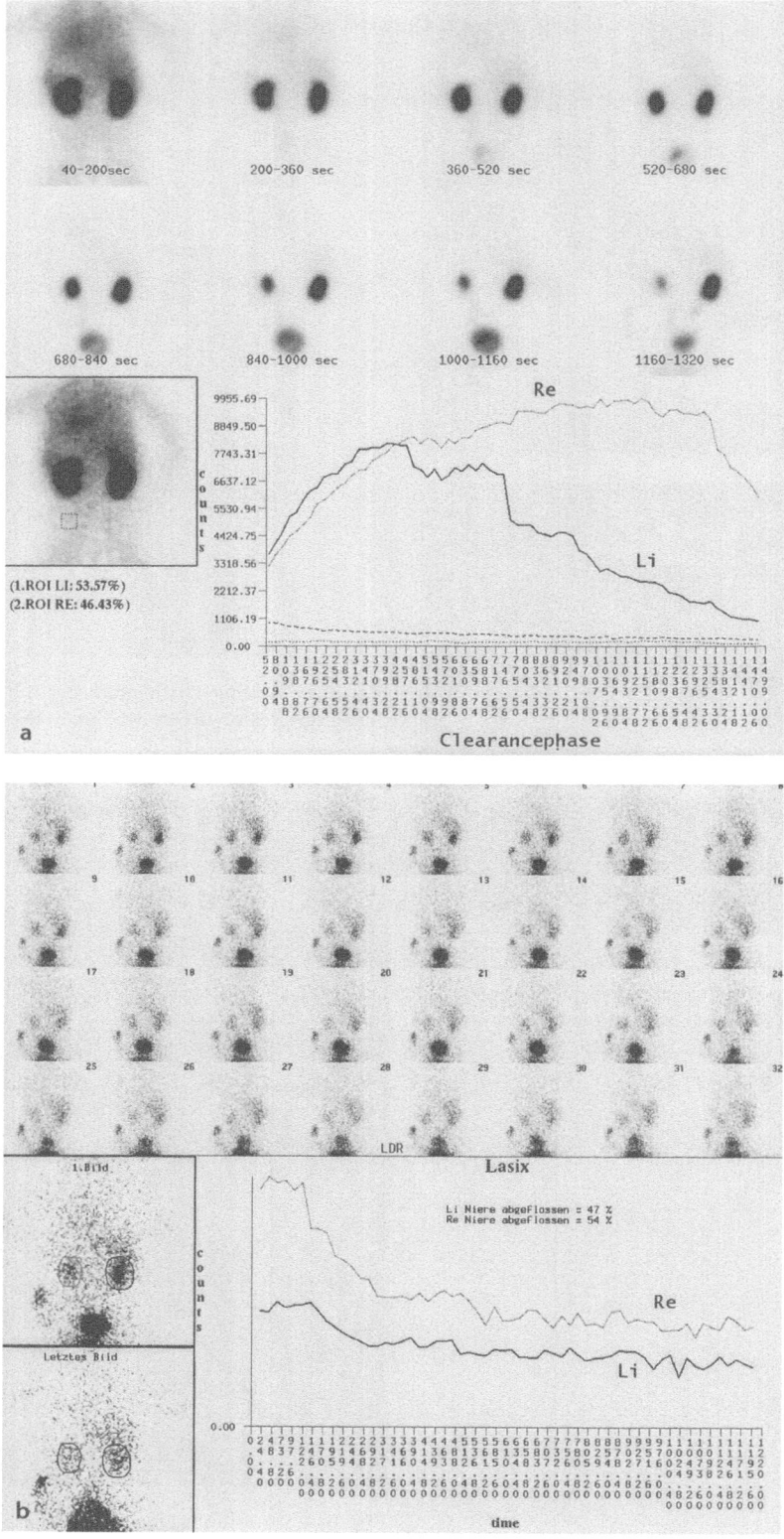

Fig. 20.5. a On ^{99m}Tc-MAG$_3$ scintigraphy the global function of the right kidney is seen not to be impaired (46% of the global tubular function). The tracer has accumulated in the renal pelvis. **b** On diuretic scintigraphy the furosemide response indicates the absence of obstruction in the lower part of the right kidney

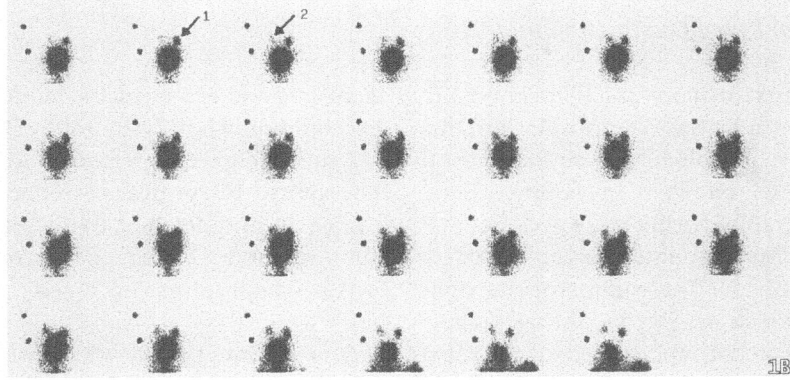

Fig. 20.6. Direct voiding scintigraphy detects bilateral (*arrows 1* and *2*) moderate VUR

CASE 21 ▶ *Bilateral Renal Duplication and VUR*

Clinical Course: A first urinary tract infection occurred in this boy when he was 4 years old. Until this time he had been free of urological symptoms. Renal malformations were not known in his family.

On the first sonography during acute pyelonephritis a hyperechoic mass was noted in a moderately filled bladder (Fig. 21.1a). The volume of the right kidney was 106 ml, which was beyond the age-adapted range, and a hyperechoic appearance of the renal parenchyma was noted (Fig. 21.1b–d). The urinary drainage system looked normal on both sides.

Surprisingly, bilateral grade-III VUR into four drainage systems was found during voiding cystourethrography. The ureters were in orthotopic positions, and there were no signs of any subvesical obstruction (Fig. 21.2). During the further clinical course, the child's parents refused prophylactic antibiotic therapy. Nine months later we saw the boy

again and found persistent moderate reflux during direct radionuclide cystography (Fig. 21.3).

Again the parents refused antibiotic therapy, but they agreed to surgical correction, which was performed in another hospital according to Lich-Gregoir's method. During postoperative follow-up no further complications occurred.

Comment: Sonography was misleading in this patient, because the method can exclude neither a duplex system nor a moderate VUR definitively. In this child further investigations were indicated after the first occurrence of a febrile urinary tract infection. In a duplex system, the possibility of spontaneous maturation is poor, even if the ureteral orifices are in orthotopic positions. We therefore performed surgical correction, especially in view of the noncompliant family of the patient.

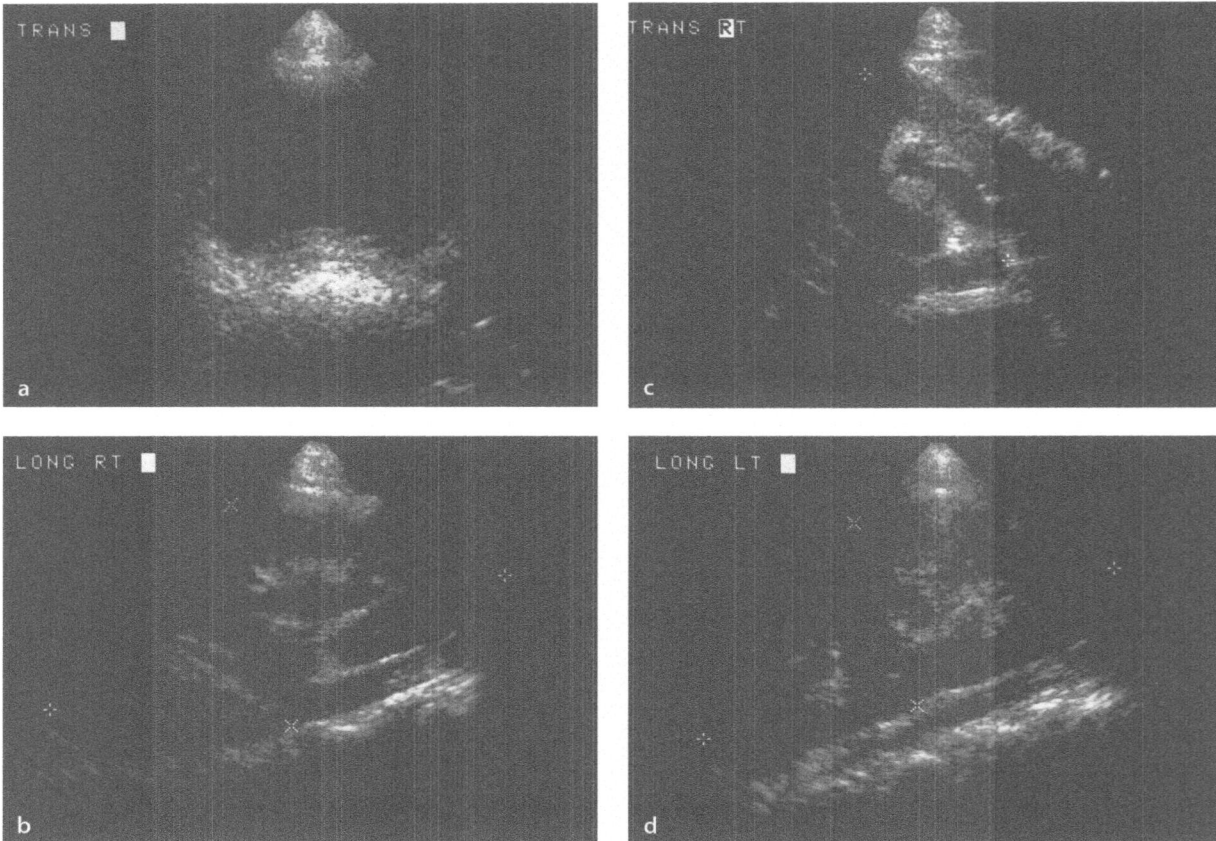

Fig. 21.1 a–d. On the first sonography **a** a hyperechoic mass in a moderately filled bladder was noted. **b–d** Note the hyperechoic parenchyma on the longitudinal view of both kidneys (**b, d**) and of the transverse view of the right kidney (**c**). The urinary drainage system looked normal on both sides

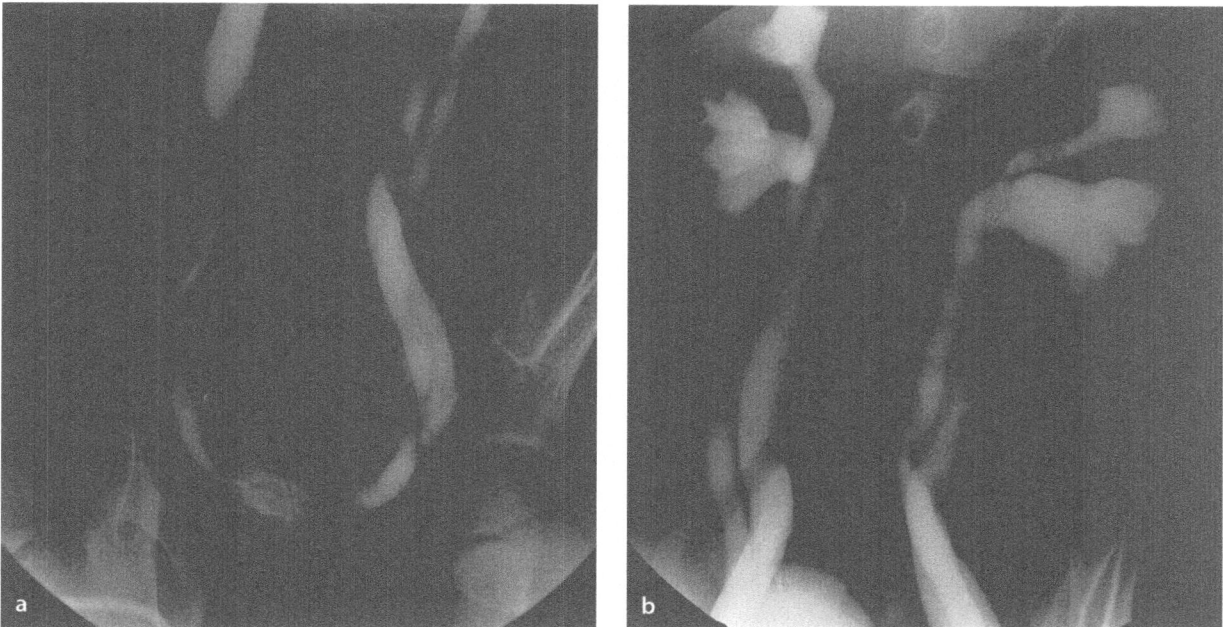

Fig. 21.2. Grade-III VUR into four ureters during the voiding cysto-urethrography. The pelvicalyceal system of both kidneys looked somewhat deformed and there was a suspicion of bilateral duplicated ureter

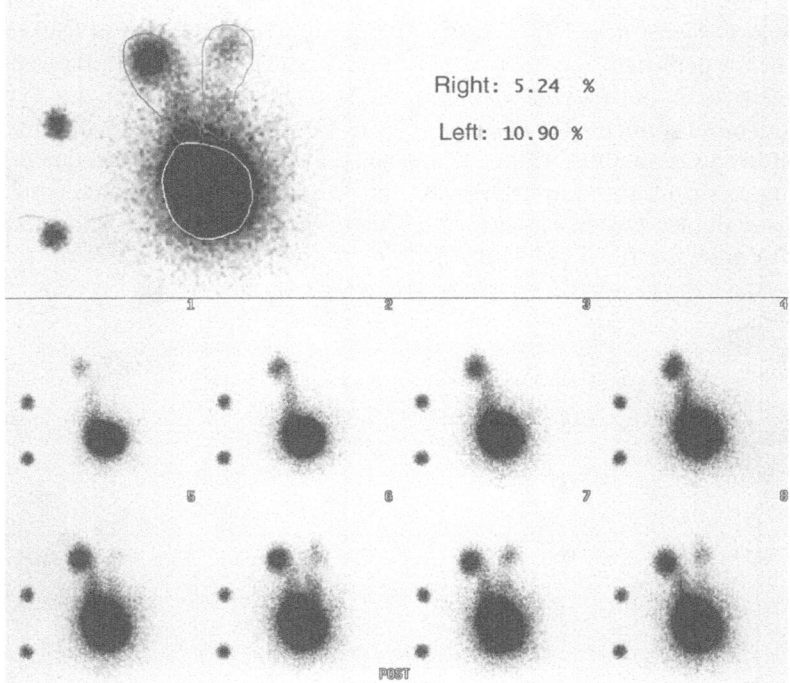

Fig. 21.3. Persistent vesico-renal reflux seen on direct radionuclide micturating cytography during follow-up 9 months later

CASE 22 ▶ *Duplex-System with Dysplastic-Lower Pole and Reflux Nephropathy*

Clinical Course: This child suffered from primary nocturnal enuresis. Enuresis by day began when he was 4 years old and started attending kindergarten. Previously, at the age of 1 he had been seen by a paediatrician who found no abnormalities on clinical examination, which also included a urine culture. On sonography he noted signs of a right-sided duplex kidney with slight dilatation of the drainage system of the lower pole, but said it further diagnostic steps were not urgently needed.

The boy was admitted to our department at the age of 4 years with fever of unknown origin (FUO). During 4 days of clinical evaluation and investigation no further episodes of fever occurred. Again the urine cultures were sterile. During his further clinical course the child developed a severe emotional disturbance with regressive behaviour tendency. He was finally admitted to the psychosomatic department of our university, where he stayed for 10 weeks without relief of the symptoms. During this time the boy developed asymptomatic pyuria, but no further urological investigations were performed. After his discharge, the child's mother again noted episodes of fever and the incontinence persisted.

We saw the boy again as an out-patient when he was $4^{1}/_{2}$ years old. Ultrasound confirmed the findings of previous sonographic examinations (Figs. 22.1, 22.2). During voiding cysto-urethrography, which was performed because a duplex system was suspected, a high-grade reflux into the renal pelvis of the lower dysplastic pole of the right kidney was found (Fig. 33.3). In this kidney the intravenous pyelogram demonstrated that there were two ureters draining the pelvicalyceal system. (Fig. 22.4). At the lower pole the calyces of the dilated drainage system were deformed, while no major abnormalities were noted in these structures at the upper pole. The ^{99m}Tc-MAG$_3$ scan showed that the global split function of the right kidney was well preserved but the function of the lower pole was diminished to 12% (Fig. 22.5).

Taken together, these findings precipitated the decision to perform ureterocystoneostomy with preservation of the lower pole of the right-sided duplex kidney. The sonography in the early postoperative period showed marked dilatation of the right drainage system (Fig. 22.6), which had completely resolved when ultrasound was repeated 6 months later (Fig. 22.7). During the further clinical course the enuresis stopped and no further urinary tract infection occurred.

Comment: In this child the initial sonographic findings unfortunately did not lead to further investigations because urinary cultures were found to be sterile. FUO in childhood is often due to occult urinary tract infections. The serious incontinence of the child and the pertinacity and perseverance of the child's family in demanding further diagnostic procedures finally led to the true diagnosis and successful therapy.

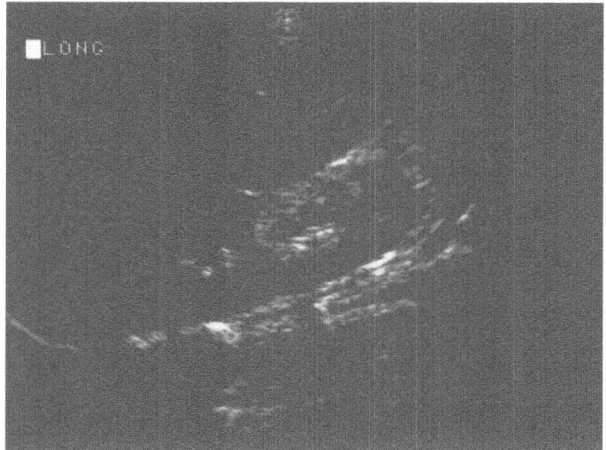

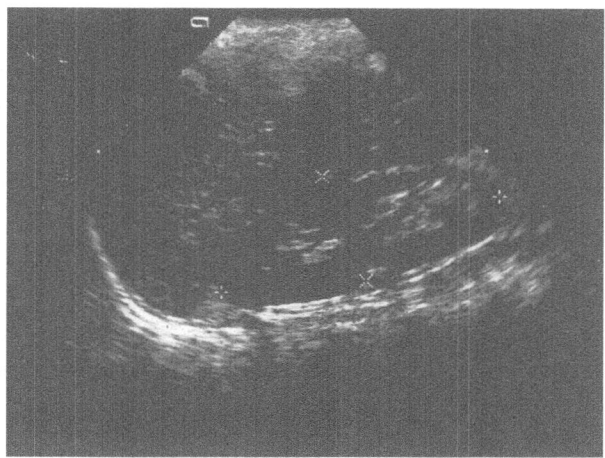

Fig. 22.1. Initial sonography (right kidney, longitudinal section). Hyperechoid appearance of the parenchyma of the lower pole of the duplex kidney

Fig. 22.2. Sonography 3 years later (right kidney, longitudinal section). Again signs of a duplex system are present. Thinning of the parenchyma of the lower pole

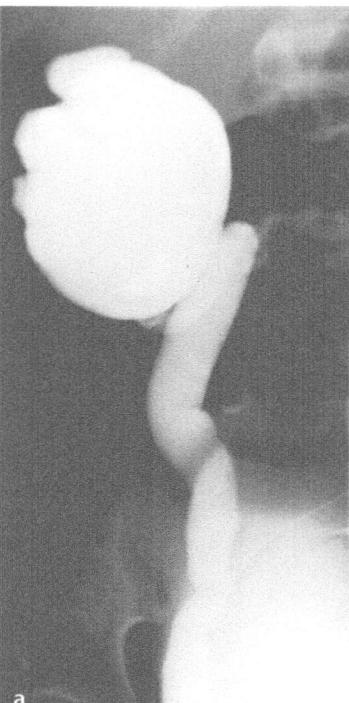

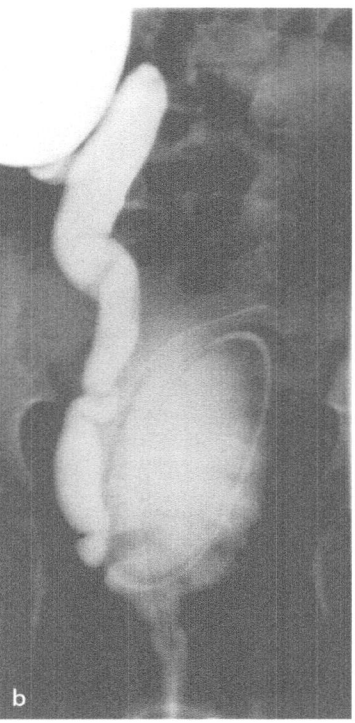

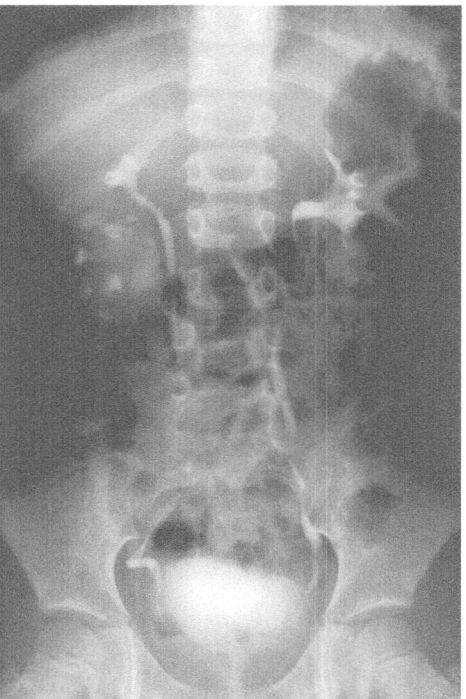

Fig. 22.3a, b (*left, middle*). On the voiding cysto-urethrogram grade-IV reflux is seen at the lower pole of the right kidney

Fig. 22.4 (*right*). The intravenous pyelogram demonstrates that two ureters are draining the pelvicalyceal system of the right kidney. At the lower pole the calyces of the dilated drainage system are deformed. No major abnormalities can be noted at the upper pole

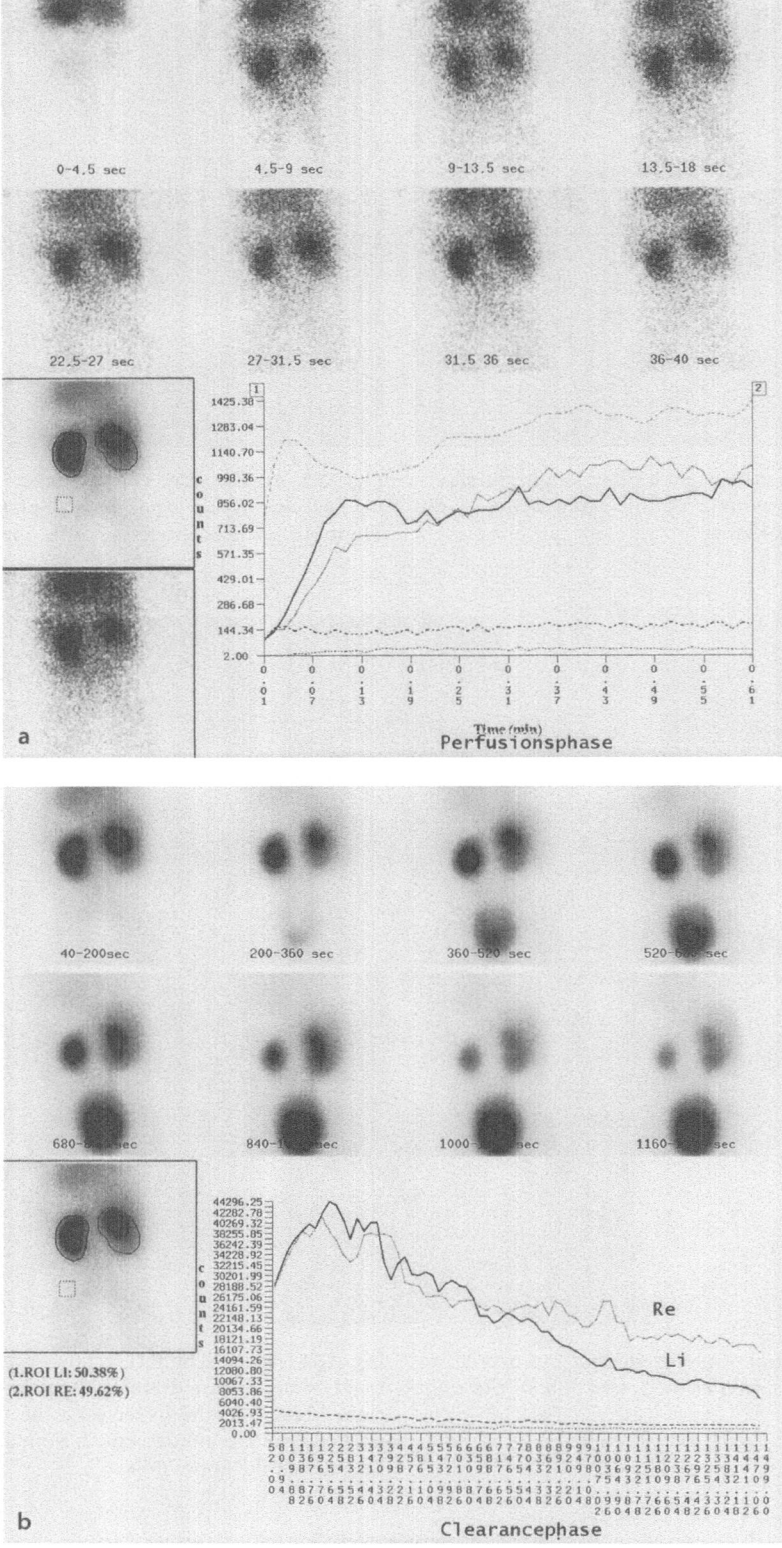

Fig. 22.5 a–c. On the ^{99m}Tc-MAG$_3$ scan (**a** perfusion phase, **b** function and excretion phase) the global split function of the right kidney is seen to be well preserved, but the function of the lower pole (**c**) is diminished to 12%. **c** see on p. 199

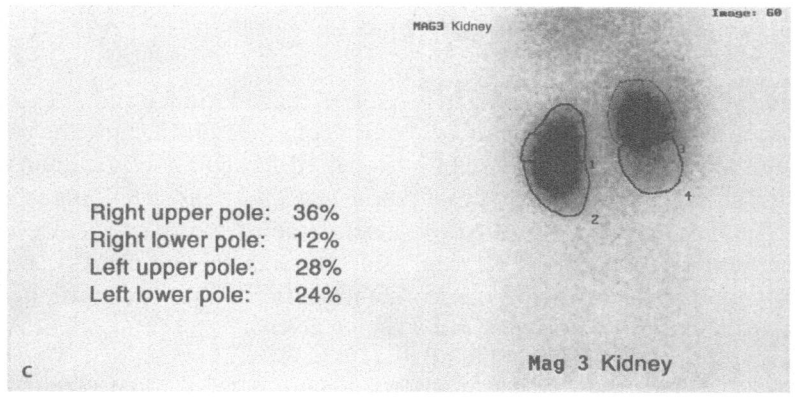

Right upper pole: 36%
Right lower pole: 12%
Left upper pole: 28%
Left lower pole: 24%

Fig. 22.5 c. Legend see p. 198

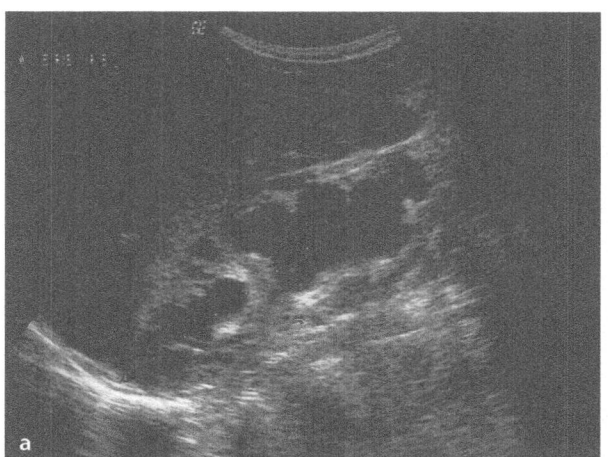

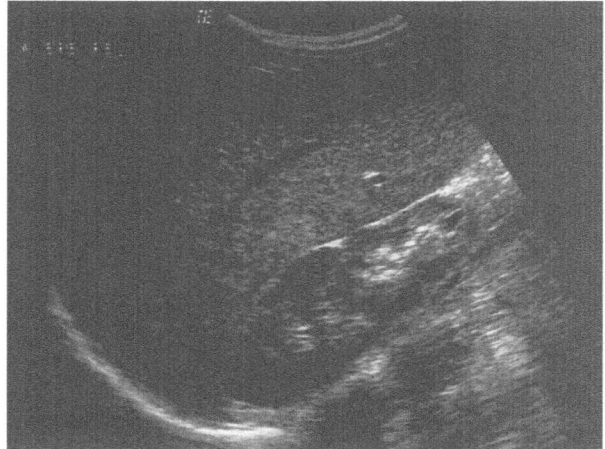

Fig. 22.7. The dilatation seen in Fig. 22.6 hat completely disappeared when ultrasound was repeated 6 months later (right kidney, longitudinal section)

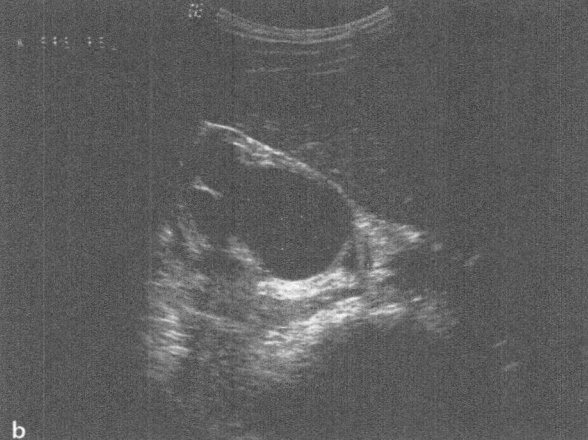

◀

Fig. 22.6 a, b. Sonography of the right kidney (**a** longitudinal, **b** transverse sections). Dilatation of the right drainage system. Note the parenchymal bridge between the upper and lower parts of the kidney

CASE 23 ▶ *Dysplastic Kidney with Severe VUR*

Clinical Course: During newborn renal screening hydronephrosis of the left urinary tract was diagnosed. A urinary tract infection was suspected and antibiotic treatment was started although there was no proof for this assumption. The boy was then admitted to our hospital for further investigation.

During the first sonography in our department (Fig. 23.1), paravesical dilatation of the ureter and marked hydronephrosis on the left side were noted. The left kidney looked substantially smaller than the right kindney. The voiding cysto-urethrography (Fig. 2) demonstrated a grade-III VUR on the left side, with kinking of the subpelvic ureter and deformed renal calyces. Suspecting a primary dysplastic kidney combined with high-grade VUR, we decided to start antibiotic prophylaxis. During his further clinical course the boy remained free of urinary tract infections.

When the boy was 10 months old we performed ^{99m}Tc-MAG$_3$ scintigraphy to evaluate the split func-tion of the left kidney and to exclude any additional obstruction. While the function of the left kidney was impaired, no signs of obstruction were present on the scan (Fig. 23.3). Direct voiding scintigraphy 2 months later demonstrated persistent severe VUR on the left side (Fig. 23.4). The child's parents agreed to the continuation of antibiotic prophylaxis, which is still being given.

Comment: It is essential to differentiate a primary dysplastic kidney from renal damage resulting from upper urinary tract infection attributable to reflux or obstruction. In this case urinary tract infection had never been confirmed, although left-sided renal impairment and reflux were present and dysplasia was therefore the most likely diagnosis. In such a case a conservative strategy with antibiotic prophylaxis over several years and waiting for spontaneous remission of the VUR is indicated.

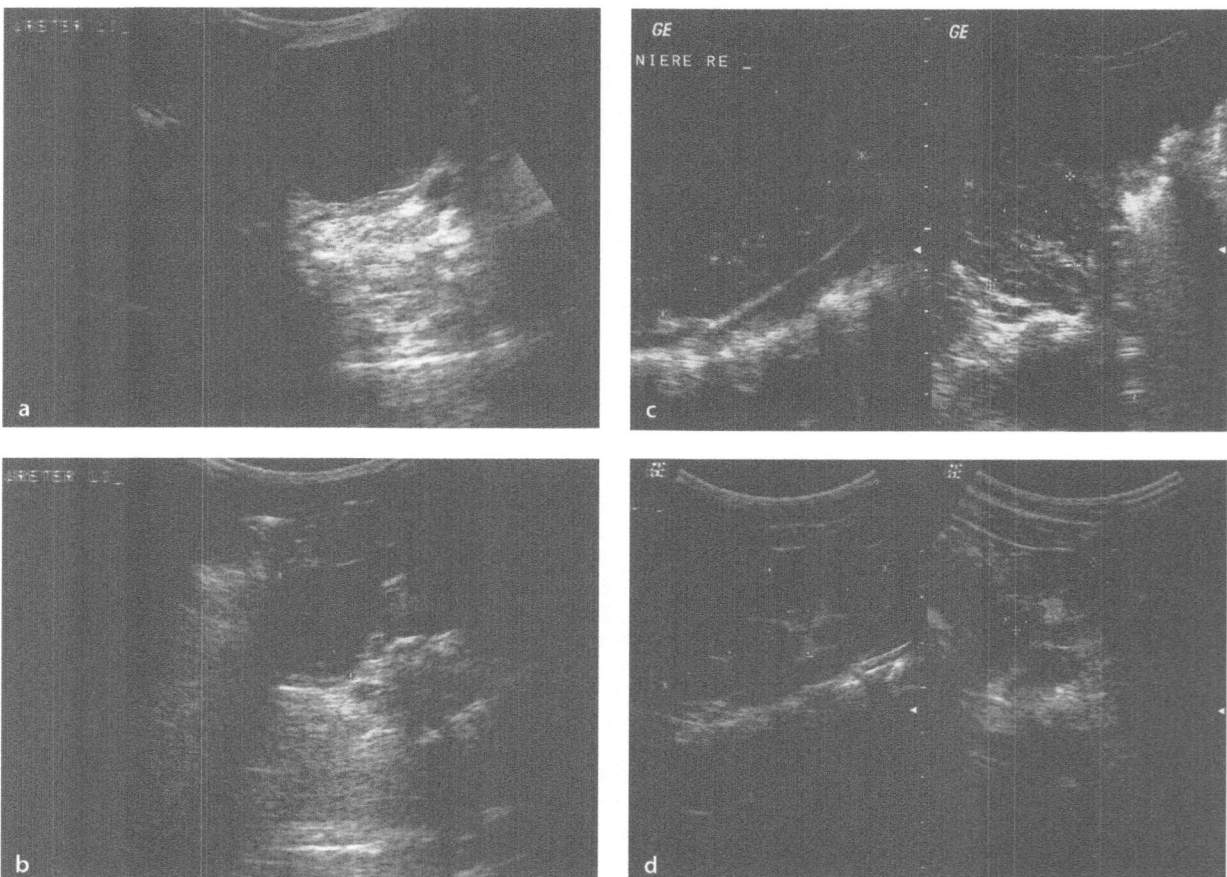

Fig. 23.1 a–d. Initial sonography. **a** Paravesical dilatation of the left ureter. **b** Hydronephrosis of the left kidney. **c** The right kidney shows no abnormalities (volume: 24 ml). **d** The volume of the left kidney is reduced (to 14 ml)

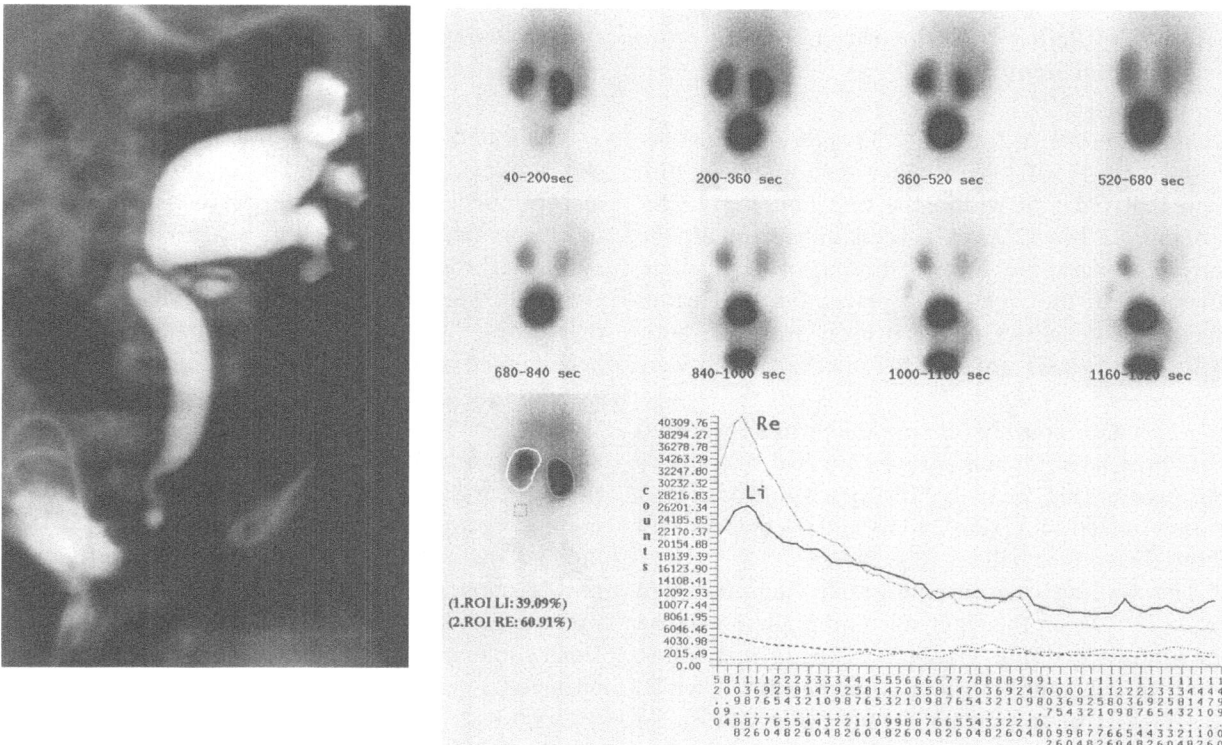

Fig. 23.2. Voiding cysto-urethrography, demonstrating a grade-III VUR on the left side, with subpelvic kinking and dilatation of the subpelvic ureter and deformed calyces

Fig. 23.3. On ^{99m}Tc-MAG$_3$ scintigraphy the function of the left kidney is seen to be impaired (39% of the global tubular function). Obstruction was excluded

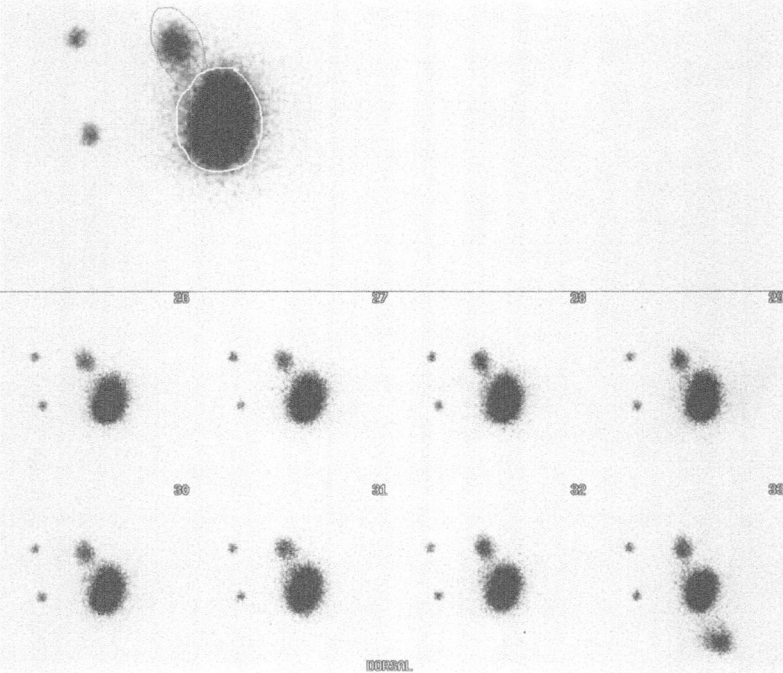

Fig. 23.4. Direct voiding scintigraphy during the early filling phase demonstrates the persistence of severe VUR on the left side

CASE 24 ▶ *Reflux Nephropathy After Two Episodes of Pyelonephritis Caused by Secondary Reflux and a Meatal Stenosis*

Clinical Course: At the age of $5^1/_2$ years this girl developed her first febrile urinary tract infection with high ESR (94 mm within the first hour) and CRP (18 mg/dl) levels. After successful treatment, the initial sonographic investigation showed a slight dilatation of the right renal pelvis, but no further major abnormalities of the urinary tract. No antibotic prophylaxis and further investigations were performed.

A second episode of pyelonephritis occurred 3 months later. On sonography no hydronephrosis was present (Fig. 24.1 a, b). The upper pole of the left kidney looked small (Fig. 24.1 b), and the bladder wall showed no abnormalities (Fig. 24.1 c).

The voiding cysto-urethrography demonstrated grade-II VUR on the right side and grade-I VUR on the contralateral side (Fig. 24.2 a). During micturition a conical dilatation of the urethra was noted, which was suggestive of a meatal stenosis (Fig. 24.2 b). No residual urine was present, and the urodynamics were normal. It was decided to start antibiotic prophylaxis with trimethoprim, which successfully prevented further infections.

The ^{99m}Tc-MAG$_3$ scan performed 8 months later showed a focal cortical defect suggestive of scarring at the lower pole of the left kidney (Fig. 24.3).

A repeated direct radionuclide cysto-urethrogram was normal, and the antibiotic prophylaxis was discontinued. Soon after, two further urinary tract infections occurred. The third direct radionuclide cysto-urethrogram verified a persistent VUR on the right side (Fig. 24.4). This finding strongly suggested that during the second cysto-urethrogram reflux had been missed because only one cycle of bladder filling was monitored.

Renal scarring combined with persistence of VUR and the recurrence of pyelonephritis is a clear indication for surgical treatment. We performed meatotomy and cystoscopic submucosal instillation of Deflux. Following these procedures the antibiotic prophylaxis was stopped. A direct radionuclide cysto-urethrogram showed no persistent reflux (Fig. 24.5). During follow-up, no further urinary tract infections occurred.

Comment: In this girl the rare occurrence of a meatal stenosis was combined with a disturbance of micturition. She developed renal scarring after two episodes of pyelonephritis in the presence of low-grade reflux.

VUR can be missed on cysto-urethrogram owing to the highly variable nature of this condition.

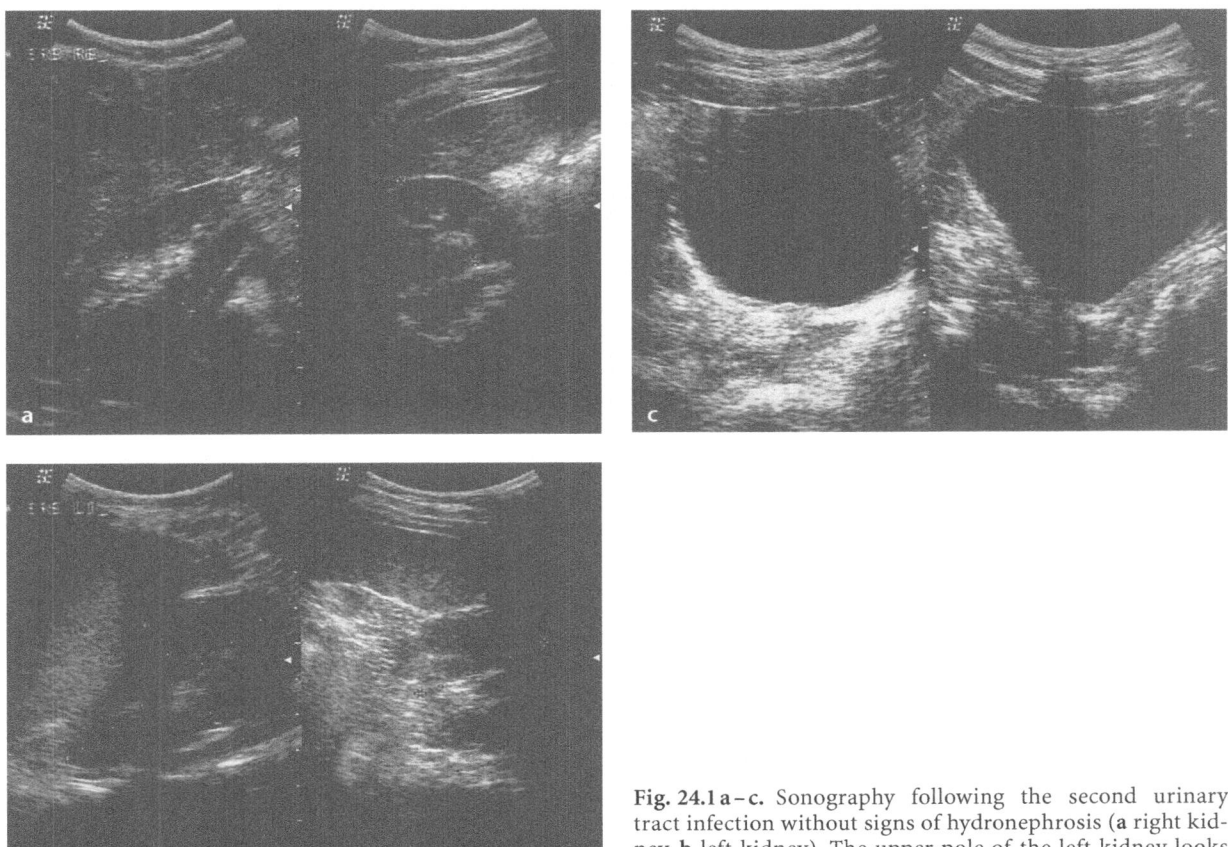

Fig. 24.1 a–c. Sonography following the second urinary tract infection without signs of hydronephrosis (**a** right kidney, **b** left kidney). The upper pole of the left kidney looks small (**b**), and the bladder wall (**c**) shows no abnormalities

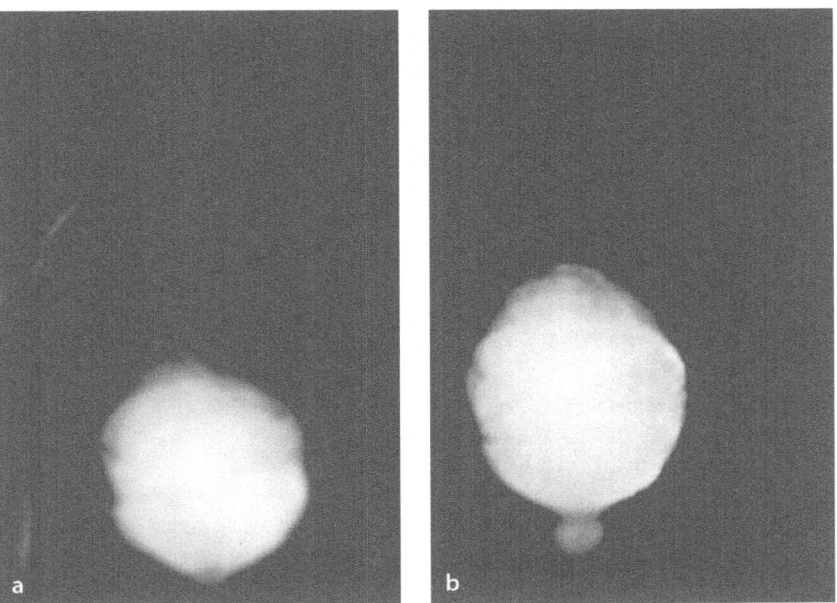

Fig. 24.2 a, b. Voiding cysto-urethrography demonstrates a grade-II VUR on the right side and a grade-I VUR on the left side. During micturition a conical dilatation of the urethra can be noted, suggesting a meatal stenosis

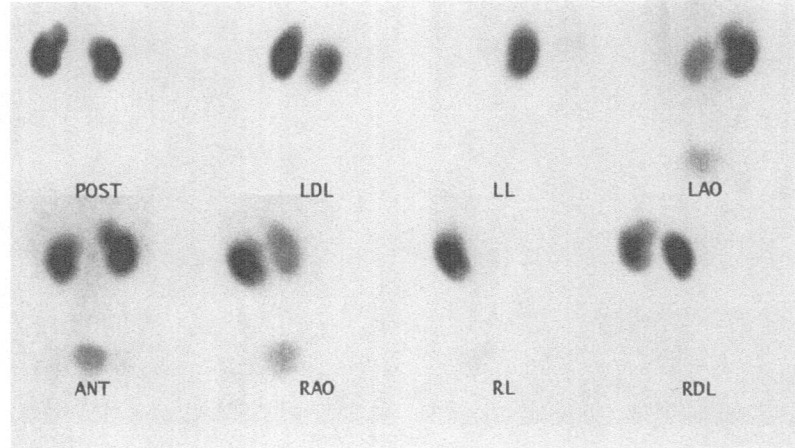

Fig. 24.3. The planar ^{99m}Tc-DMSA$_3$ scan shows a focal defect on the upper pole of the left kidney, while the uptake of the tracer in the contralateral kidney is undisturbed

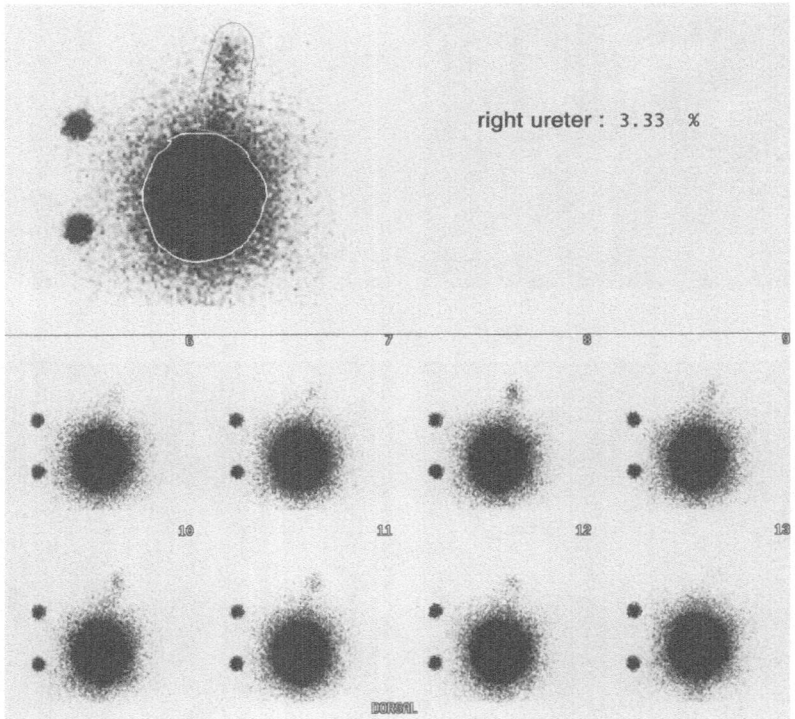

Fig. 24.4. Moderate VUR on the right side, seen during the third direct radionuclide cysto-urethrogram

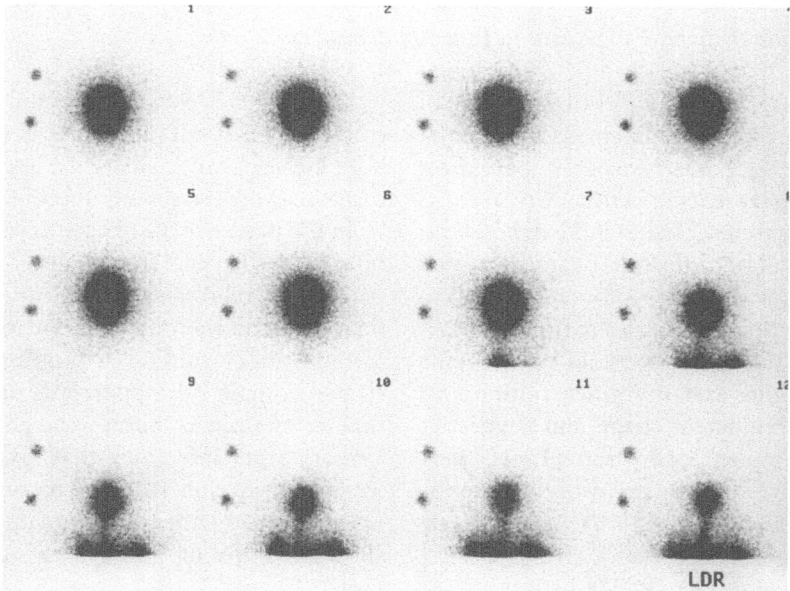

Fig. 24.5. Direct radionuclide cysto-urethrogram following therapy with Deflux: no VUR is present

CASE 25 ▶ *Hig-grade Bilateral VUR and Reflux Nephropathy*

Clinical Course: This 2-year-old girl presented with a retardation of motor development as a result of rickets. Further investigations revealed impaired renal function and urinary tract infection (*Streptococus pneumoniae*). The parents of the child did not remember any urinary tract infection or undiagnosed fever in the past, so that the asyptomatic infection may have been present for quite a long time.

On sonography (Fig. 25.1) the renal parenchyma looked inhomogeneous and the outer contours of the kidneys were irregular in shape and suggestive of renal scarring. No signs of hydronephrosis were present. Surprisingly, voiding cysto-urethrography (Fig. 25.2) demonstrated a grade-IV VUR on the right and a grade-V VUR on the left side.

This child's rickets therefore had to be interpreted as secondary to renal insufficiency caused by reflux nephropathy and successful treatment with high dosages of vitamin D was possible. While the clinical symptoms of vitamin D deficiency disappeared during the course, the renal insufficiency did not. The serum creatinine persisted at a level of 0.8 mg/dl and the creatinine clearance (55 ml/min), which was determined according to the method of Schwarz, remained impaired.

On the ^{99m}Tc-DMSA scan, reflux nephropathy was confirmed by multiple photopenic cortical areas on both kidneys, especially at the upper poles, which indicated severe renal scarring (Fig. 25.3).

In the presence of this combination of high-grade bilateral VUR, renal insufficiency and reflux nephropathy, surgical treatment was indicated and was performed some months later. Postoperatively we performed direct voiding scintigraphy, which demonstrated complete disappearance of the reflux. During further vitamin D therapy the child developed well. Urinary tract infections that occurred sporadically were afebrile. Renal impairment persisted but did not progress further. A follow-up sonography, again showing signs of renal scarring, is illustrated in Fig. 25.4.

Comment: In this girl asymptomatic chronic urinary tract infection was diagnosed after some delay. Severe reflux nephropathy with renal impairment and renal rachitis was found. This condition usually cannot be fully compensated. The girl remains at risk of progressive deteroration of renal function and renal hypertension.

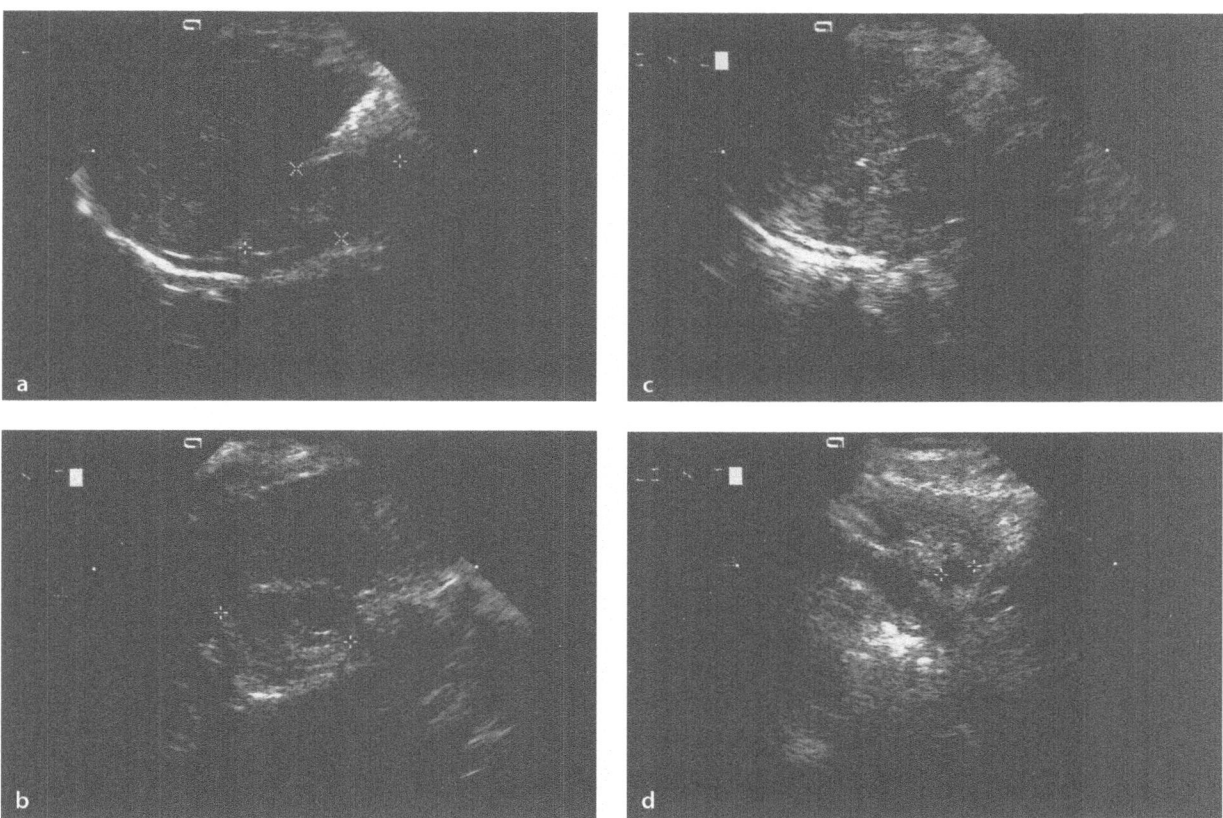

Fig. 25.1. **a, b** Right kidney; **c, d** left kidney. On initial sonography the renal parenchyma looks inhomogeneous and the outer contours of the kidneys are irregularly shaped and suggestive of renal scarring

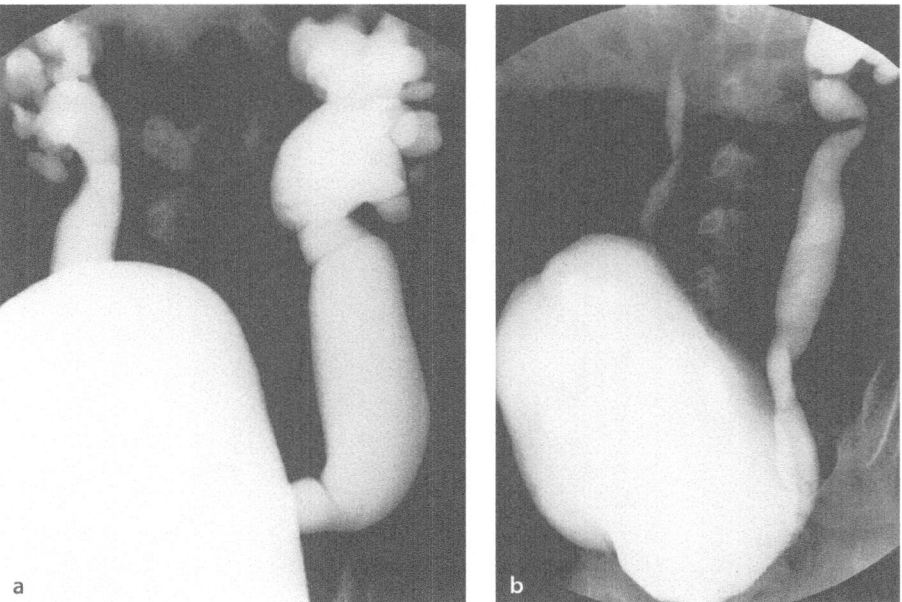

Fig. 25.2. Voiding cysto-urethrography demonstrating **a** grade-IV VUR on the right and **b** grade-V VUR on the left

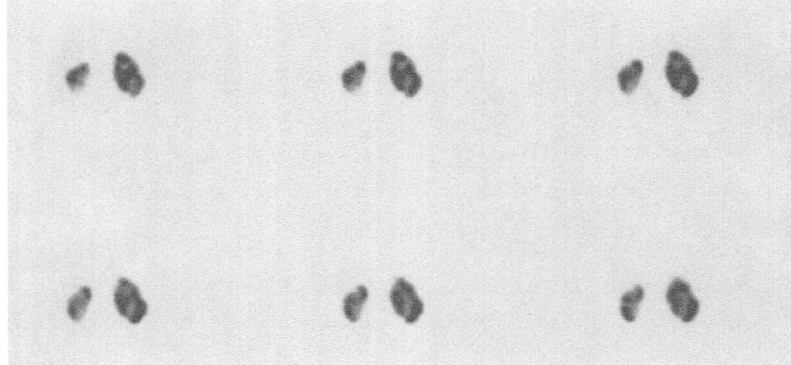

Fig. 25.3. On the ⁹⁹ᵐTc-DMSA SPECT (coronal slices from right to left), reflux nephropathy is confirmed by multiple photopenic cortical areas on both kidneys, indicating severe renal scarring. The split function of the right kidney was 39%

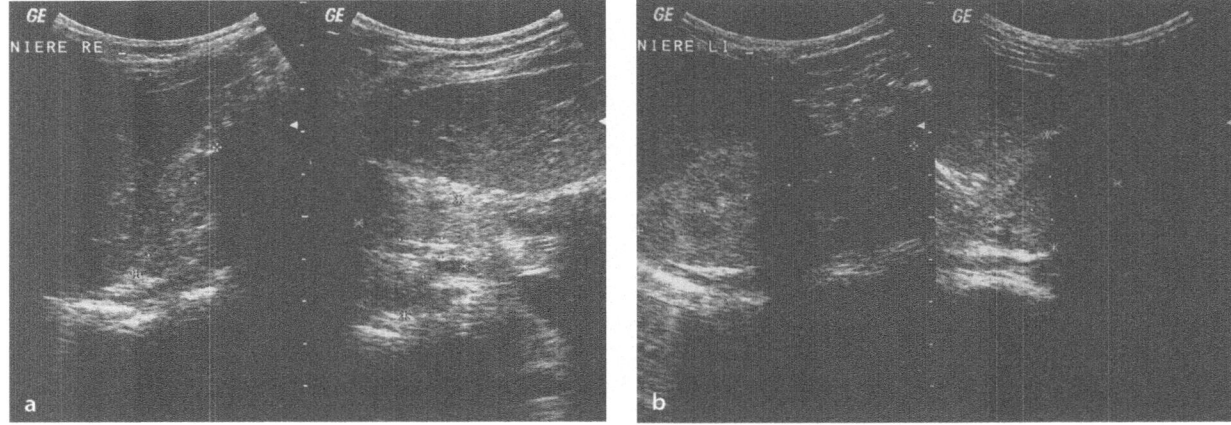

Fig. 25.4. a Right kidney; **b** left kidney. The signs of renal scarring are still present during sonographic follow-up

CASE 26 ▶ *Functional Disturbance of Micturition with Secondary Bilateral VUR*

Clinical Course: This girl was admitted to our institution when she was 7 years old. During the previous few years she had had several urinary tract infections. The initial ultrasound was suggestive of renal scarring. The renal pelvis seemed to be dilated, and the ureters on both sides could be visualized during bladder filling. These findings were highly suggestive of bilateral vesico-ureteral reflux (Figs. 26.1, 26.2).

Laboratory examinations revealed elevated serum creatinine levels of 1 mg/dl (GFR approximately 70 ml/min according to the method of Schwarz). No hypertension was present. During the first examination urinary tract infection with significant bacteriuria (*E. coli*) was diagnosed. The ESR and the CRP level were elevated (49 mm during the first hour and 7.2 mg/dl, respectively). After initial treatment of the urinary tract infection, we started antibiotic prophylaxis.

During voiding cysto-urethrography grade-III VUR was present (Fig. 26.3). We also found markedly deformed calyces. The urinary bladder looked trabeculated, which suggested a functional disturbance of micturition. On the ^{99m}Tc-DMSA scan the split function of the left kidney was diminished (32%). Focal cortical defects on both kidneys could also be diagnosed (Fig. 26.4).

An impairment of the global renal function combined with bilateral significant VUR and renal scarring was a clear indication for surgical correction in this 7-year-old girl. During surgery the typical findings of a cystic cystitis were noted. Reimplantation of the ureters, which were found in an orthotopic position, was performed according to Cohen's method. Postoperatively the urinary tract infections completely disappeared. The renal function remained stable, but is still moderately impaired. No renal hypertension developed. Sonographic follow-up demonstrated a smaller right kidney on the right side (39 ml). The contralateral kidney was considerably larger (78 ml). Both kidneys exhibited multifocal hyperechoic lesions suggestive of scarring in the renal cortex (Fig. 26.5).

Comment: In this girl a functional disturbance of micturition led to recurring urinary tract infections and a secondary bilateral VUR. Throughout the years before she was referred to our hospital severe reflux nephropathy with impaired renal function developed. The clinical symptoms and signs of urinary tract infection disappeared postoperatively, and the impairment of renal function did not progress further although renal function remained below the age-related normal range. Late complications such as renal hypertension are to be feared.

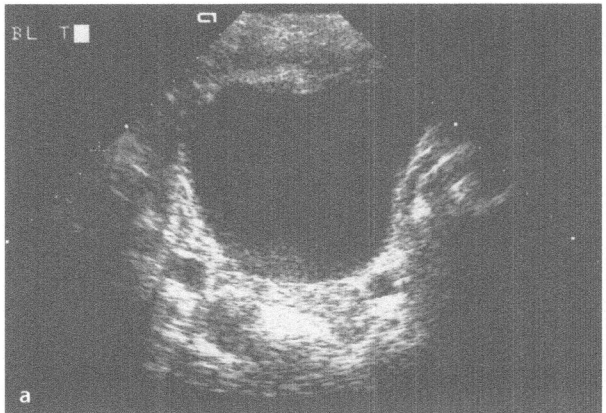 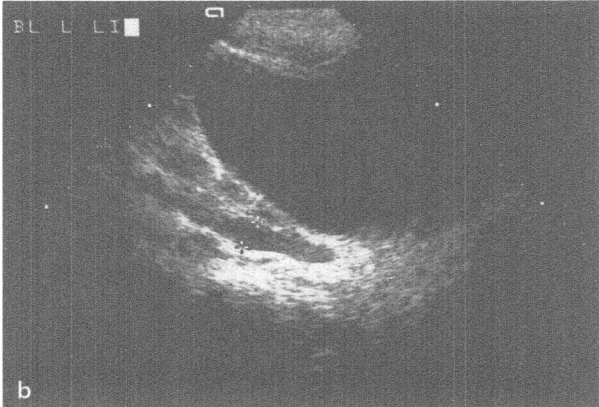

Fig. 26.1 a, b. Sonography during the first examination (**a** transverse, **b** longitudinal sections). Dilated ureters can bei seen bilaterally near the urinary bladder

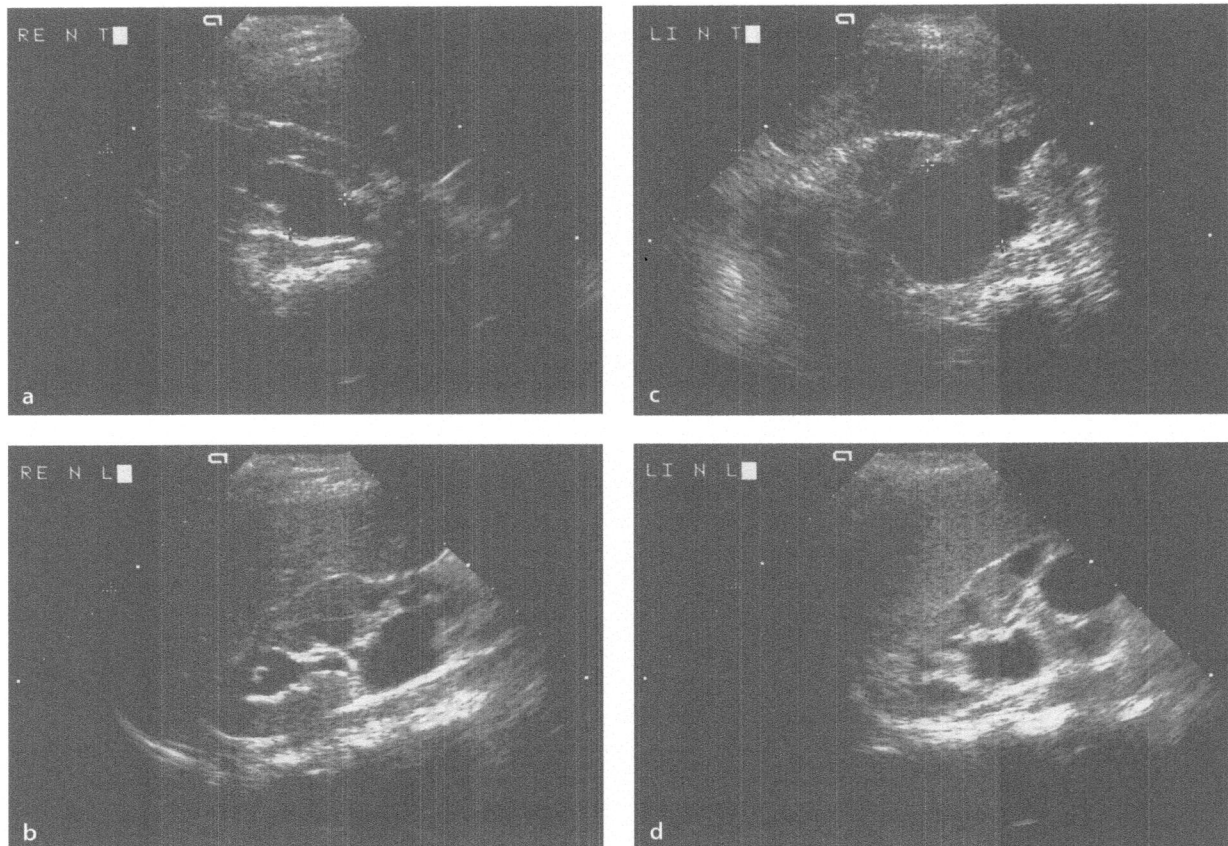

Fig. 26.2 a–d. Sonography of the kidneys (**a** transverse, **b** longitudinal sections of the right kidney, **c** transverse, **d** longitudinal sections of the left kidney). The pelvicalyceal system is dilated on both sides (hydronephrosis grade II on the right and grade III on the left). There are signs of cortical thinning, which is suggestive of scarring

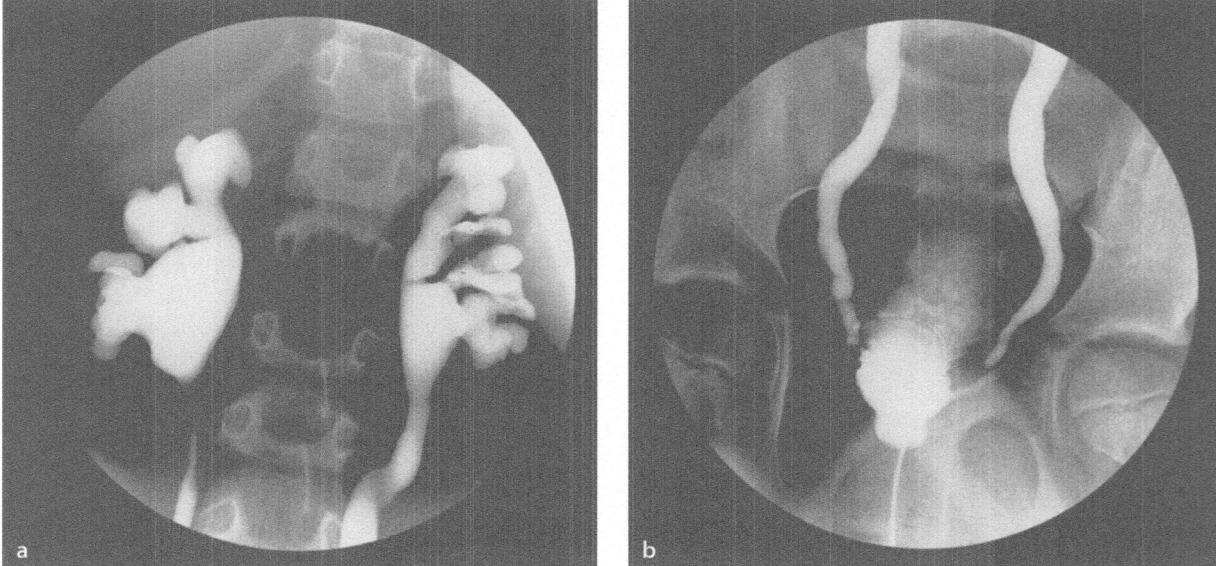

Fig. 26.3 a,b. On the voiding cysto-urethrogram grade-II reflux is present on both sides. The urinary bladder wall looks trabeculated

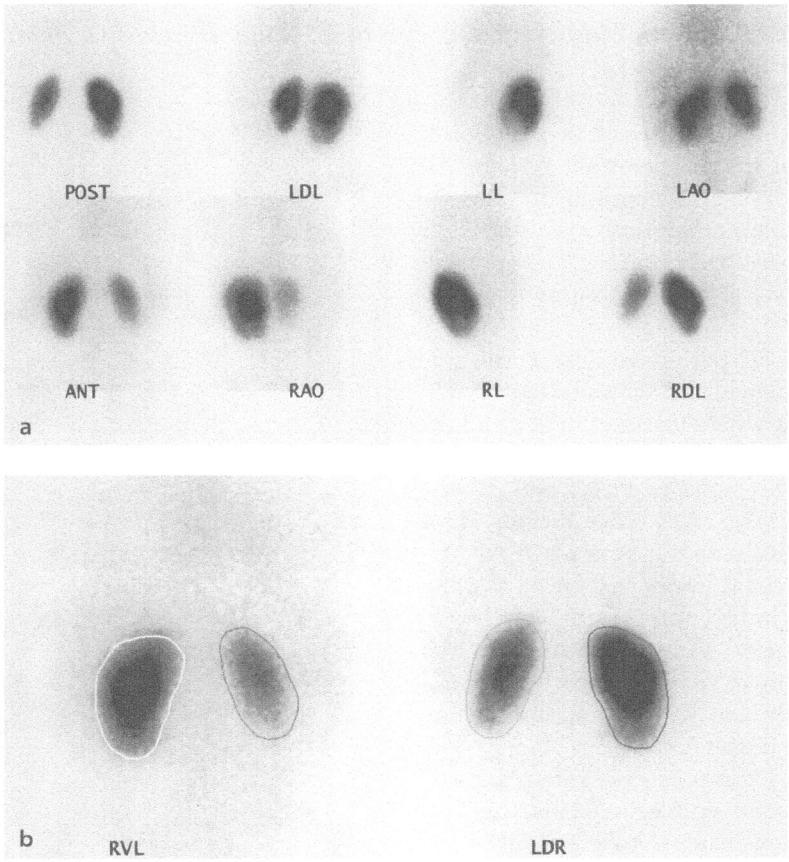

Fig. 26.4 a, b. ^{99m}Tc-DMSA scan. **a** Planar scan shows cortical defects, especially at the lower poles, on both kidneys. The tubular function is impaired on the left side. **b** The split renal function of the left kidney is 32 %, of the right kidney is 68 %

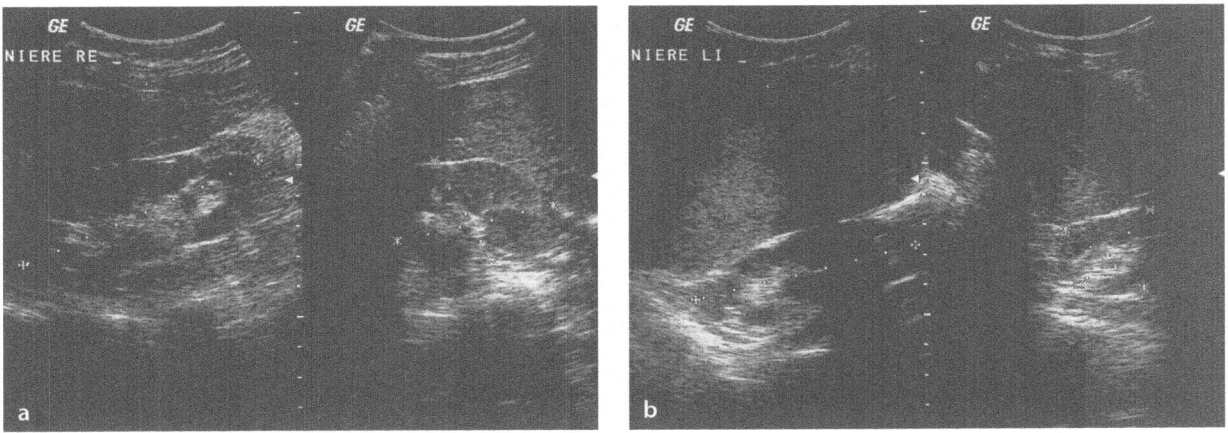

Fig. 26.5 a, b. Sonography during postoperative follow-up: signs of cortical scarring on both kidneys. The right kidney (**a**) is considerably larger than the left one (**b**). No signs of obstruction can be found

CASE 27 ► *Left-sided Dysplastic Multicystic Kidney and Testicular Dysplasia Combined with Contralateral High-grade VUR*

Clinical Course: During the 34 week of gestation a bilateral dilatation of the urinary tract system had been recognized on prenatal sonography in this boy. The first postnatal sonography raised the suspicion of a multicystic-dysplastic left kindney. The drainage system of the contralateral kidney was grossly dilated (Fig. 27.1).

During the neonatal period voiding cysto-ure-thrography was performed and showed a high-grade VUR on the right side with a tortuous ureter, and dilatation of the renal pelvis combined with deformation of the calyces. No signs of an infravesical obstruction were noted (Fig. 27.2). When the boy was 4 weeks old a ^{99m}Tc-MAG$_3$ scan was performed. On this scan the left kidney could not be visualized and the function of the right kidney was seen to be well preserved. The right ureter was seen throughout the drainage phase, but there were no signs of obstruction. Antibiotic prophylaxis was started, and the boy was discharged from hospital.

When the boy was 1 year old he was referred to our institution for a second opinion. During the first physical examination a painless enlargement of the left testicle was noted. Testicular sonography revealed a marked difference in volume between the right and left testicles (Fig. 27.3) and an inhomogenous pattern combined with multicystic degeneration of the lower pole on the left side. As a testicular tumour was suspected, orchidectomy was performed. Histologically, cystic dysplasia of the left testicle was diagnosed. Besides well-differentiated tubules in some regions, the histological slices showed highly atrophic and dilated tubules in other sections of the specimen. No abnormality was found in the rete testis.

Comment: This boy had testicular dysplasia combined with an ipsilateral multicystic renal degeneration. Similar cases, which indicate a common ontogenetic background for this coincidence, have been described in the literature. In addition, a high-grade VUR on the contralateral side with well-prserved renal function was noted in our case. Surgical correction will be mandatory if the reflux persists during follow-up.

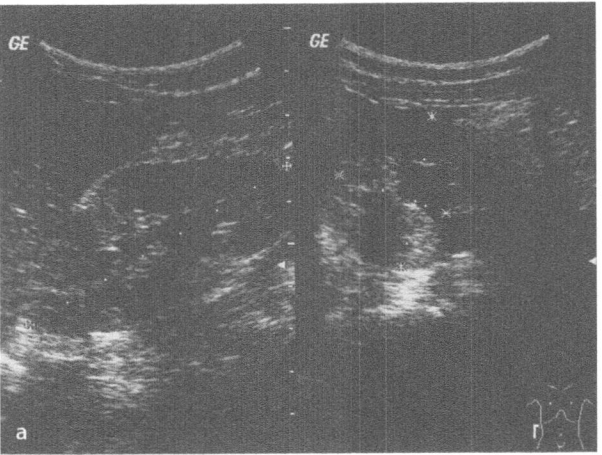

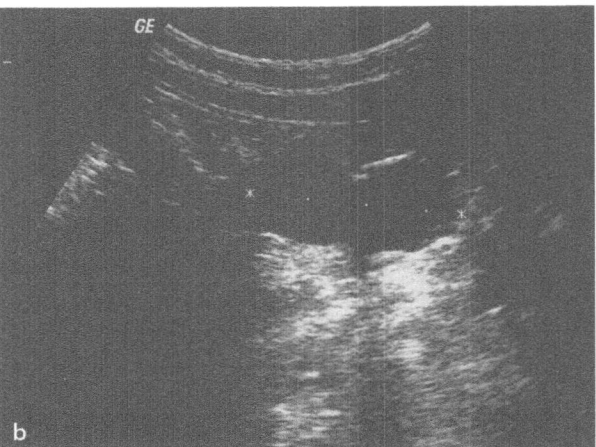

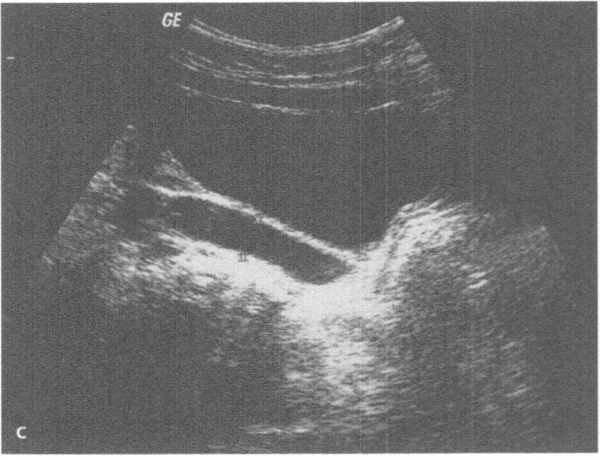

Fig. 27.1a–c. Initial sonography. **a** Sonography of the right kidney (longitudinal and transversal sections): normal thickness of the parenchyma and slight dilatation of the drainage system. **b** Sonography of the left kidney region, demonstrating two cystic structures without evidence of a normally developed parenchyma. **c** Dilatation of the right distal ureter

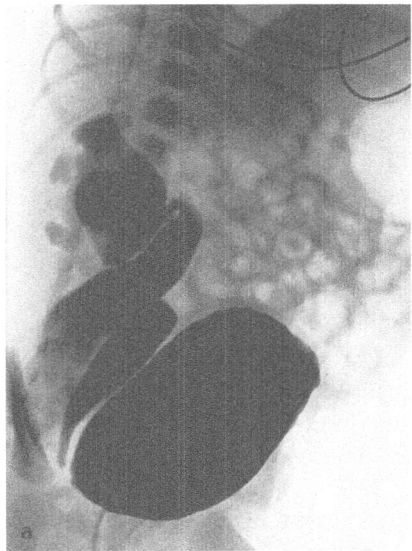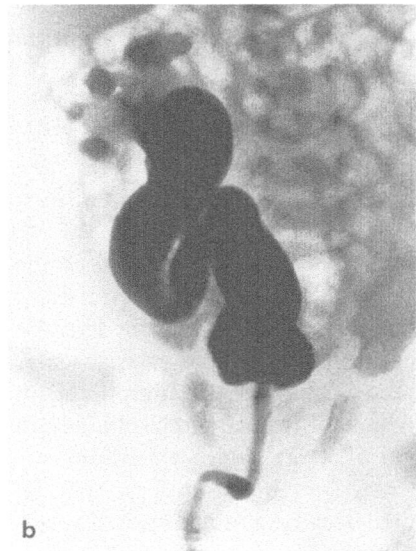

Fig. 27.2a,b. Voiding cysto-urethrography. **a** High-grade VUR on the right side with tortuous ureter and dilatation of the renal pelvis combined with deformation of the calyces. **b** During micturition the urethra shows no abnormalities, and an infravesical obstruction can be excluded

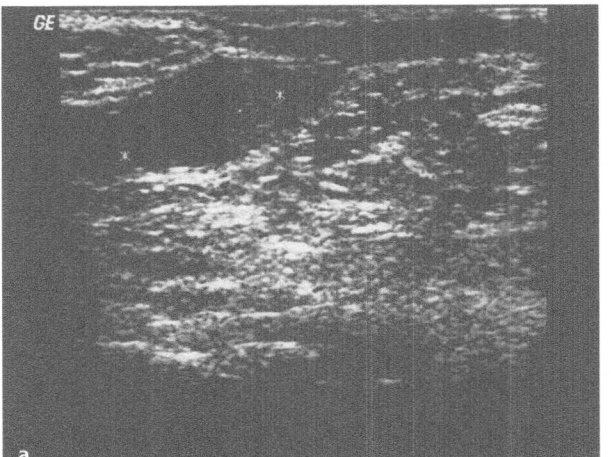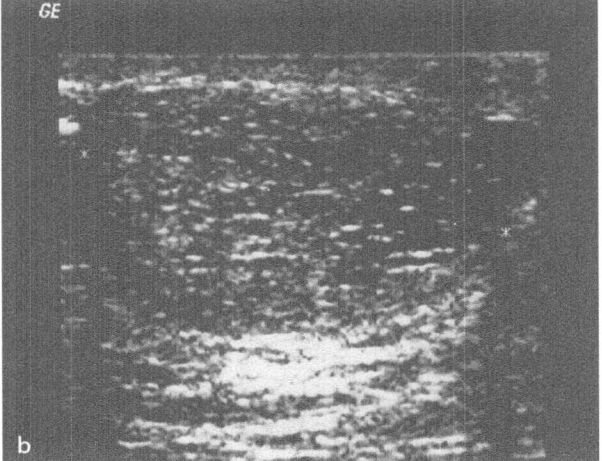

Fig. 27.3a,b. Testicular sonography. **a** Normal appearance and volume of the right testicle. **b** The left testicle shows a hyperechoic inhomogeneous pattern combined with multicystic degeneration of the lower pole

CASE 28 ▶ *Polycystic Kidney (Autosomal Dominant Type)*

Clinical Course: In this girl a tumour was palpated in the left upper quadrant of abdomen by the paediatrician when she was 6 weeks old. The child was then admitted to our university hospital for further investigations.

The first sonography (Fig. 28.1) showed multiple cysts in a large and ireegularly structured left kidney, which extended from the abdomen into the left side of the pelvis. Cavography revealed a regular vascular supply to the kidney, and the pyelogram again demonstrated a considerably enlarged left kidney, in which the excretion of X-ray contrast medium was delayed but preserved. Computed tomography (CT), which was performed because a tumour was suspected, confirmed the diagnosis of cystic degeneration of the left kidney and was suggestive of additional renal cysts on the contralateral kidney, as was a follow-up songraphic investigation 2 years after the first (Fig. 28.2). During diagnostic laparotomy the suspicion of a tumour was subsequently ruled out and the diagnosis of a bilateral cystic renal disease was established. The parents and other members of the family were found to be free of renal abnormalities. The asymmetric involvement of the kidneys, the absence of cystic lesions in the liver and a well-preserved function of the left kidney seemed to make autoso-

mal recessive polycystic renal disease or multicystic renal degeneration unlikely in this child. In addition, there were no signs of renal involvement as part of an underlying syndrome (tuberous sclerosis, von Hippel-Landau's disease). The most probable diagnosis was therefore an early manifestation of an autosomal dominant polycystic renal degeneration due to a spontaneous germline mutation.

During the next 12 years the child was only infrequently seen in our institution. The girl's global renal function remained stable. When she was 14 years old she developed unselective proteinuria with a protein excretion of 4 g/day. At the same time we diagnosed mild hypertension, which disappeared after weight reduction without further medical treatment. When the patient was seen again at the age of 18 years, the sonography revealed a pattern similar to that seen in the preceding investigations (Fig. 28.3).

Comment: A clear classification of the underlying cystic renal disease was not possible in this child. The most probable diagnosis was an autosomal dominant polycystic renal degeneration due to a spontaneous germline mutation. Molecular genetic confirmation of this assumption was not obtained, because of a lack of specific molecular markers in this family.

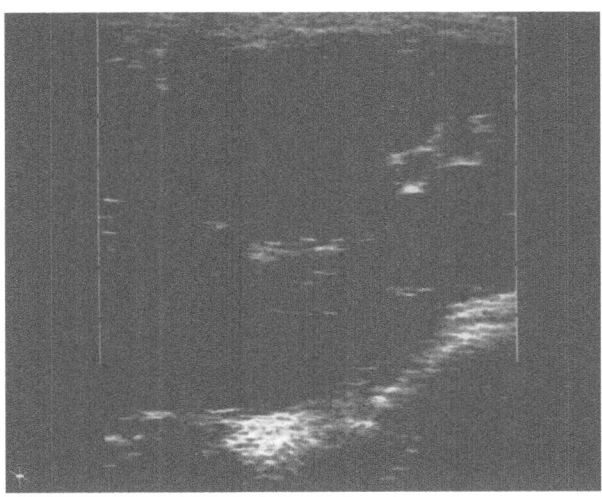

Fig. 28.1. The initial sonography in the 6-week-old girl shows a irregularly structured large kidney on the left side, with multiple cysts

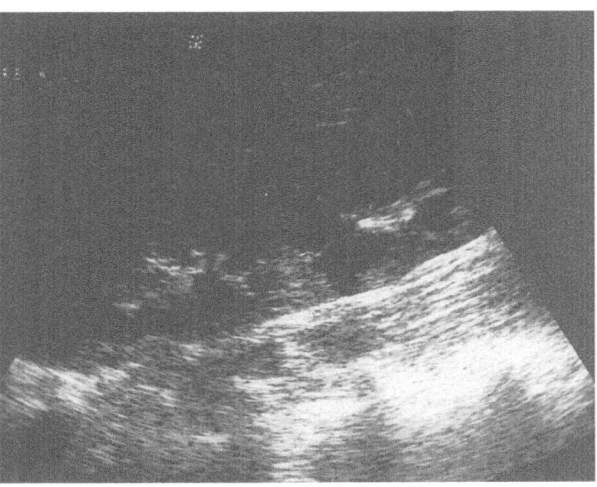

Fig. 28.3. Sonographic appearance of the right kidney when the girl was 18 years old.

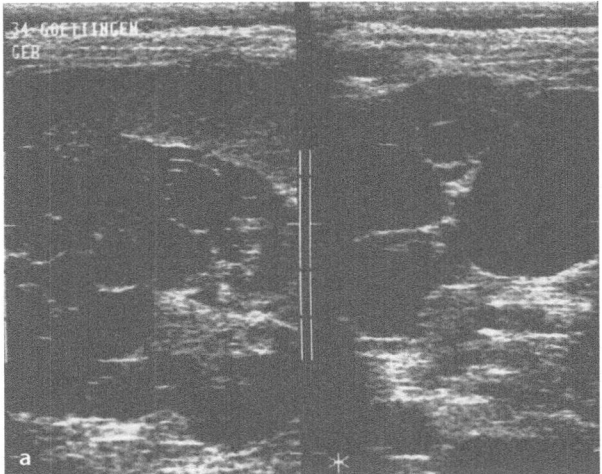

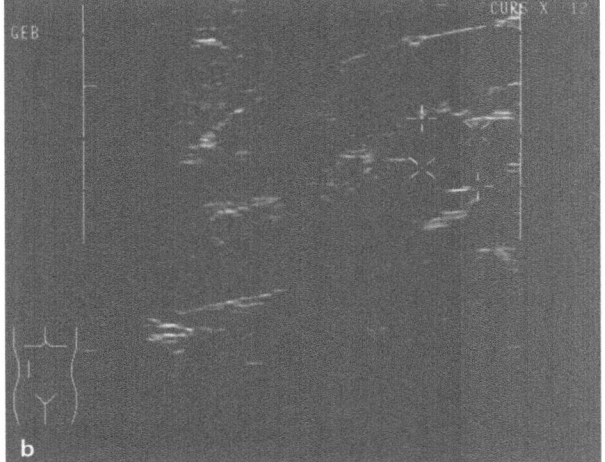

Fig. 28.2. During sonographic follow-up 2 years later, cystic lesions are also found on the right kidney (**a** left kidney, **b** right kidney)

CASE 29 ▶ *Tuberous Sclerosis – Cystic Renal Disease*

Clinical Course: This female sibling developed seizures when she was 6 months old. Clinical examination revealed foci of cutaneous depigmentation ("ash-leaf" sign: Fig. 29.1), which are typical stigmata of tuberous sclerosis. Another feature of this disease is adenoma sebaceum, which usually develops later in childhood, and the caracteristic paraventricular protuberances (Fig. 29.2), which were diagnosed on the CT scan when the girl was 8 years old.

Half the children affected with this disease suffer from additional renal pathology, such as polycystic renal disease and harmartomas. During her clinical course, our patient also developed sonographic features of renal involvement. Small cystic lesions (maximum diameter 4 mm) and an inhomogeneous parenchymal pattern of both enlarged kidneys can be seen in Fig. 29.3.

Throughout our patient's entire childhood, medical therapy was focused on control of the seizures. In addition, the girl developed marked mental retardation. Up to now there has been no deterioration in renal function.

Comment: Tuberous sclerosis is an autosomal dominant disease caused by mutations on chromosomes 6 and 13. In 50% of cases spontaneous new mutations occur. Children with tuberous sclerosis should be screened for polycystic renal disease. If features of renal involvement are found invasive confirmation (biopsy) is not necessary.

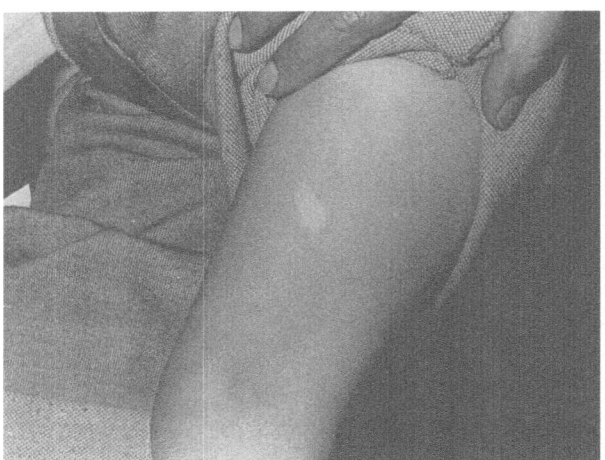

Fig. 29.1. Typical depigmentation ("ash-leaf spot")

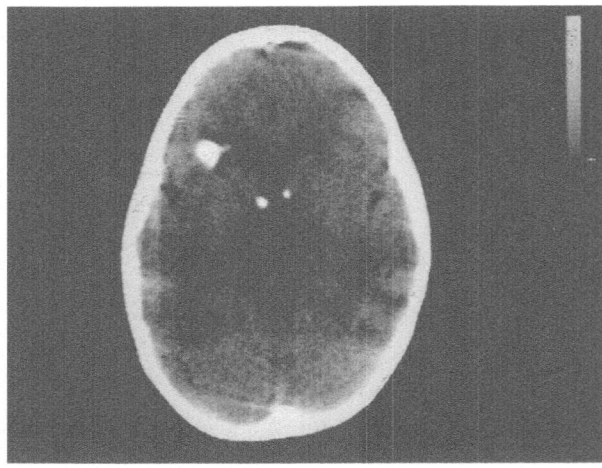

Fig. 29.2. Chracteristic paraventricular protuberances seen on the CCT

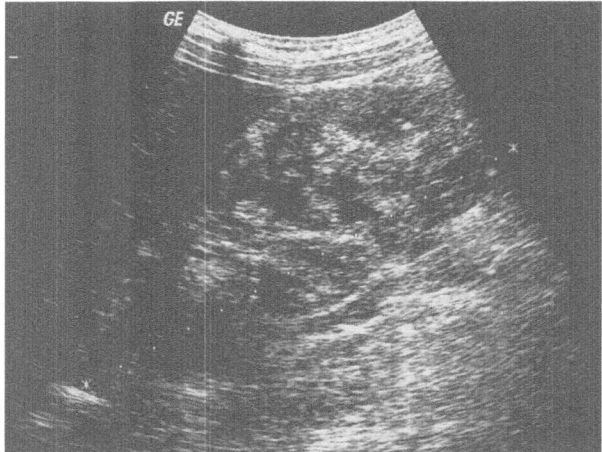

◀

Fig. 29.3. Sonographic findings: small cystic lesions and hyperechoic spots are seen

CASE 30 ▶ *Urethral Valve – Severe Secondary Reflux*

Clinical Course: On the 5th day after birth this boy developed fulminant urosepsis. On the first sonography the kidneys and both collecting systems looked abnormal, a thickening of the urinary bladder wall (Fig. 30.1 a) and bilateral hydronephrosis, which was more pronounced on the left side, were recognized (Fig. 30.1 b, c). In addition, the left kidney looked to be smaller than the right one (Fig. 30.1 c) and to have a thinned parenchyma and a dilated pelvicalyceal system (Fig. 30.2). The first voiding cysto-urethrography was performed on the assumption that an infravesical obstruction (urethral valve) was present, which was subsequently confirmed by the typical dilatation of the prostatic urethra and a sudden change in the diameter of the urethra at the prostatic-penile junction (Fig. 30.3). The urinary bladder wall exhibited multiple pseudodiverticula. A bilateral VUR was recognized. Both ureters looked massively dilated. In addition, the right ureter was twisted and there was marked intrarenal reflux on the same side (Fig. 30.3).

We performed valvotomy on the 25th day after birth. No persistent reflux was detected on the postoperative voiding cysto-urethrography (Fig. 30.4). The diameter of the urethra had substantially decreased. On the cystogram the pseudodiverticula persisted.

We performed a ^{99m}Tc-MAG$_3$ scan when the boy was 4 weeks old, as we assumed there was acquired renal failure or renal dysplasia on the left side. Complete loss of left renal function was noted (Fig. 30.5).

There were no more complications in the further clinical course under antibiotic prophylaxis. The thickening of the urinary bladder decreased (Fig. 30.6a), and while mild hydronephrosis persistent in the right kidney renal parenchyma looked normal (Fig. 30.6b). When the child was 15 months old the ^{99m}Tc-DMSA scan showed that there had been no recovery of the left renal function (Figs. 30.7, 30.8), and nephrectomy of the left kidney was subsequently performed.

Comment: Urethral valves are among the most severe abnormalities of the male urinary tract and may be followed by severe renal damage in utero. In our case the prenatal diagnosis failed. A complete loss of the left renal function occurred due to secondary VUR. Although severe VUR was also present on the right side, early valvotomy made it possible to preserve this kidney.

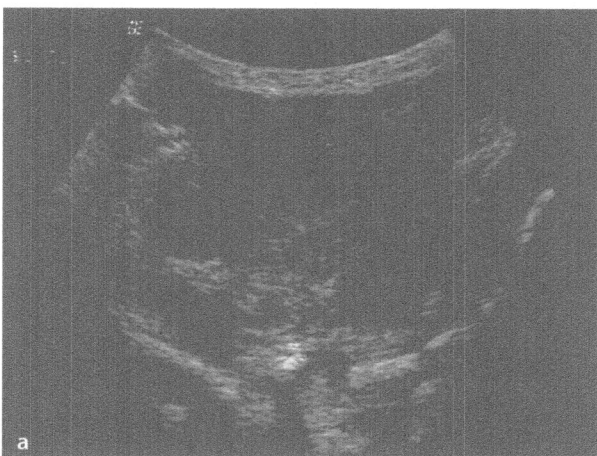

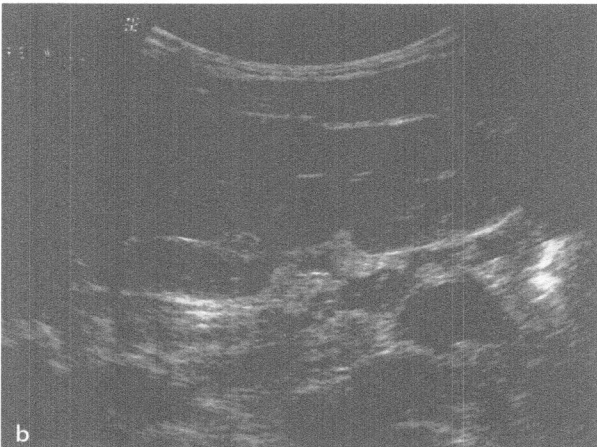

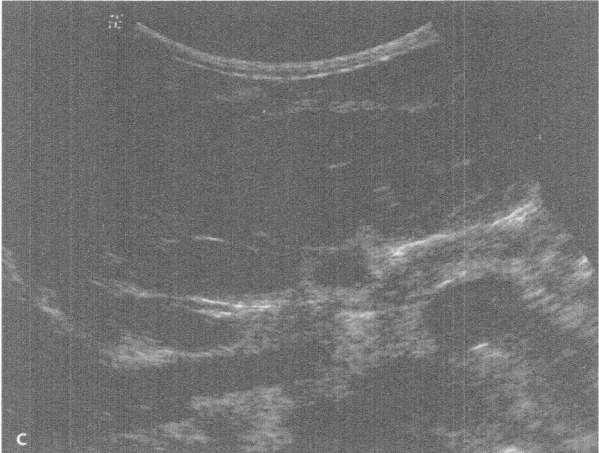

Fig. 30.1 a–c. Sonography. **a** Thickening of the urinary bladder wall. **b** Right kidney: normal echogenicity of the parenchyma, dilated calyces. **c** Left kidney: dilatation of the collecting system. The parenchyma appears to be small

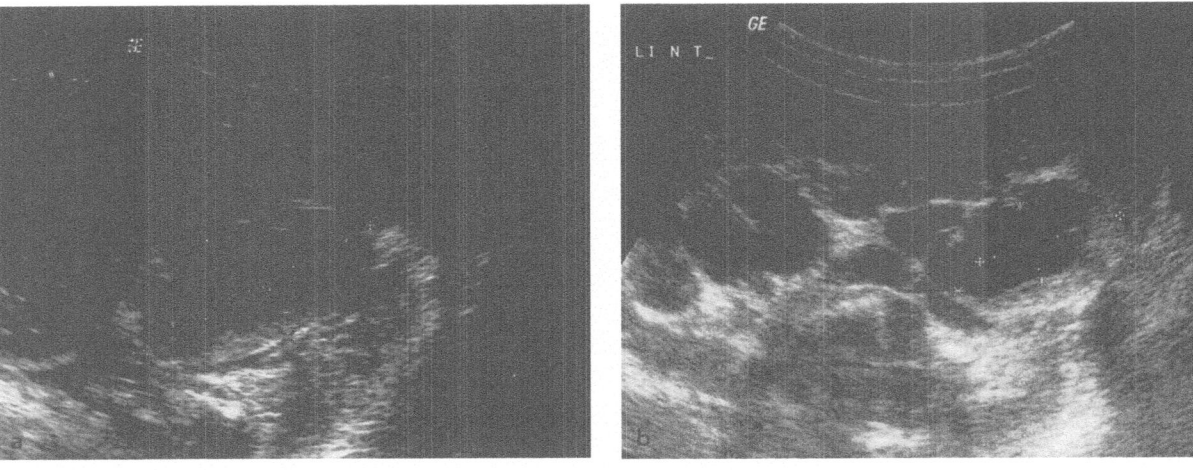

Fig. 30.2 a, b. Left kidney with thinned parenchyma and dilatation of the pelvicalyceal system

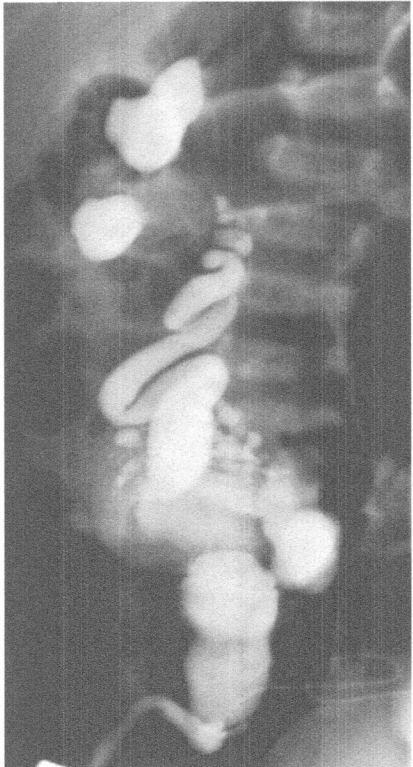

Fig. 30.3. Voiding cysto-urethrography: massive dilation of the prostatic urethra and stenosis in the junction to the penile part of the urethra. Multiple pseudodiverticula in the urinary bladder wall. Massively dilated left ureter. Twisting of the right ureter and intrarenal reflux on the right side

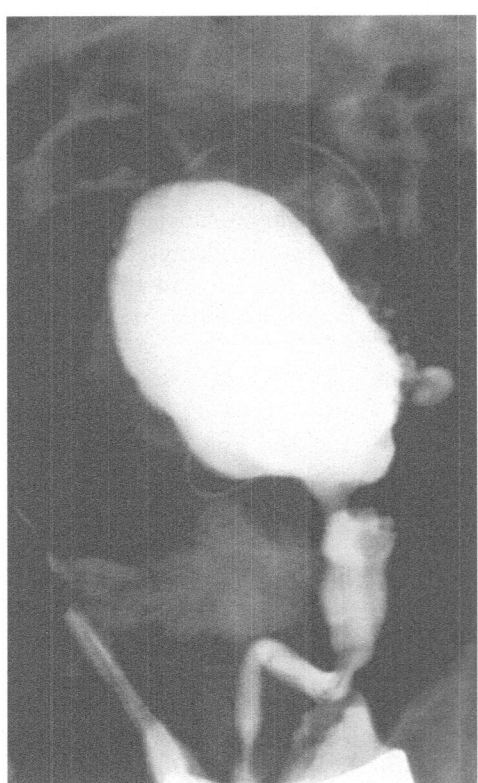

Fig. 30.4. Partial normalization of the voiding cysto-urethrography in the postoperative phase. Absence of persistent urethral stenosis and VUR. Para-ureteral diverticulum on the left side. Irregularities of the urinary bladder wall contour

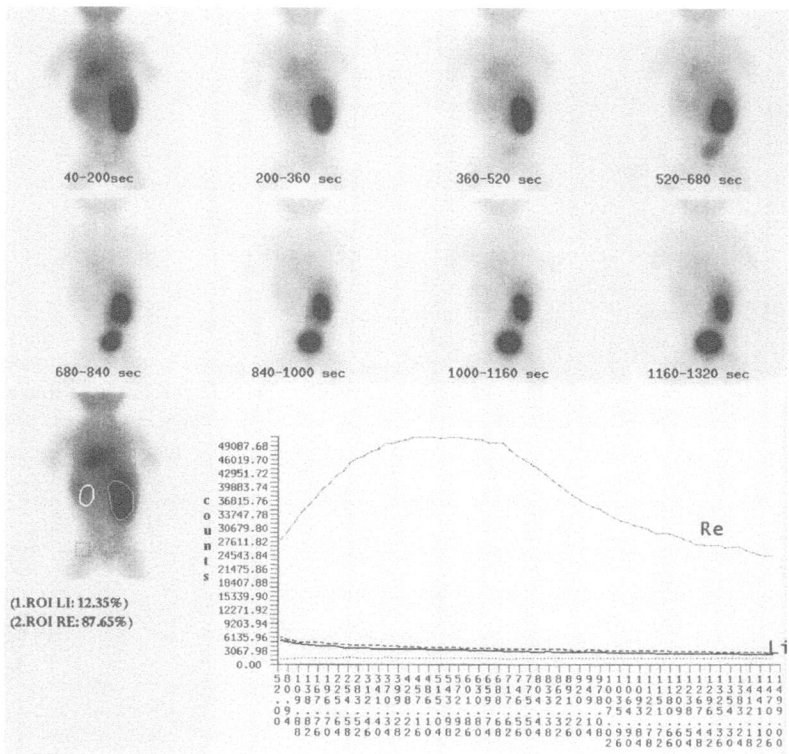

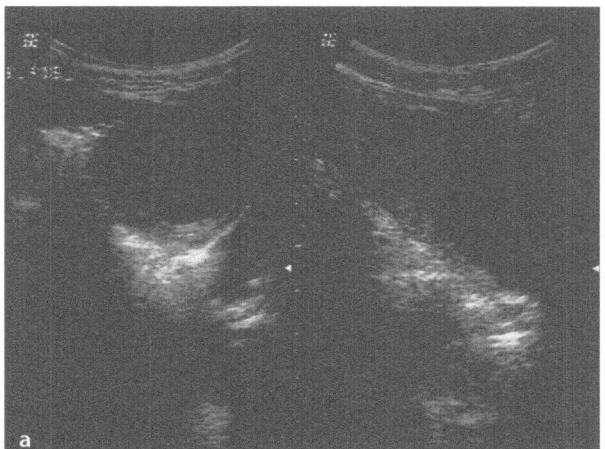

Fig. 30.5 (*above*). ^{99m}Tc-MAG$_3$ scan: complete loss of the left kidney's function. The transit of the tracer on the right side is somewhat delayed, but still normal for a 4-week-old child

Fig. 30.6a–c (*below*). Sonographic follow up. **a** Normalization of the thickened wall of the urinary bladder. **b, c** Moderate dilation of the collecting system of the right kidney

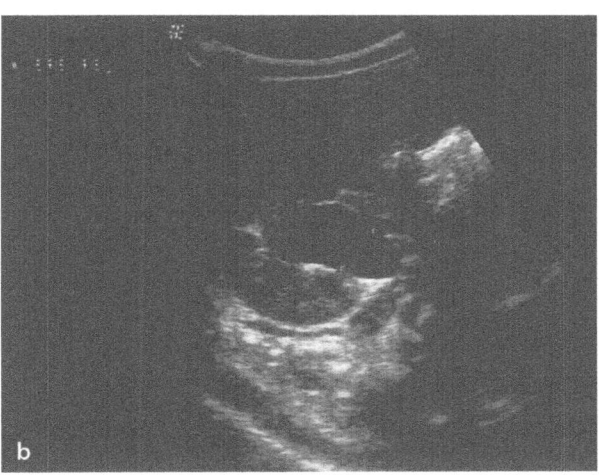

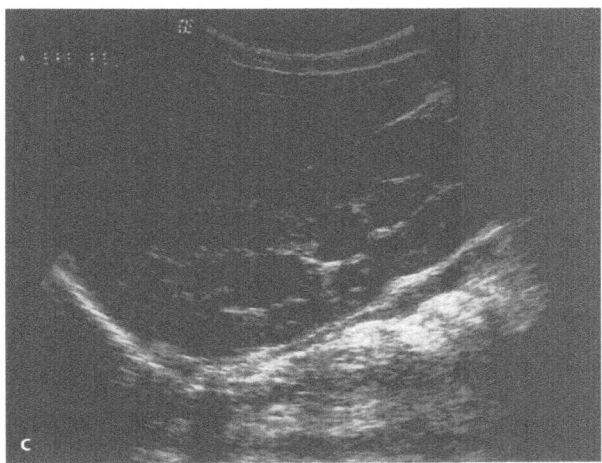

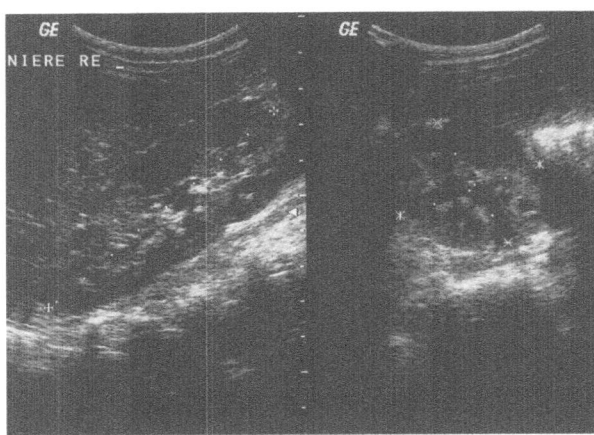

Fig. 30.7. The hypertrophic right kidney during follow-up
◀

Fig. 30.8. The planar ^{99m}Tc-DMSA scan shows there has been no recovery of the left renal function, while the uptake of the tracer in the contralateral kidney is undisturbed
▼

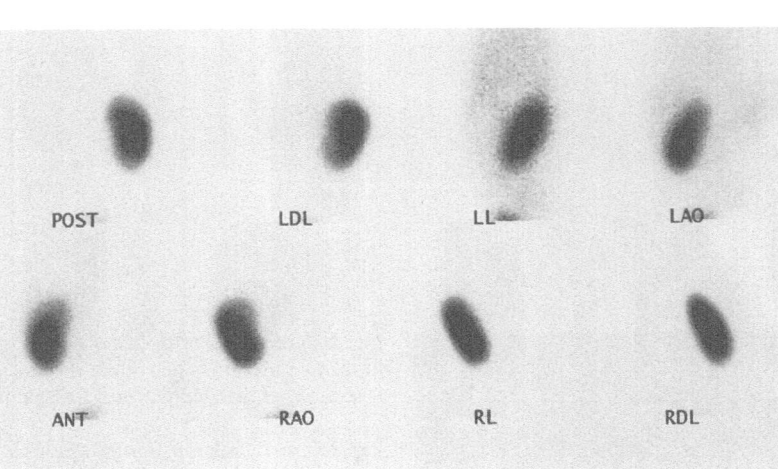

CASE 31 ▶ *Terminal Renal Insufficiency Due to Obstructive Uropathy Caused by a Urethral Valve: Renal Transplantation at 2¹/₂ Years of Age*

Clinical Course: During the 18th week of gestation dilatation of the drainage system was recognized in this male patient. Because hypertrophy of the urinary bladder wall was also present, an obstructive uropathy caused by a urethral valve was suggested at an early stage. An oligohydramnion was know to have been present since the 31st week of gestation, and a caesarian section was therefore performed during the 32nd week. After the birth the child was in good general condition.

The first sonography revealed a small urinary bladder (Fig. 31.1 a) with a hypertrophic wall, combined with bilateral hydronephrosis and thinning of the renal parenchyma (Fig. 31.1 b, c).

The voiding cysto-urethrography exhibited the typical pattern of a urethral valve in the prostatic–penile junction of the urethra. A bilateral secondary vesico-ureteral reflux was recognized. Both ureters looked tortuous and were massively dilated. On the left side pyeloparenchymal reflux into a dysplastic renal pelvis was seen (Fig. 31.2).

We performed percutaneous ureterostomy on the boy's 2nd day. Resection of the urethral valve was performed 2 months later. During the further clinical course the child showed progressive deterioration of renal function (Fig. 31.3). Percutaneous endoscopic gastrostomy was performed due to progessive failure to thrive when the boy was 1 year old, and for the first time renal transplantation was considered. Hyperalimentation was given to normalize the boy's weight and growth. Renal transplantation was performed when the boy was 30 months old and has so far proved successful (Fig. 31.4). During transplantation the right kidney was removed, followed by the removal of the contralateral kidney 2 weeks later.

Comment: In this boy a high-grade obstructive uropathy due to a urethral valve was diagnosed prenatally. During his postpartal course the child developed progressive renal insufficiency. Successful renal transplantation was performed when the child was 30 months old.

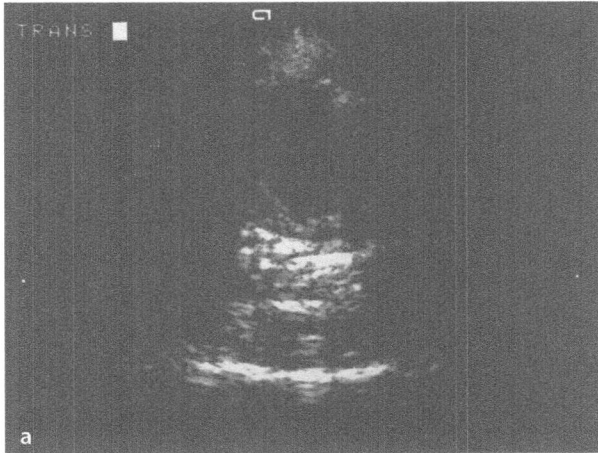

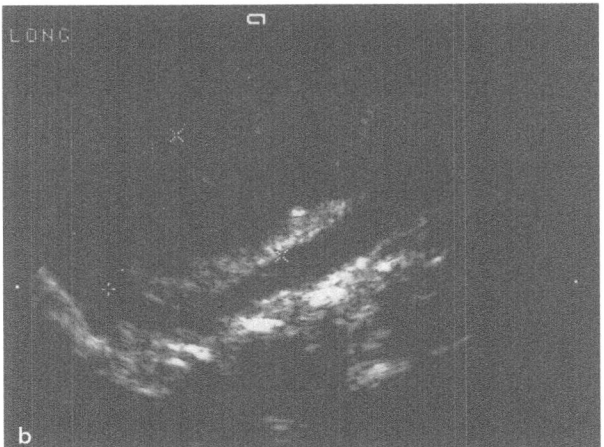

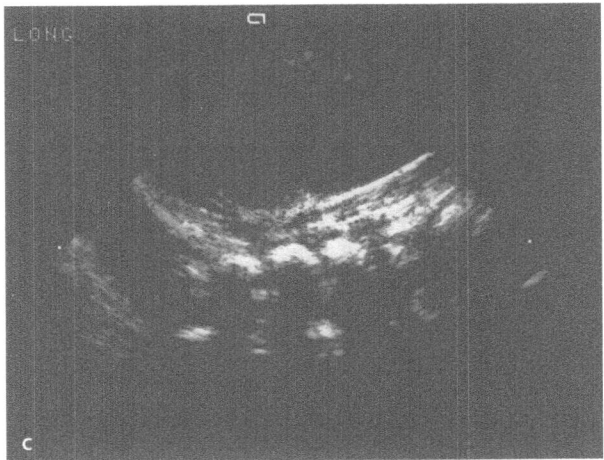

Fig. 31.1 a–c. First postpartal sonography. **a** Thickening of the urinary bladder wall. **b** Left kidney (longitudinal section): dilatation of the intrarenal collecting system. The parenchyma appears to be hyperechoic and thin. **c** In the right kidney a similar pattern can be observed

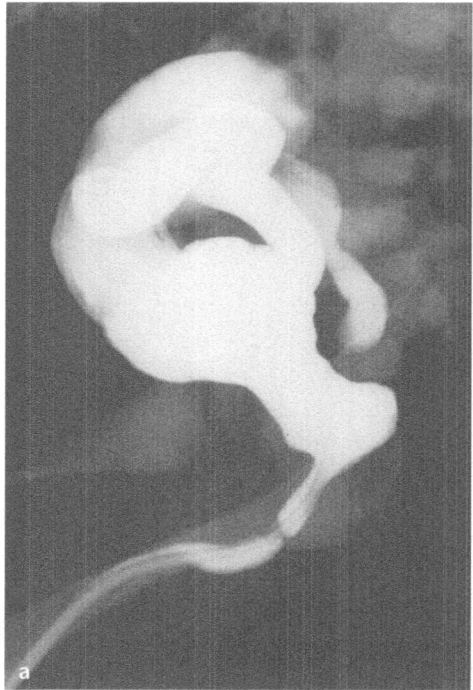

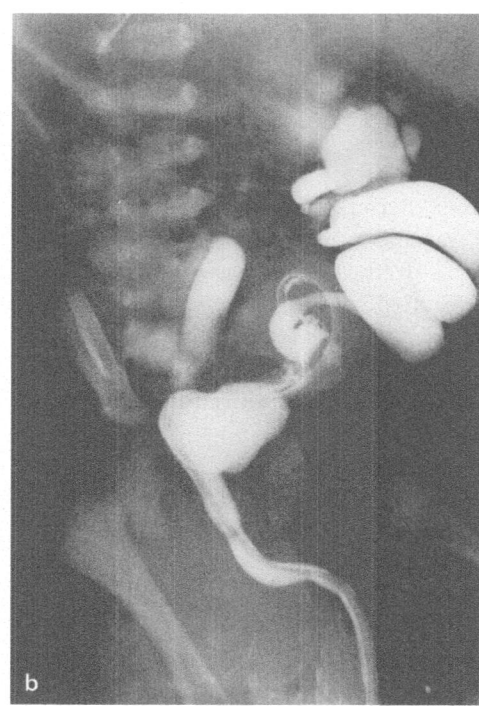

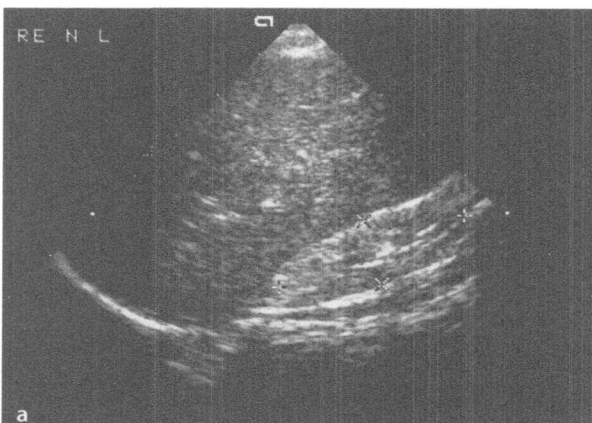

Fig. 31.2a, b (*above*). During voiding cysto-urethrography a narrowing between the prostatic and penile part of the urethra can be observed. The urinary bladder wall looks irregular. VUR into both ureters, which are dilated and tortuous, and pyeloparenchymatous reflux on the left side can be seen. As a sign of massive dypslasia on the left side the parenchyma is very small

Fig. 31.3a, b (*left*). Sonography at the child's 6th month. Both kidneys (**a** right, **b** left) are hyperechoic and small (longitudinal sections)

Fig. 31.4 (*below*). The transplanted kidney in the right pelvis. The echogenicity is normal. The parenchyma is well preserved and there are no signs of hydronephrosis

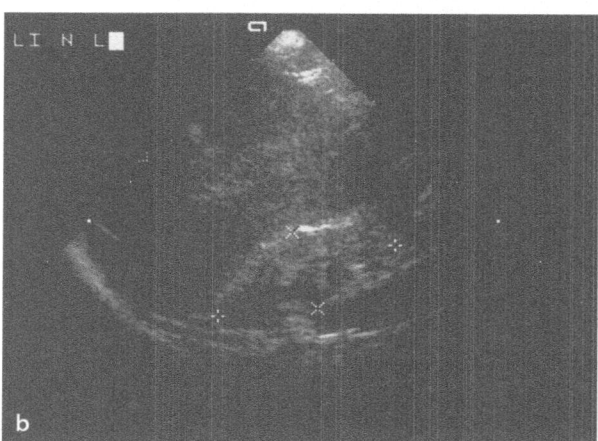

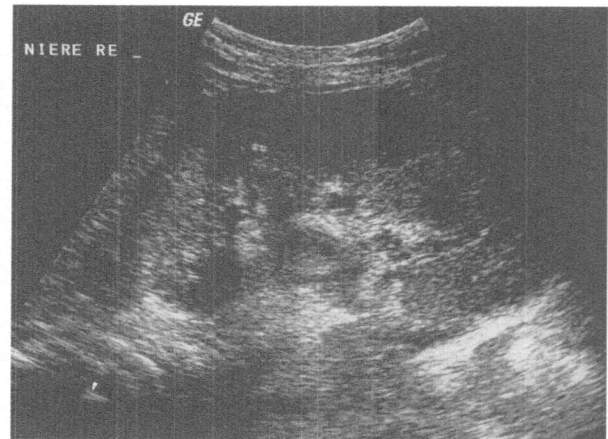

CASE 32 ▶ *Bladder Exstrophy and Uretero-enterostomy (Mainz Pouch II)*

Clinical Course: A full-term newborn girl with bladder exstrophy was referred to our department immediately after birth. Figure 32.1 shows the split pelvis and the bipartite clitoris without further abnormalities. The child's urinary bladder was closed during the 1st day after delivery, and the split pelvis was surgically fixed. Figure 32.2 shows the girl at 5 weeks of age. Besides the bipartite clitoris, scarring of the skin from the umbilical region to the pubic symphysis can be seen.

Postoperatively we started antibiotic prophylaxis. During the further clinical course we diagnosed an increasing dilatation of the upper urinary tract and hypertrophy of the urinary bladder wall, which are indicative of infravesical obstruction (Fig. 32.3 a–c). On the ^{99m}Tc-MAG$_3$ scan we found the typical pattern of bilateral obstruction, with no response after furosemide (Fig. 32.4).

We performed cystoscopy when the child was 9 months old. A percutaneous supravesical catheter was used for voiding cysto-urethrography, which revealed a bilateral 4th grade vesico-ureteric reflux (Fig. 32.5). During the second operation, dilatation of the scarred urinary bladder neck and urethra was performed. Intraoperatively a polypoid transformation of the bladder mucosa was seen.

Following the second correction, the infravesical obstruction improved, but the girl had occasionally recurring upper urinary tract infections with *Pseu-domonas aeruginosa*. These infections were treated with intravenous antibiotics. We therefore decided to perform uretero-enterostomy when the child was $3^1/_2$ years old. During this procedure the ureters were implanted into a pouch constructed from the girl's recto-sigmoid (Mainz pouch II).

Postoperatively the child developed well and no further urinary tract infections occurred. The dilatation of the upper urinary tract showed subsequent improvement on ultrasound. Sonographically we found no signs of scarring and a normal thickness of the parenchyma (Fig. 32.6). On the pyelogram (Fig. 32.7) the calyces were seen to be only slightly deformed, especially on the left side. The left ureter was dilated from the renal pelvis to the pouch, while the right ureter looked normal. The ^{99m}Tc-MAG$_3$ scan excluded an obstruction (Fig. 32.8).

Comment: Bladder exstrophy is a rare but severe malformation of the lower urinary tract and a therapeutic challenge. Reconstructive surgery is necessary to prevent complications, especially urinary tract infections and helps to avoid permanent incontinence.

In this child early surgical correction led to infravesical obstruction and secondary VUR followed by urinary tract infections. Uretero-enterostomy protected the child against further infections and enabled adequate continence during the further clinical course.

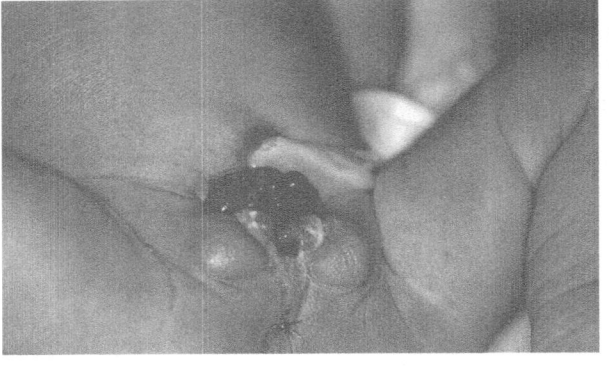

Fig. 32.1. Bladder exstrophy on the girl's 1st day

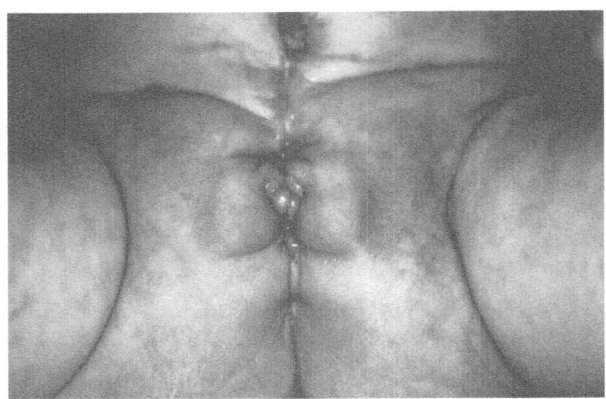

Fig. 32.2. The girl postoperatively during her 5th week

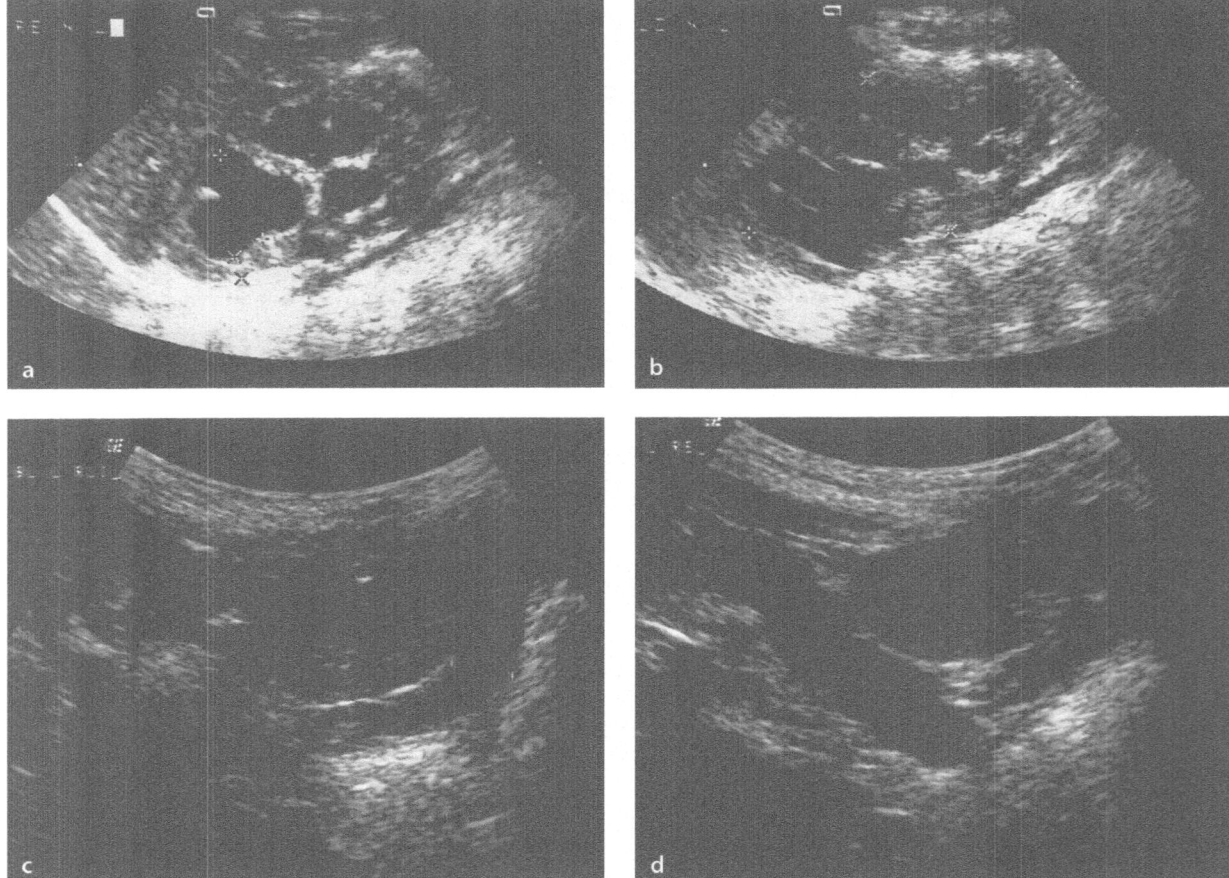

Fig. 32.3a–d. Sonography. **a** The right kidney, with dilatation of the calyces. **b** The left kidney, with dilatation of the calyces. **c** Hypertrophic urinary bladder wall. **d** The dilated retrovesical ureters

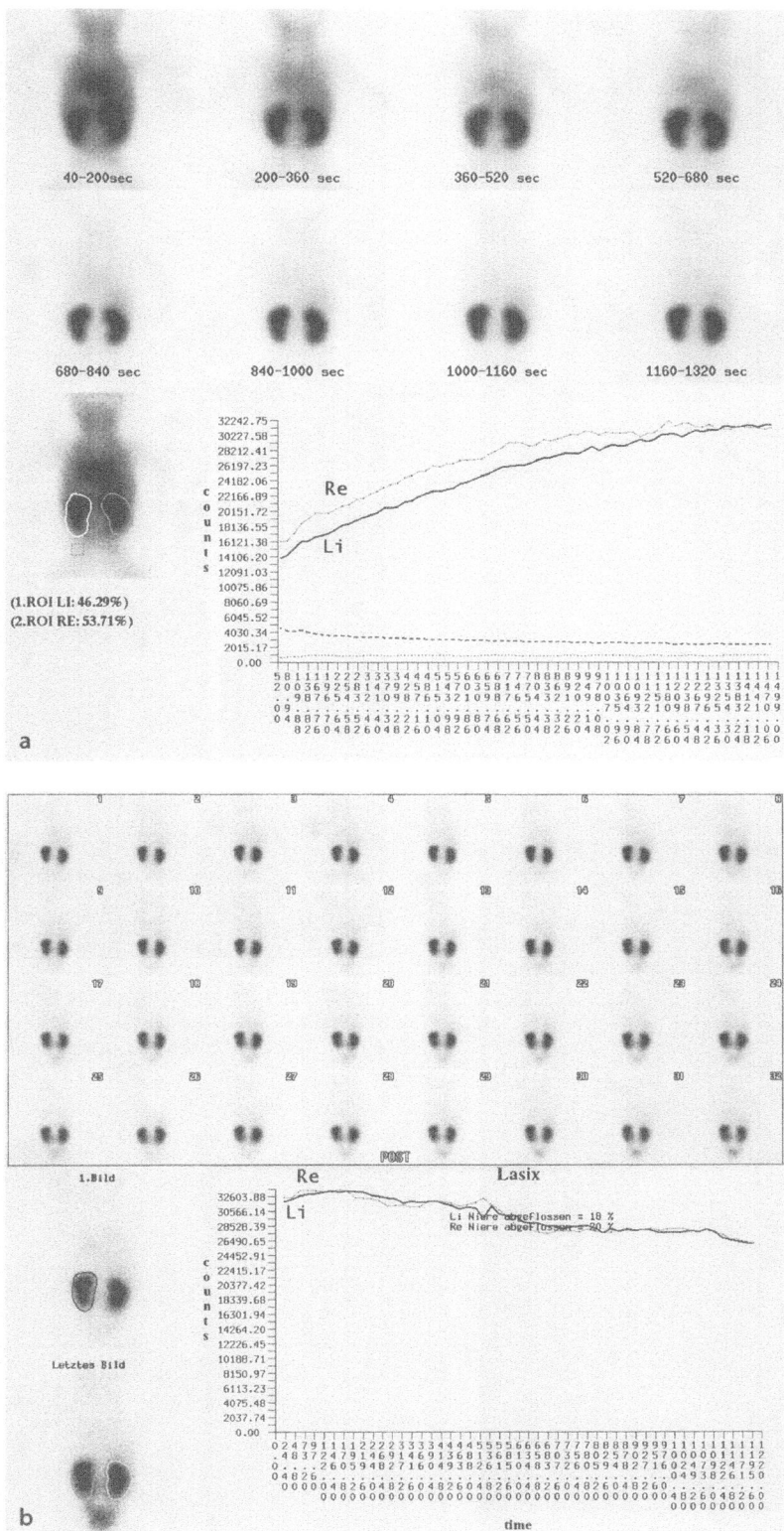

Fig. 32.4a,b. On the ⁹⁹ᵐTc-MAG₃ scan the renal function on both sides is preserved. **a** During the parenchymal phase there is a continuous accumulation of the tracer in the drainage system. **b** No significant response to furosemide can be observed

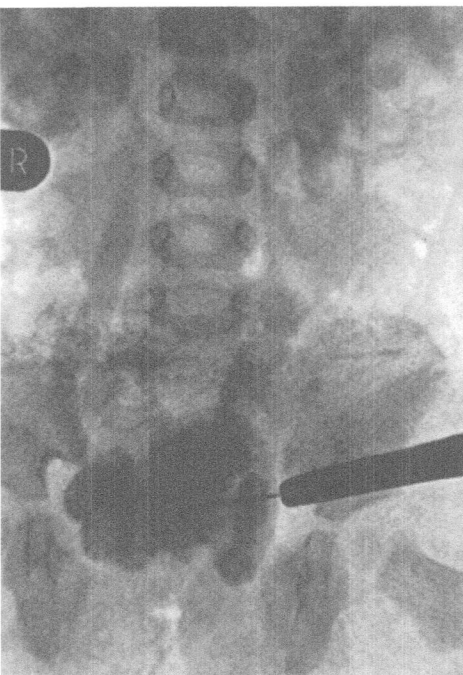

Fig. 32.5. Voiding cysto-urethrography demonstrating a bilateral grade-IV vesico-ureteric reflux and an irregular shape of the urinary bladder wall

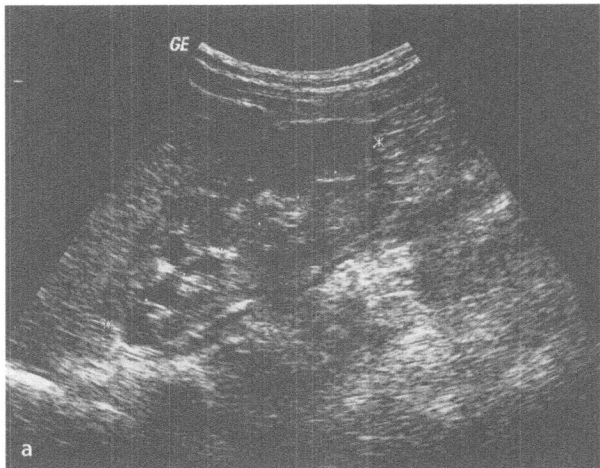

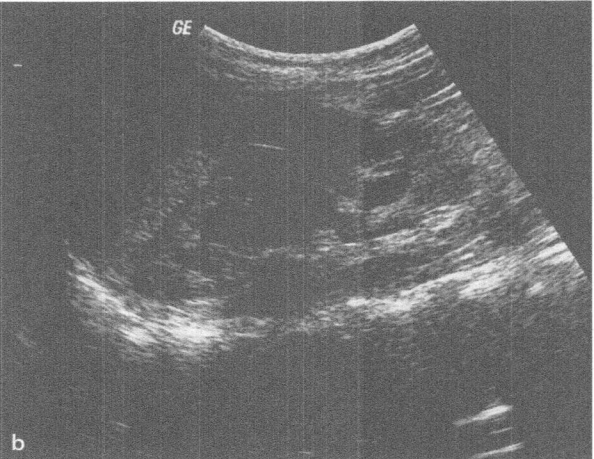

Fig. 32.6a, b. Sonography of the upper urinary tract (longitudinal sections): the calyces are only slightly dilated, and the parenchyma looks normal (**a** right kidney, **b** left kidney)

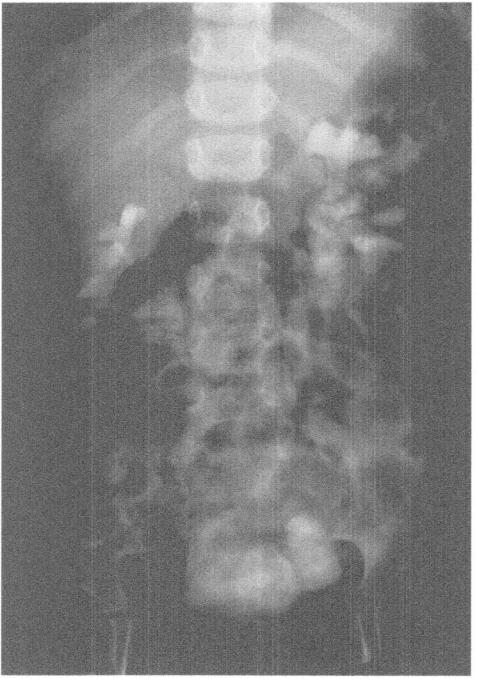

Fig. 32.7. On the postoperative pyelogram the calyces are only slightly deformed, especially on the left side. The left ureter is dilated from the renal pelvis to the pouch, while the right ureter looks normal

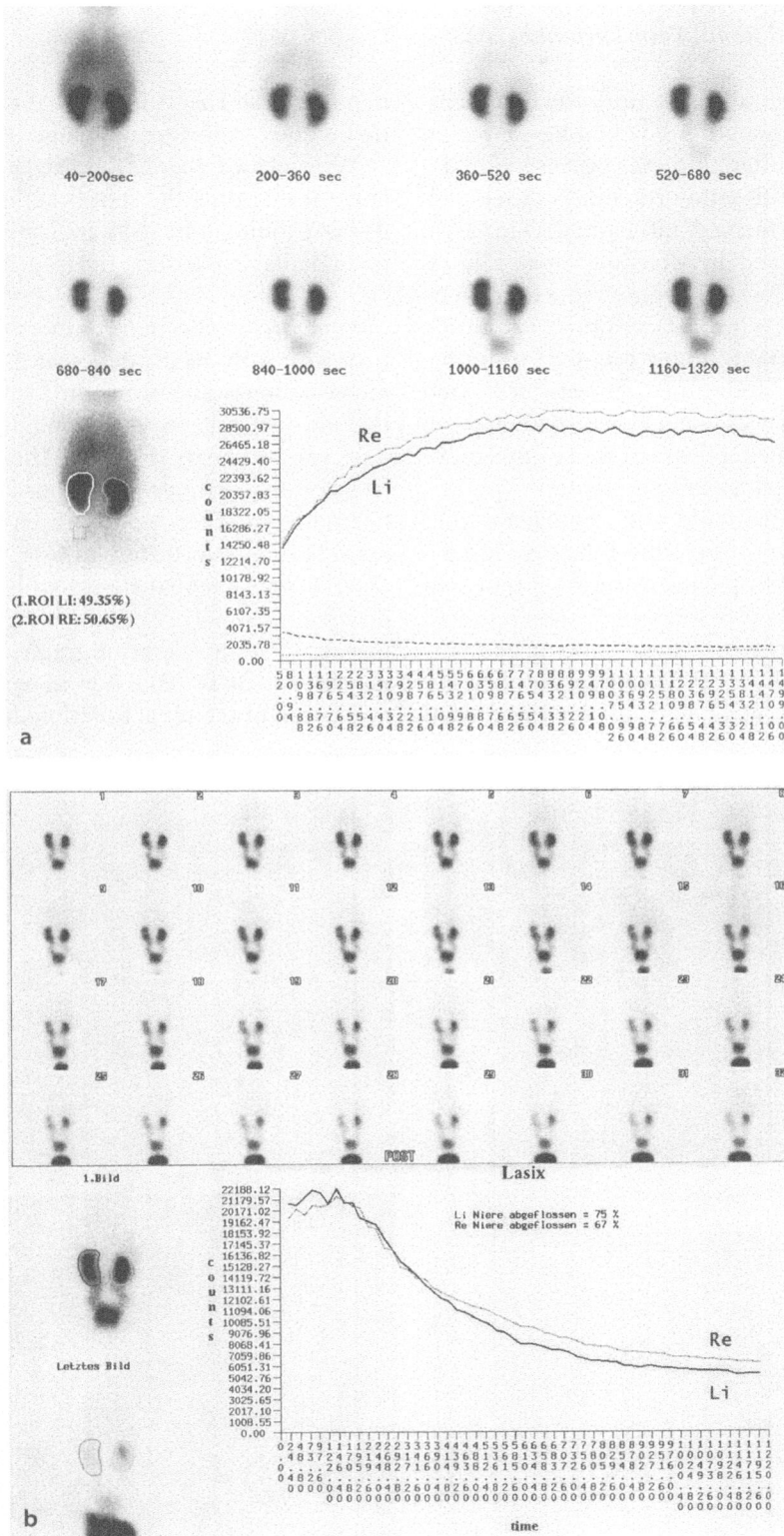

Fig. 32.8. a On the postoperative ^{99m}Tc-MAG$_3$ scan the renal function on both sides is preserved. **b** Obstruction is excluded by a significant fall of the time-activity curve following furosemide

CASE 33 ► *Neonatal Renal Vein Thrombosis*

Clinical Course: Due to respiratory distress syndrome (RDS III) a premature boy had be ventilated for 4 days. On day 15 after his birth, macroscopic haematuria combined with mild proteinuria developed. We immediately performed ultrasound (Fig. 33.1) and found an enlarged hyperechoic right kidney. Arterial and venous flow were preserved, as shown by Doppler sonography (Fig. 33.2). On the ^{99m}Tc-MAG$_3$ scan (Fig. 33.3) the right kidney was seen to be hypoperfused and the split function was decreased (42%). The findings were suggestive of renal vein thrombosis, and following the exclusion of thrombophilia the child was treated with heparin.

The condition of the child was improved within the following 2 weeks. The volume of the right kidney decreased and macroscopic haematuria disappeared within 2 days. The Doppler sonography was repeated several times, but further no signs of disturbed perfusion were found (Fig. 33.2). Sonographic follow-up showed decreasing echogenicity of the right renal parenchyma. The volume of the kidney decreased further below the normal range (Fig. 33.4).

We repeated the ^{99m}Tc-MAG$_3$ scintigraphy 1 year later. At that time the split function of the right kidney was found to be 28%, indicating that irreversible renal damage had occurred (Fig. 33.5).

Comment: Renal vein thrombosis is a rare disease in neonates, with an incidence of 2.2/100000, and it is more common in premature infants. Risk factors include dehydration, sepsis, poliglobulia and congenital cyanotic heart diseases. The prognosis of unilateral renal venous thrombosis is usually good, but subsequent renal parenchymal damage must be expected in two-thirds of the affected children. Macroscopic haematuria is highly suggestive for the disease, especially if concomitant risk factors are present. ^{99m}Tc-MAG$_3$ scintigraphy may be helpful in the assessment of renal flow in early cases and in the evaluation of the renal function during follow-up.

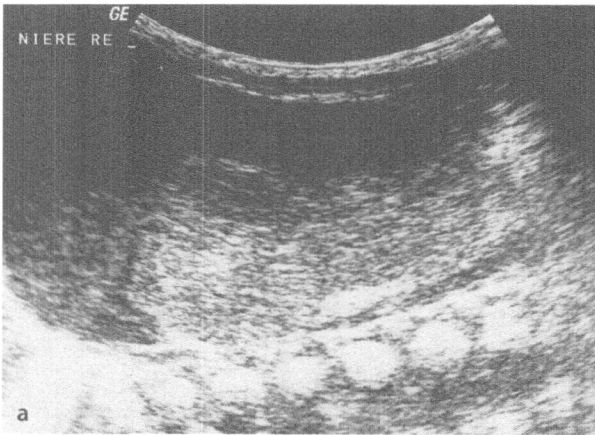

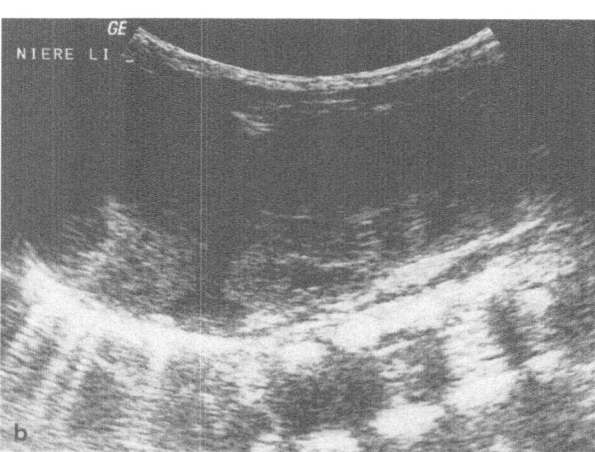

Fig. 33.1 a, b. Sonography. Enlargement of the right hyperechoic kidney (**a**) compared with the contralateral kidney (**b**)

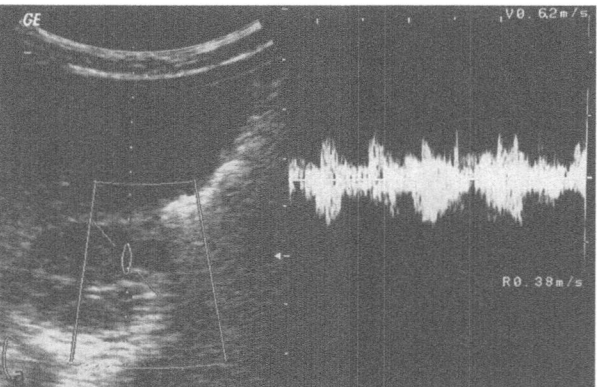

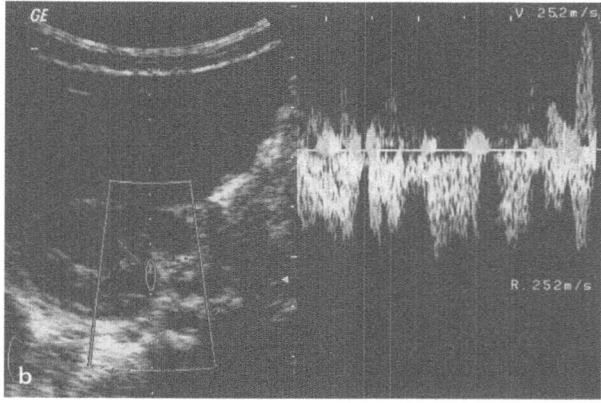

Fig. 33.2 a, b. Doppler sonography. Preserved venous (**a**) and arterial (**b**) flow in the hilus of the right kidney

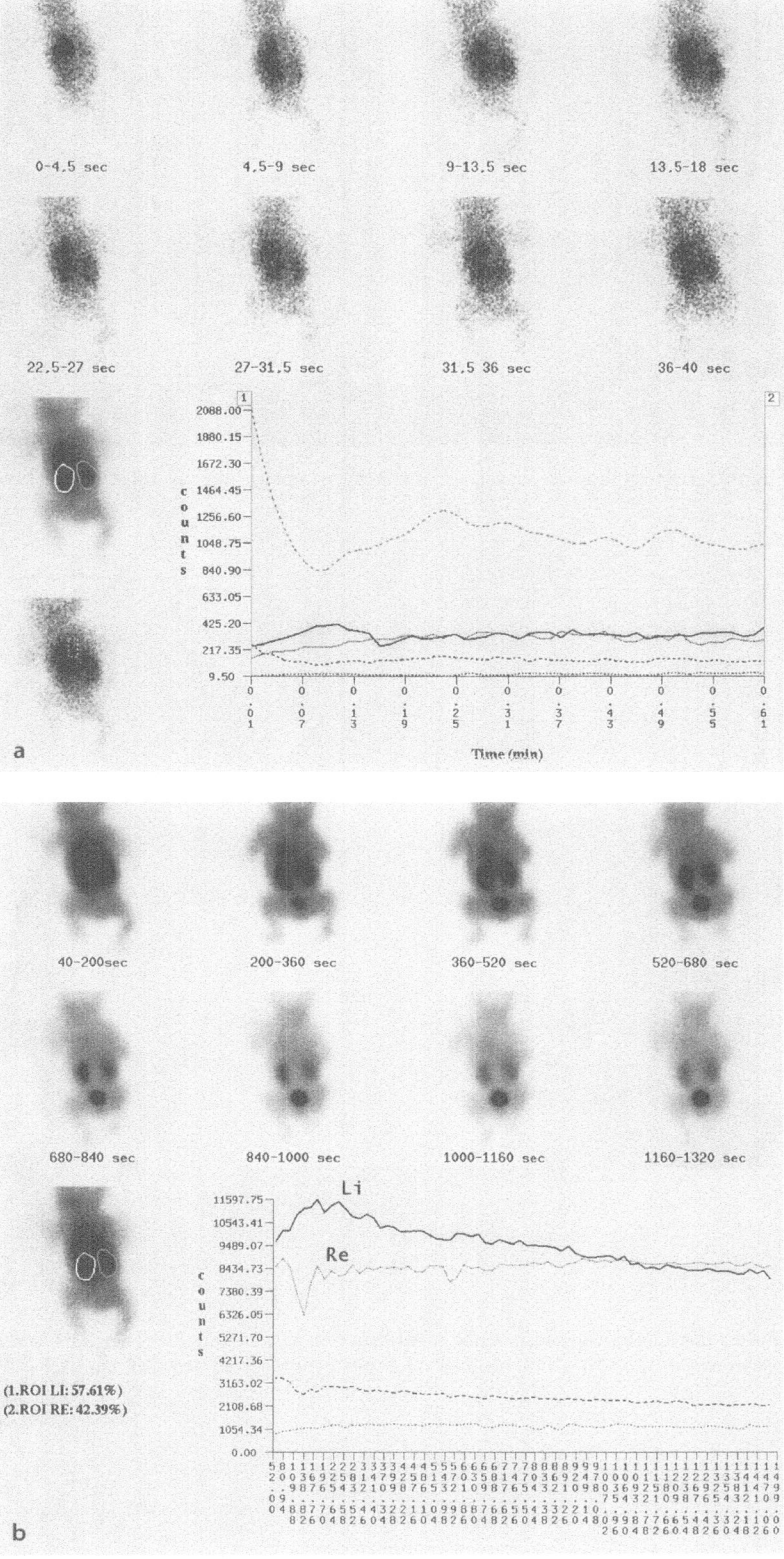

Fig. 33.3 a, b. ^{99m}Tc-MAG$_3$ scan during the early phase of venous thrombosis. Decreased renal perfusion (**a**) and function (**b**) of the right kidney

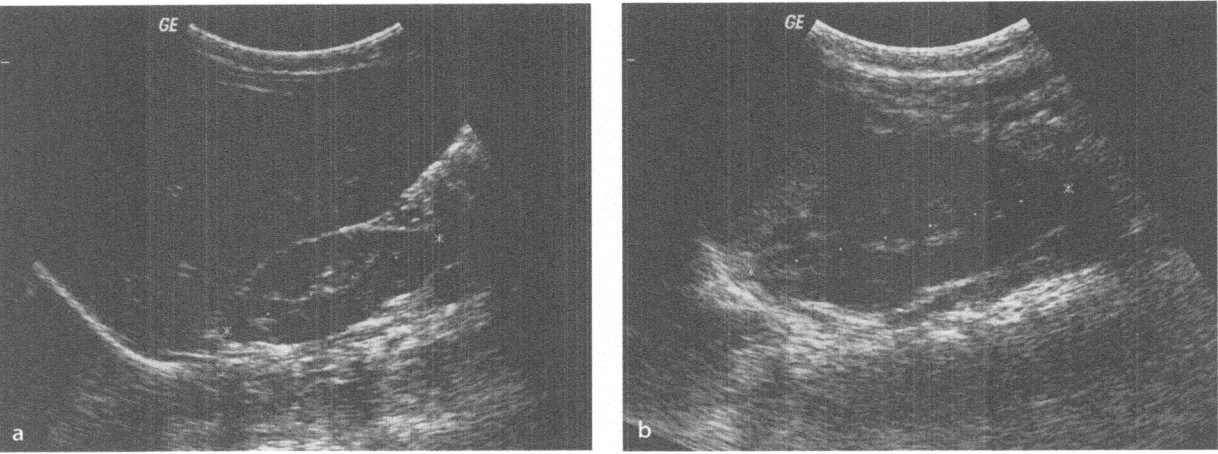

Fig. 33.4a,b. Sonography 1 year after the acute disease. The volume of the kidney (**a**) decreased below the normal range (**b**)

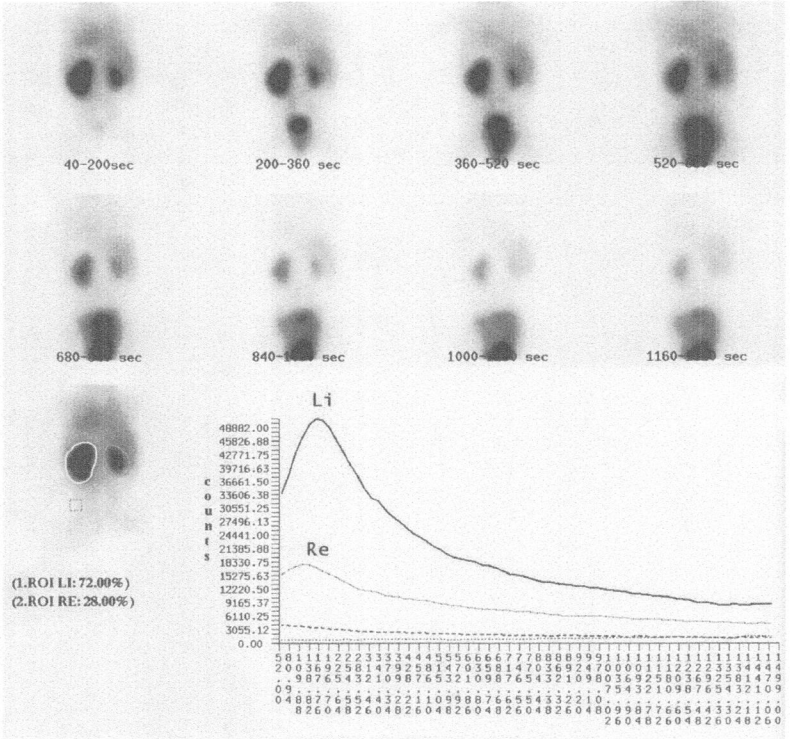

Fig. 33.5. Within 1 year after the acute disease the right renal function deteriorated further. The calculated right split function on the ^{99m}Tc-MAG$_3$ scan was only 28%, which indicated further progressive parenchymal damage

CASE 34 ▶ *Nephrolithiasis, Cystinuria*

Clinical Course: At the age of 5 this boy, who was a refugee from the former Yugoslavia was diagnosed with a urinary tract infection with *Proteus mirabilis*. The initial sonography showed multiple nephroliths in the calyces and the pelvis of the right kidney. The parenchyma of the affected kidney looked slightly thinned. No stones were observed in the left kidney, which was considerably larger than the right one (Fig. 34.1). During further laboratory investigations we diagnosed cystinuria from the elevation of cystine, ornithine, lysine and arginine in the urine.

On the plain abdominal radiograph we found multiple stones in the calyces and one large nephrolith in the pelvis of the right kidney (Fig. 34.2). We started antibiotic prophylaxis and increased the child's fluid intake. On the intravenous pyelogram the parenchyma of the right kidney was thinner than that of the contralateral kidney, the calyces looked dilated, and there were filling defects in the renal pelvis owing to nephrolithiasis. The parenchyma on the left kidney looked normal (Fig. 34.3).

On the ^{99m}Tc-MAG$_3$ scan the function of the right kidney was impaired (25%) with no signs of obstruction (Fig. 34,4). We performed seven sessions of extracorporeal lithotripsy without achieving complete removal of all the stones. This procedure was stopped when we noted a substantial decrease in the right kidney function on the ^{99m}Tc-DMSA scan, where the calculated split function was only 10% (Fig. 34.5).

During the further clinical course two nephroliths persisted on the right side. In addition, the contralateral kidney remained stone free and became hypertrophic (Fig. 34.6). In view of the stable condition, nephrectomy has not appeared to be urgently indicated up to now.

Interestingly, a shrunken kidney with multiple nephroliths was diagnosed in the child's father, who also suffered from cystinuria. Cystinuria is an autosomal recessive disease leading to a failure in the renal resorption of dibasic amino acids. The underlying mutations have been located in the *CLC7A9* and *CLC3A1* genes encoding a renal cystine transporter protein. In our patient and his father we found a mutation in the T216M region on the *SLC3A1* gene. Because cystinuria is an autosomal recessive disease these findings have to be explained either by homozygosis due to consanguinity or by hemizygosity with loss of the second copy of the gene.

Comment: In patients with nephrolithiasis, inborn errors of metabolism are relatively more frequent in children than in adult patients. This holds true especially in certain ethnic groups, such as inhabitants of the Mediterranean area.

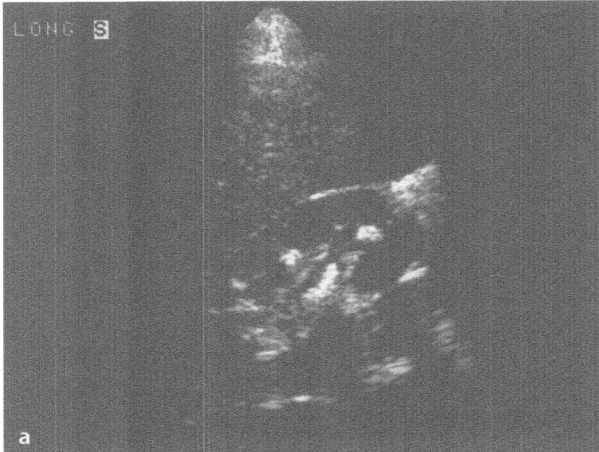

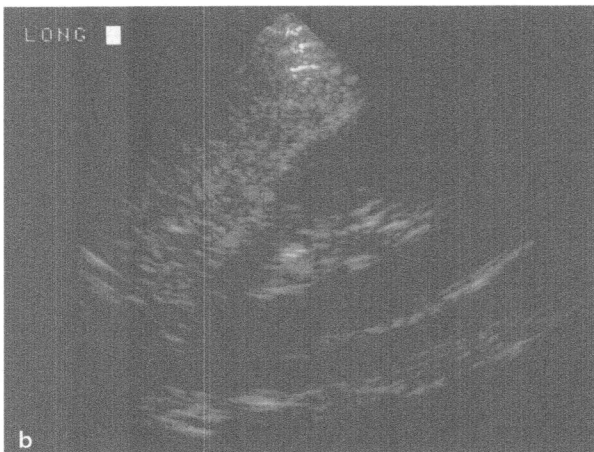

Fig. 34.1 a, b. Initial sonography shows multiple nephroliths in the calyces and the pelvis of the right kidney. **a** Thinning of the parenchyma is present. **b** The left kidney looks hypertrophic. No stones can be found

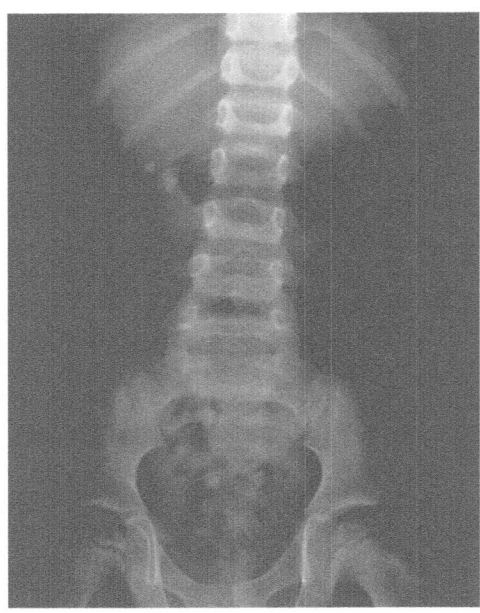

Fig. 34.2. On the plain abdominal radiograph multiple concrements are seen in the calyces and one large nephrolith in the pelvis of the right kidney

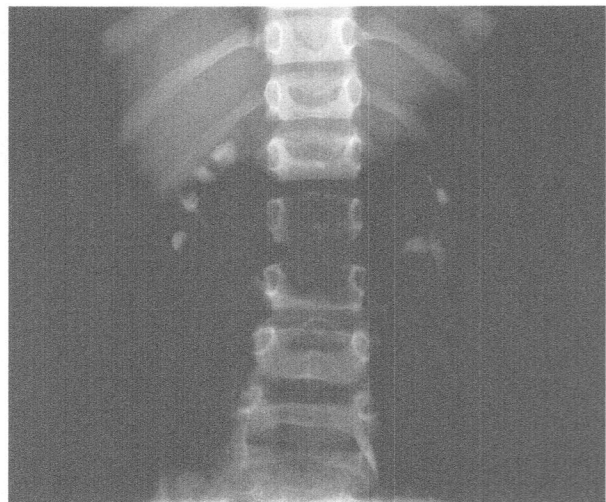

Fig. 34.3. Intravenous pyelography showing a thinner parenchyma of the right than of the left kidney; the calyces of the right kidney look to be dilated with folling defects in the renal pelvis caused by nephrolithiasis. The parenchyma of the left kidney looks normal

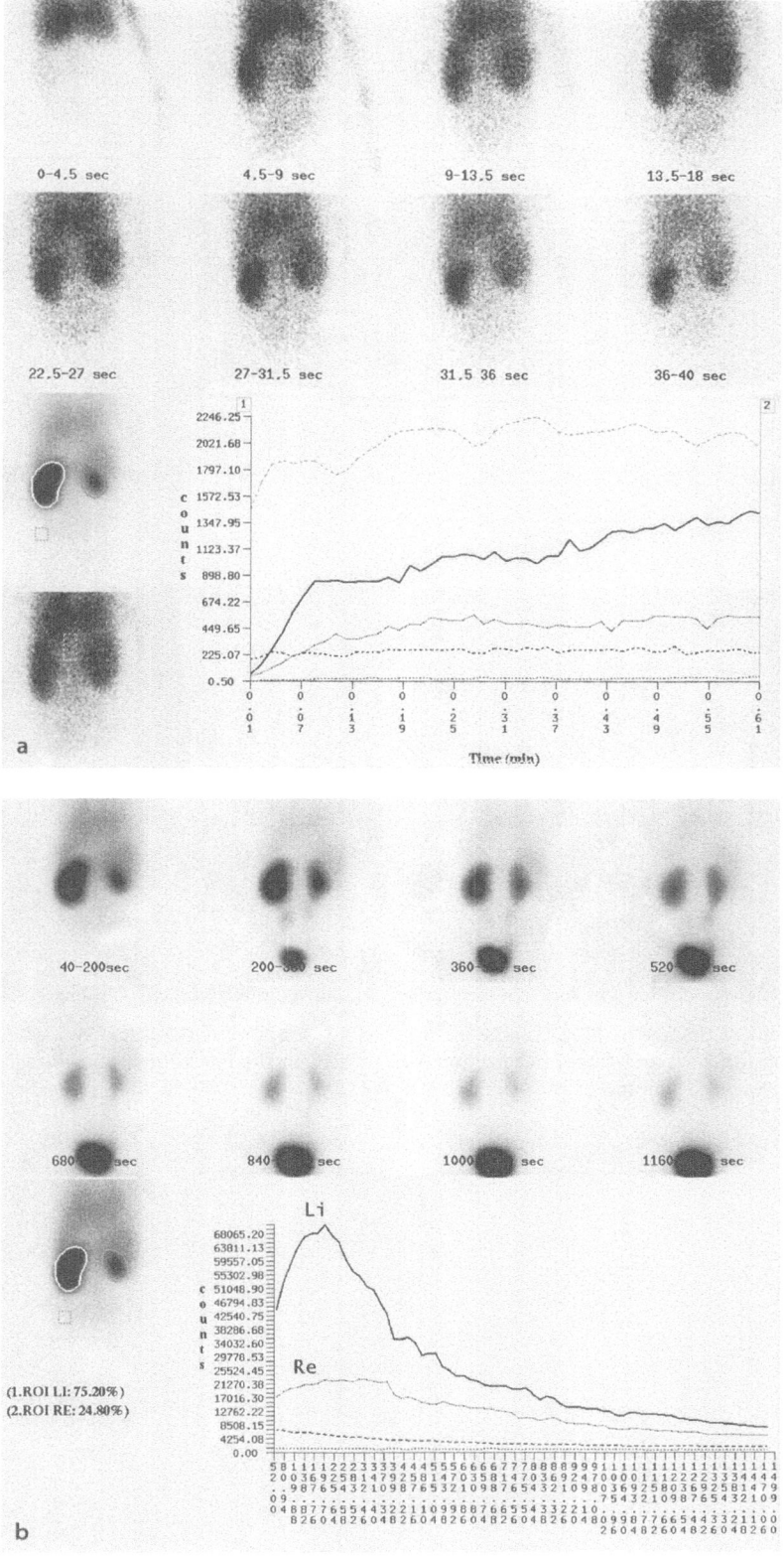

Fig. 34.4 a, b. ^{99m}Tc-MAG$_3$ scan. The perfusion (**a**) and function (**b**) of the right kidney are impaired (25%). No signs of obstruction are present

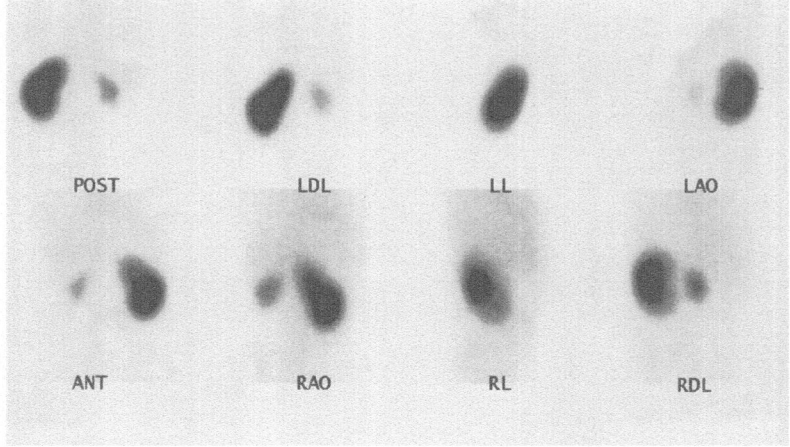

Fig. 34.5. Planar ^{99m}Tc-DMSA-scan: calculated split function of the right kidney is only 10%; appearance of the left kidney is normal

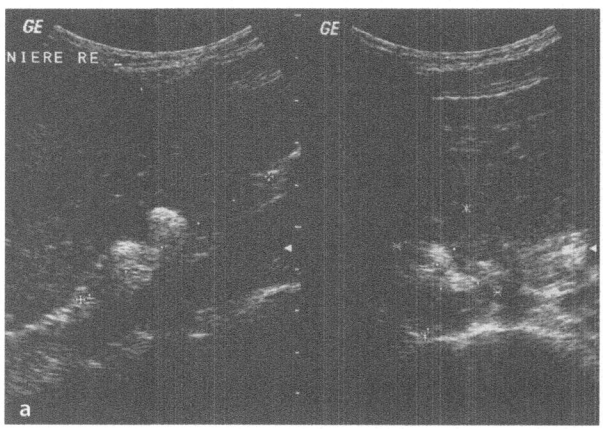 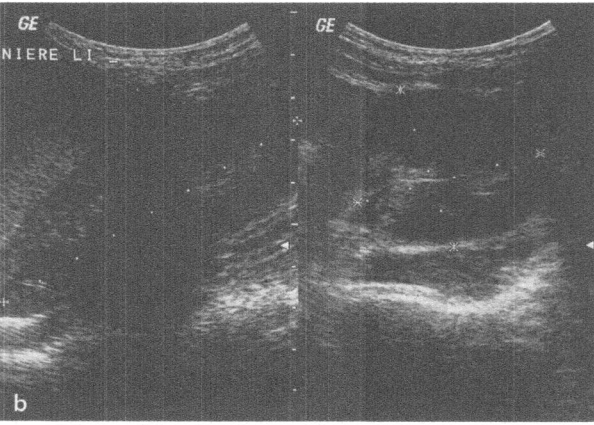

Fig. 34.6a, b. Sonography at the age of 10. **a** Volume of the right kidney: 21 ml (longitudinal and transverse sections). Two large stones are present. **b** Volume of the left kidney: 68 ml (longitudinal and transverse sections). No stones are present in the left kidney, and the parenchyma is well preserved

CASE 35 ▶ *Hereditary Nephrolithiasis Due to Hyperresorptive Hypercalciuria*

Clinical Course: This 6-month-old sibling of an index patient was admitted to the paediatric department for further investigations during an episode of acute gastroenteritis with haematuria. Large amounts of erythrocytes and calcium oxalate, some leucocytes and protein were found in the urine. The urinary excretion of calcium (321 µg calcium/mg creatinine) and the serum calcium (10.7 mg/dl) was elevated by absence of other laboratory abnormalities. A urinary tract infection was not present at that time.

On sonography (Fig. 35.1) we noted multiple hyperechoic structures suggestive of nephroliths on the left kindney. Interestingly, calcium oxalate nephroliths were already known to be present in an older sister of the boy.

During diagnostic work-up we excluded a vitamin D intoxication and hyperparathyroidism. We performed a PAK test and there obsurved a rise of the serum calcium and of the urinary calcium excretion following oral calcium loading. These features were diagnostic of hereditary resorptive hypercalciuria.

As a consequence we modified the diet of the boy by reducing the content of calcium in the nutrition. We avoided giving milk products if possible, hydrated the child and stopped vitamin D prophylaxis. During the next weeks the serum calcium values did fall and the child gained weight.

When the child was 15 months old, he had a relapse of macrohaematuria with renal colic. On ultrasound a significant dilatation of the left renal pelvis was seen (Fig. 35.2). In addition, a nephrolith in his left side was found by sonography (Fig. 35.3) and later confirmed on the pyelogram (Fig. 35.4). Following hydration and analgesic therapy the nephrolith was passed. The analysis revealed that it was a calcium oxalate concrement.

Comment: In most cases nephroliths in childhood are caused by inborn errors of metabolism. In this boy we found hyperresorptive hypercalciuria. This condition causes problems especially in early childhood, because of the large amount of alimentary calcium.

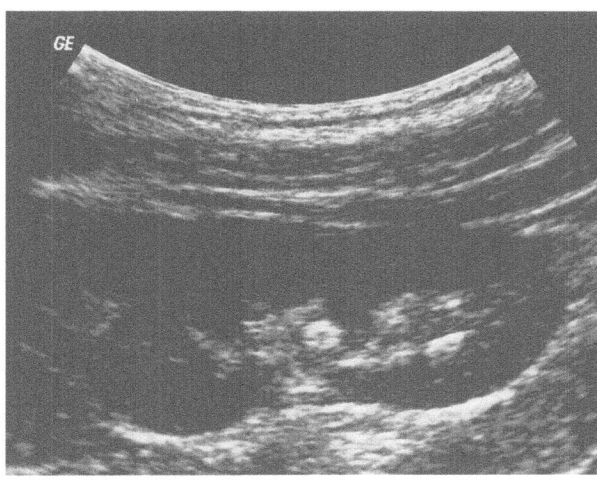

Fig. 35.1. Sonography of the left kindney (longitudinal section), with a hyperechoic mass centrally and at the lower pole. This finding is suggestive of a pelvic nephrolith

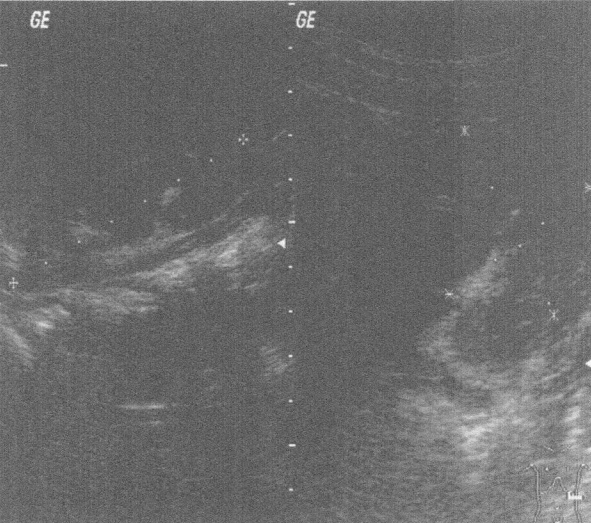

Fig. 35.2. Left kidney (longitudinal and transverse sections), showing pelvic ectasia due to obstruction

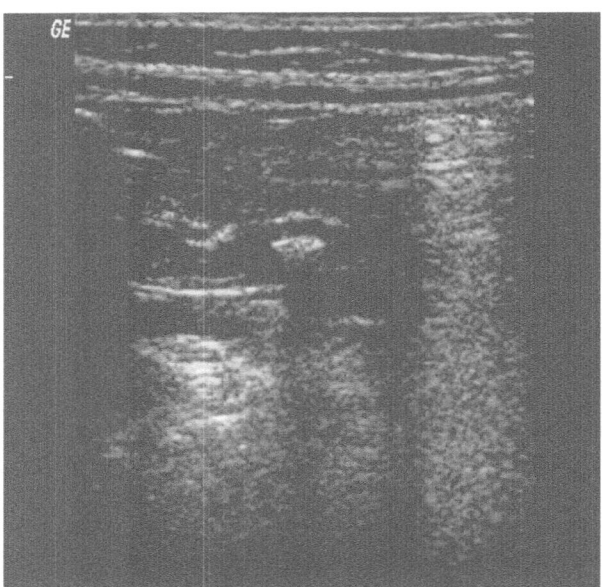

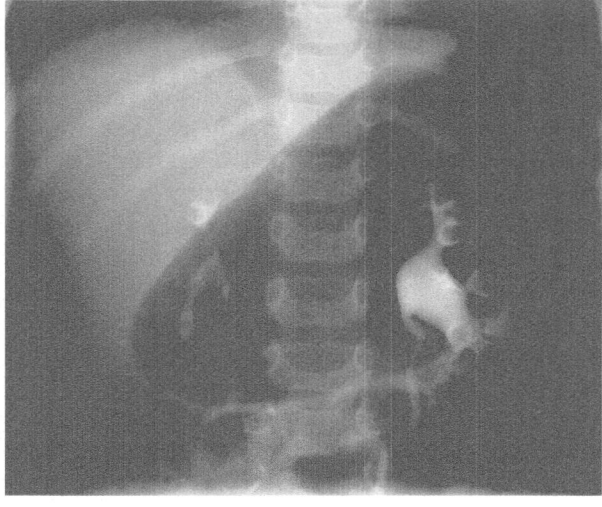

Fig. 35.3. Sonographic appearance of a nephrolith in the proximal ureter

Fig. 35.4. On the pyelogram 20 min after intravenous injection of the X-ray contrast medium an obstruction is seen on the left side, with narrowing of the proximal ureter

CASE 36 ▶ *Renal Bruise on the Right Side*

Clinical Course: One day, after an accident in a swimming pool, a 5-year-old boy developed macroscopic haematuria and the clinical picture of an acute abdomen. The haemoglobinconcentration was low (7.4 g/dl), and the lower pole of the right kidney was hypoechoic on ultrasound, which further revealed a loss of corticomedullary differentiation (Fig. 36.1). These finding were highly suggestive of a renal bruise or a renal tumour. Arterial renal flow was virtually absent in the space-occupying lesion at the lower right renal pole, as shown by Doppler sonography (Fig. 36.2). Spiral CT finally confirmed that the lesion was a perirenal haematoma and excluded a tumour (Fig. 36.3). Immediately after the diagnosis was made, surgery was performed. Intraoperatively we found a large haematoma at the lower right renal pole. The hilar structures were preserved. The lower pole was successfully resected.

Comment: In this case, spiral CT and Doppler sonography made it possible to differentiate a space-occupying lesion at the right lower kidney pole.

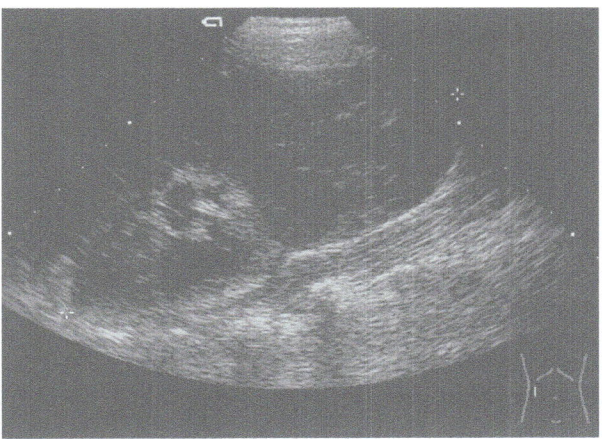

Fig. 36.1. Sonography (longitudinal section) of the right kidney demonstrates a space-occupying lesion at the lower pole of he right kidney. The upper pole shows moderate dilatation

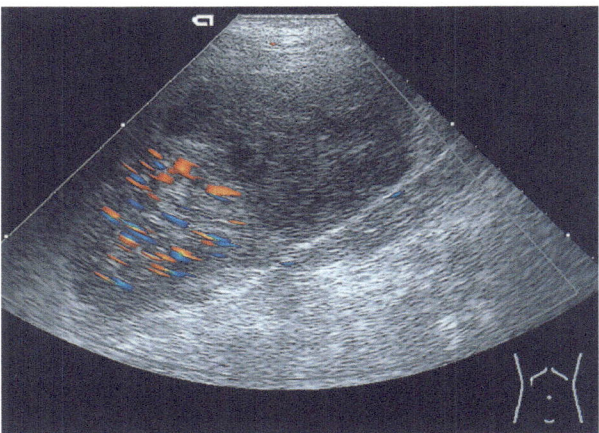

Fig. 36.2. Doppler sonography of the right kidney (longitudinal section) reveals the absence of arterial flow to the lower pole. In contrast, the flow to the upper pole appears to be normal

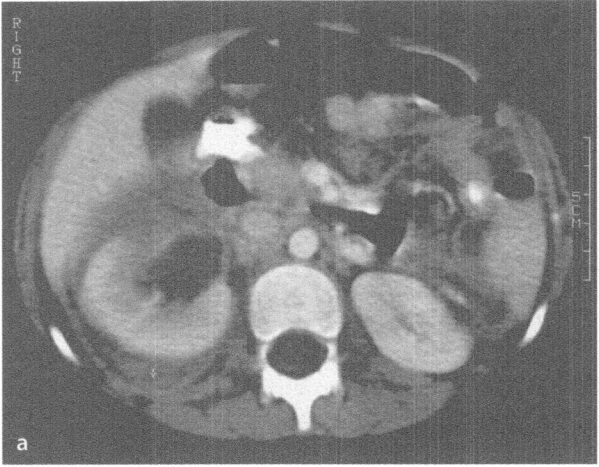

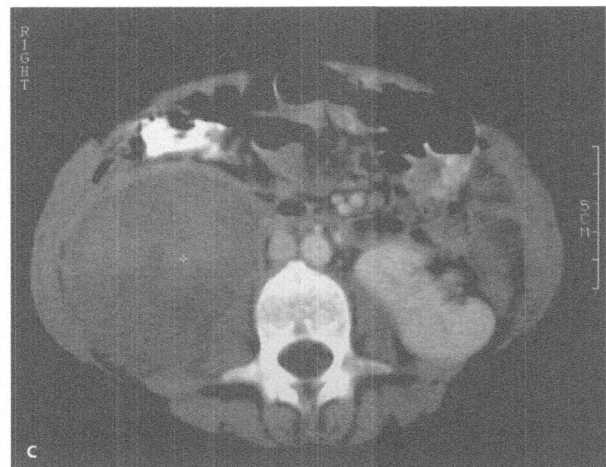

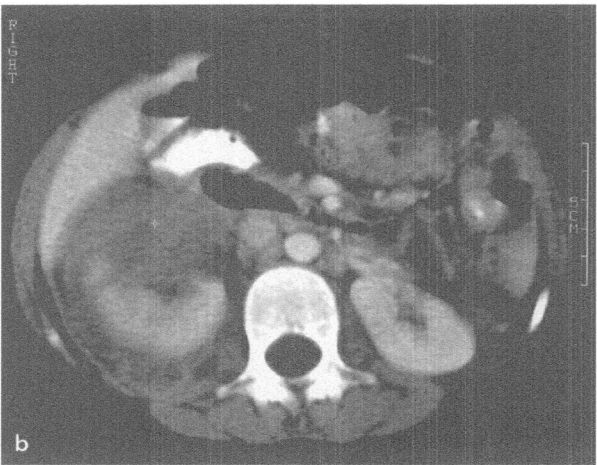

Fig. 36.3a–c. Spiral CT. **a** Significant ectasia of the pyelon on the right side. **b, c** In the middle part of the kidney a perirenal haematoma can be observed; at the lower pole solely a haematoma is seen, while the normal renal structures are absent

CASE 37 ▶ *Wilms' Tumour – Aniridia Syndrome with Deletion of 11p12*

Clinical Course: This boy from a healthy family was born by caesarian section. When he was 3 month old a failure of fixation was noted. Aniridia was diagnosed. Further ophthalmological examinatin revealed a cataract on both sides. As the one on the right eye was already in an advanced stage phacoerysis had to be performed on that side.

Within the last decade it has been recognized that about 30% of sporadic patients with aniridia develop a Wilms' tumour. Therefore, we screened the child for deletion of 11p12, which was subsequently confirmed by molecular genetics. This defect comprises not only the aniridia gene, but also the Wilms' tumour gene (*WT1*), and therefore this child carried a high risk for the development of a nephroblastoma. Until the boy was 1 year old, the sonographic findings were normal (Fig. 37.1). Thirteen months later we had the first suspicion of a tumour at the lower pole of the right kid-

ney (Fig. 37.2), with progressive growth seen on a sonogram a month later (Fig. 37.3). On the CT scan (Fig. 37.4) a large tumour of the right kidney, with only slight accumulation of the contrast medium and the suspicion of central necrosis, was diagnosed.

Following the exclusion of distant metastases we started preoperative chemotherapy according to the SIOP93/01 protocol. Successful reduction of the tumour was assessed by sonography (Fig. 37.5). Following neoadjuvant chemotherapy nephrectomy and regional lymphadenectomy were subsequently performed.

Comment: The risk of a syndromic disease (WAGR syndrome, Denis-Drash syndrome) can be assessed by molecular genetic analysis. Repeated sonographic screening is helpful in the detection of early nephroblastoma in those who carry a high risk.

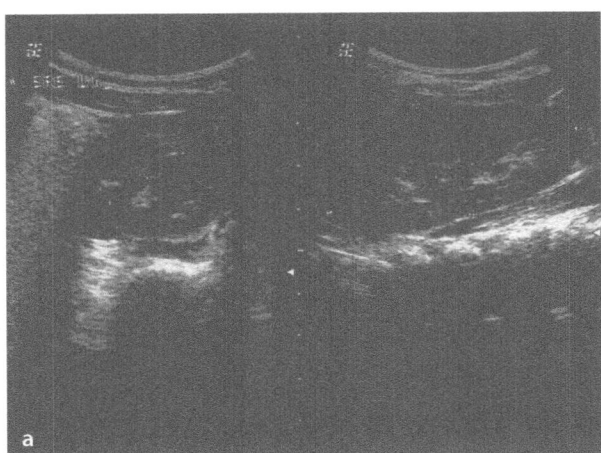

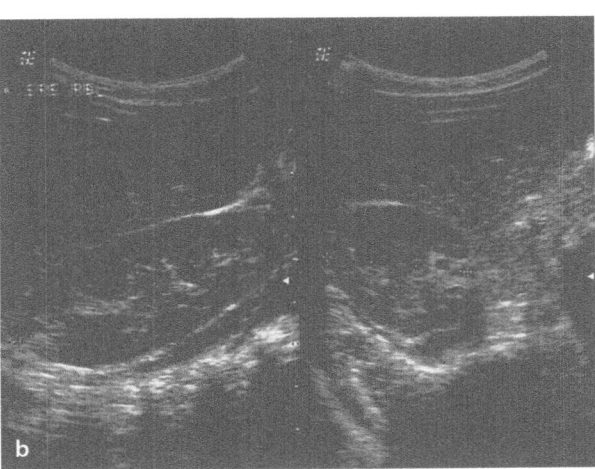

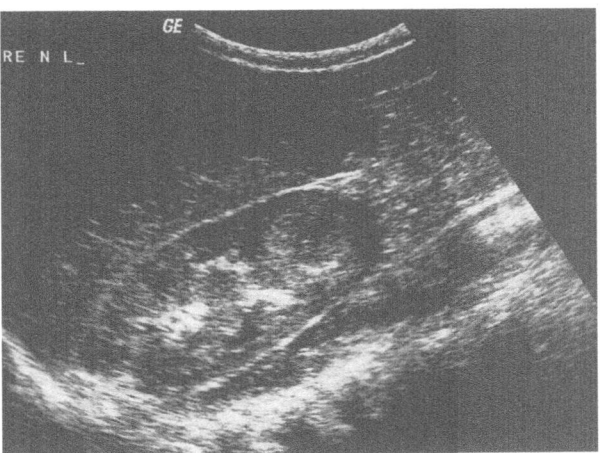

Fig. 37.2. Sonography of the right kidney during the child's 23rd month (longitudinal section) shows a nodule suggestive of a tumour at the lower pole

◀

Fig. 37.1 a, b. The initial sonography during the child's 5th month. The left (**a**) and right (**b**) kidneys look normal

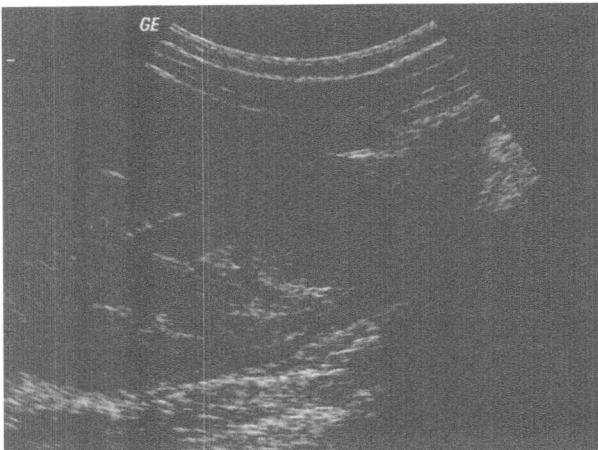

Fig. 37.3. Repeated sonography (longitudinal section) 1 month later: progressive growth of the tumour

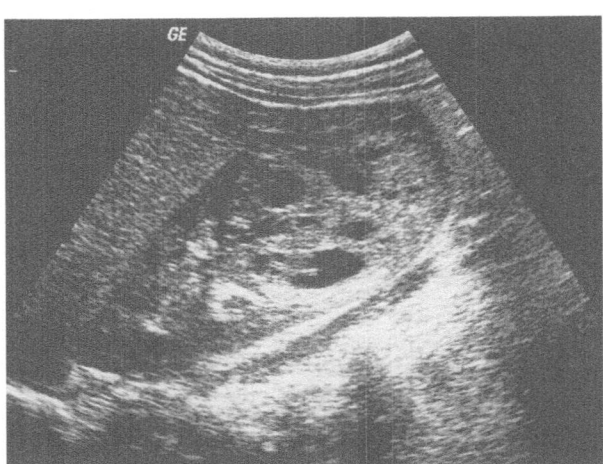

Fig. 37.5. Following neoadjuvant chemotherapy successful reduction of the tumour can be noted. The hyperechoic tumour shows cystic degeneration

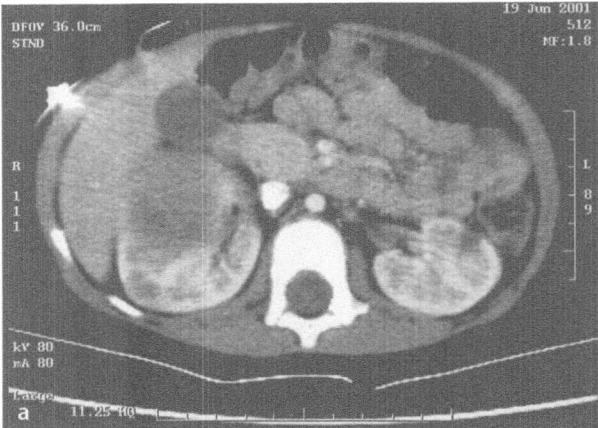

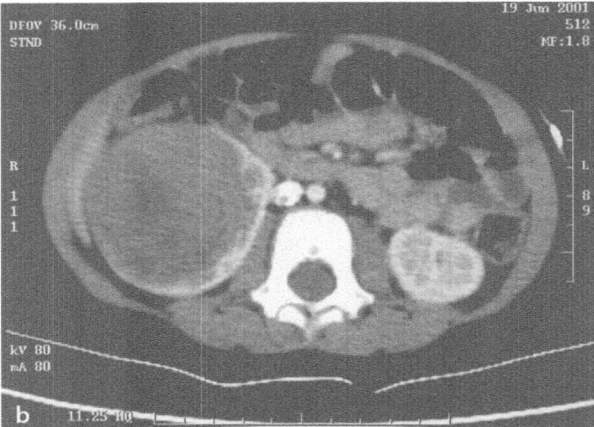

Fig. 37.4. a On the CT scan a large tumour of the right kidney, with only slight accumulation of the contrast medium, is diagnosed. The central part of the tumour consists mainly of a hypodense necrotic mass. **b** The left kidney looks normal

CASE 38 ► *Neuroblastoma*

Clinical Course: Abducens nerve palsy occurred in a 3-year-old boy, with unsteady gait and recurrent vomiting. On sonography we found a large pararenal space-occupying lesion on the left side (Fig. 38.1). This tumour led to hydronephrosis of the left kidney. On the CT scan the extension of the lesion, which involved the large abdominal vessels and led to a compression and dilatation of the left renal pelvis, could be clearly delineated (Fig. 38.2).

On the MRI a space-occupying lesion was seen in the middle cranial fossa, with infiltration of the greater wing of the sphenoid bone (Fig. 38.3).

The suspicion of a neuroblastoma was supported by elevated excretion of the urinary catecholamines, and it was subsequently confirmed by an ^{123}I-MIBG scan, which showed the primary tumour in the left abdomen and extensive involvement of the whole bone marrow, especially in the skull, and hence a stage-IV neurobalstoma (Fig. 38.4).

We started chemotherapy according to the high-risk protocol NB97. Four months later we performed nephrectomy and adrenalectomy on the left side. Renewed examination by ^{123}I-MIBG revealed residual bone marrow infiltration of the skull, and we decided to perform ^{131}I-MIBG therapy with 11.3 GBq. On the posttherapy scan, bone marrow infiltration of the mandibles and peripheral bone marrow was confirmed (Fig. 38.5). The radionuclide therapy was followed by severe bone marrow suppression and significant infection. Recovery was obtained by stem cell support. Chemotherapy was continued, and residual bone marrow infiltration persisted, as demonstrated by repeated ^{123}I-MIBG scans. According to our therapy protocol, a treatment with the chimeric antiganglioside antibody ch14.18 was performed, but had to be stopped owing to incompatibility after the second cycle. A new cerebral manifestation of the tumor led to vomiting and headache (Fig. 38.6). Unfortunately, the girl died before we were able to perform surgical excision.

Comment: So far, children with widespread neuroblastoma have a poor prognosis. Imaging with radioiodinated MIGB is sensitive and highly specific in the diagnosis of neuroblastoma and metastases and can also be used as a therapeutic agent.

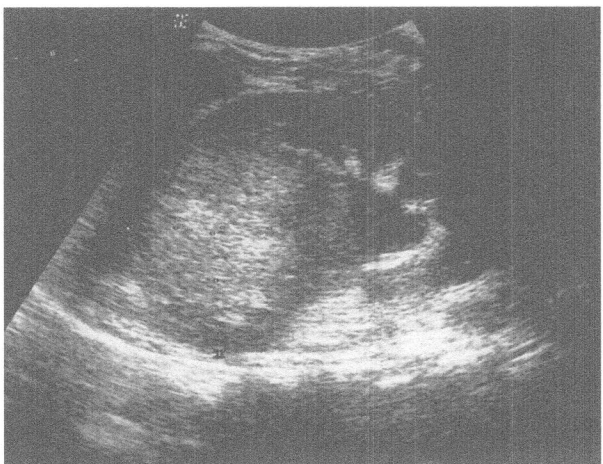

Fig. 38.1. Sonography shows a large hyperechoic pararenal space-occupying lesion near the upper pole of the left kidney, with compression of the renal pelvis and dilatation of the drainage system

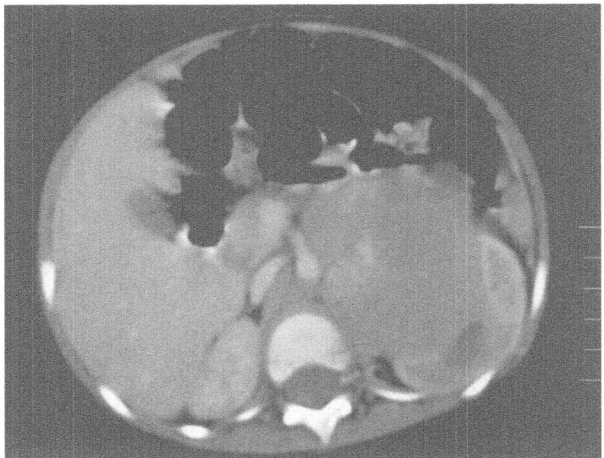

Fig. 38.2. On the CT scan the extent of lesion, which is infiltrating the large abdominal vessels leading to compression and dilatation of the left renal pelvis can be clearly delineated

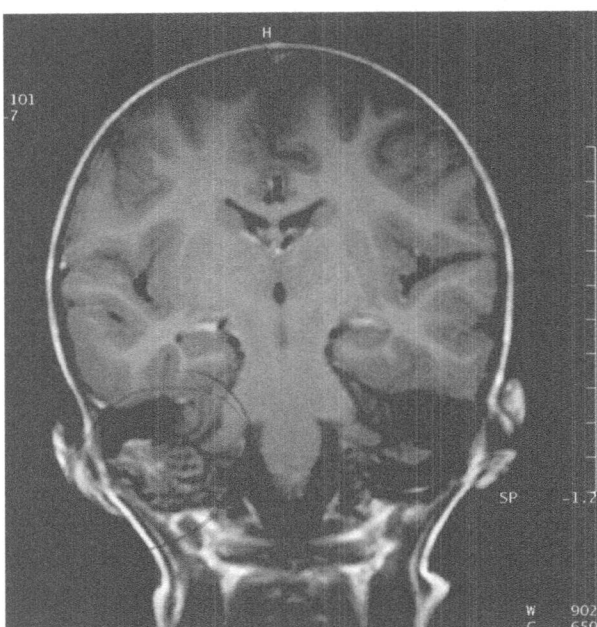

Fig. 38.3. On the MRI a space-occupying lesion in the middle cranial fossa with infiltration of the anterior wing of the sphenoid bone is seen to be present
◄

Fig. 38.4a–c. The initial ^{123}I-MIBG scan 24 h after injection shows the primary tumour in the left abdomen. **a** Dorsal view. Extensive involvement of the whole bone marrow is present. **b** Dorsal view of the pelvis and lower extremities. **c** Lateral view demonstrates the bone marrow involvement of the skull, especially in the mandibles and skull base
▼

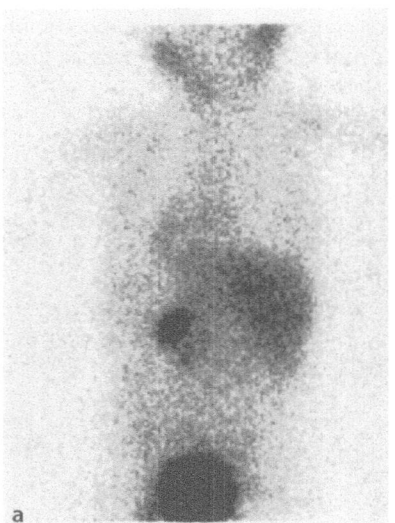
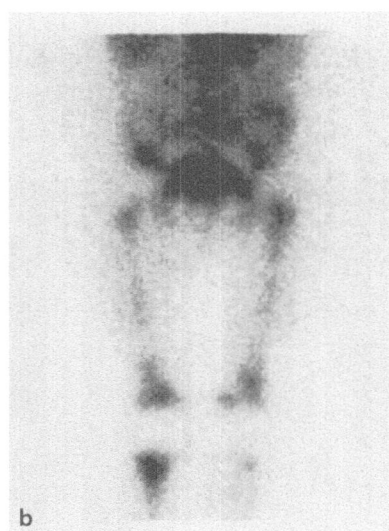
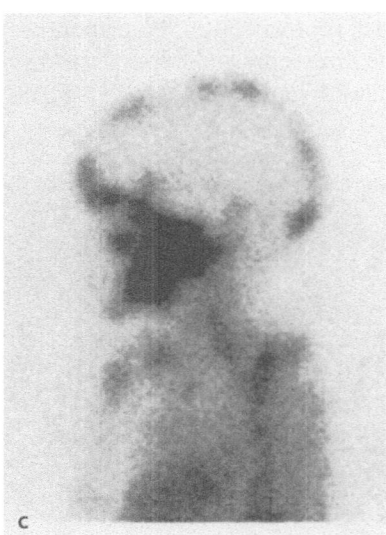

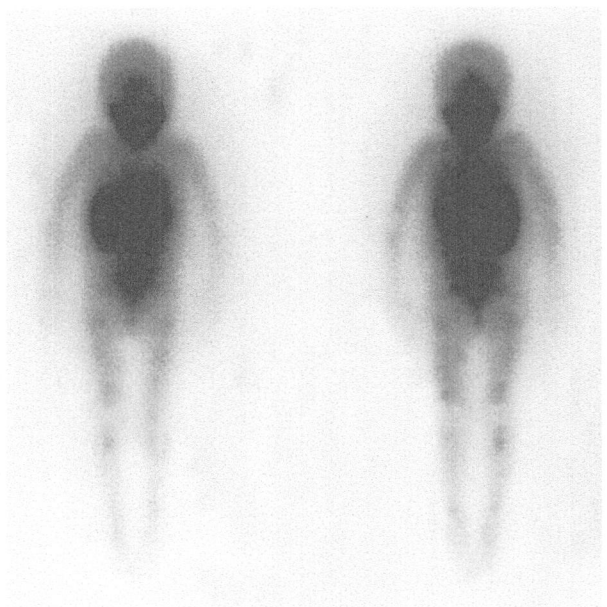

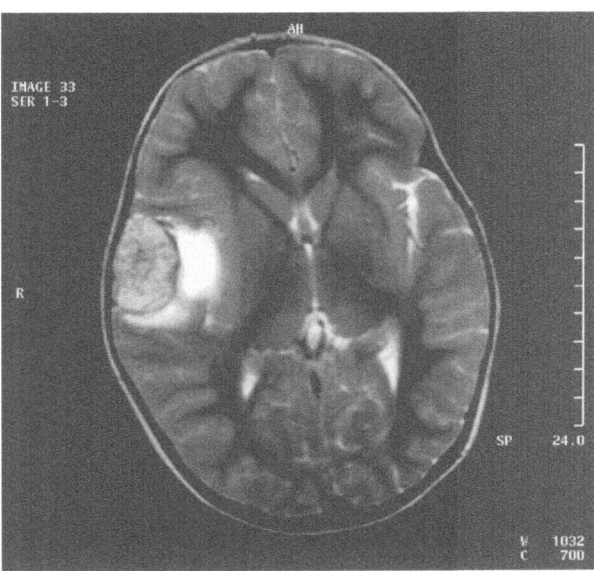

Fig. 38.5. The posttherapy whole-body ^{131}I-MIGB scan still shows residual pathologic uptake in the mandibles and lower extremities

Fig. 38.6. MRI of the skull: large tumour in the left temporoparietal region with peritumour oedema

Subject Index

Abdominal
- kidney 10
- trauma 73
- wall 29
- reconstruction 29
Abducens nerve palsy 241
Aberrant vessel 54, 152, 163
Abnormal position of the ureteral
  orifice 40
Abscess 80
Acute
- abdomen 237
- gastroenteritis 235
- obstruction 52
- pyelonephritis 143
- rejection 73
- scrotum 33
- upper urinary tract infection 143
Adenine-phosphoribosyl transferase
  36
Adenoma sebaceum 216
Adenylate cyclase 35
Adequate fluid intake 38
Adrenalectomy 241
Adult polycystic kidney disease 9
Adverse contrast reactions 78
Aesthesioneuroblastoma 60
aFP 62
Agenesis 103
- of the bladder 22
- of the internal female genitalia 6
Alanine-glycoxylate aminotransferase
  35
Alkalization 38
- of the urine 37
Allantoic duct 23
Allopurinol 38
Alpha fetoprotein (s. also aFP) 62
Alpha mercapto-propionylglycine 38
American Intergroup Rhabdo-
  myosarcoma Study (s. also IRS) 63
Aminoglycoside 33
Aminopenicillin 33
Amniorrhexis 171
Amoxicilline 143
Anderson-Hynes 130, 152
Aneurysm 9
Angiotensin II 52
Aniridia 239
- gene 239
- syndrome 239
Anorectal malformations 78
Antenatal surgical intervention 27

Anterior prostatic lobe 5
Anterior urethral valves (s. also con-
  genital urethral diverticula) 27
Antibiotic
- prophylaxis 44, 126, 136, 159, 167,
  171, 176, 200, 209, 212, 217, 231
- therapy 183
- treatment 140
Apatite 35
Apical diverticulum 167
Apoptosis 52
Arginine 36
Arreflexia
- of the detrusor muscle 24
- of the sphincter mechanism 24
Arterial hypertension 40
Arteriovascular hypertension 52
Arteriovenous fistula 74
Artificial sphincter 183
Ascensus renalis 3
Ash leaf 216
Ask-upmark kidney 7
Assisted micturition 29
Asymptomatic
- bacteriuria 31
- chronic urinary tract infection 206
- pyuria 196
Atresia of the ureter 7
Atrial septal defects 28
Augmentation of the bladder 48, 148
Autosomal dominant 9
- pattern of inheritance 15
- polycystic renal degeneration 214
Autosomal recessive polycystic
  renal disease 214
Autotransplantation 167
Auxiliary
- interventions 39
- ureteral DJ-stenting 39

Bacteriuria 140
Bartholin's glands 5
Beckwith-Wiedemann syndrome 57
Bifid
- clitoris 21
- renal pelvis 14
- scrotum in males 22
- ureter 15
Bilateral
- 4th grade vesico-ureteric reflux
  223
- agenesis of the kidney 6
- cryptorchidism 167

- cystic renal disease 214
- ectopic ureter 183
- grade-III VUR 194
- hydronephrosis 217, 221
- nephroblastoma 59
- single ectopic ureters 17
- thoracic kidneys 11
- vesico-ureteral reflux 209
Biopsy 10
Bipartite clitoris 223
Bladder 69
- development 3
- capacity 76, 167
- diverticula 49
- exstrophy 20, 223
- injury 73
- instability 78
- neck 183
- training 181
- volume 73
Bladder neck, development 3
Bolus tracking 80
Bone marrow
- aspiration 60
- suppression 241
Bourneville-Pringle syndrome 8
Bovine collagen 44
Bowel preparation 78
Bud theory 6

Caesarian section 167, 221, 239
Calcification 80
Calcium oxalate 235
Calculi 69
Calyceal
- dilatation 159
- diverticulum 14
Carboplatin 59
Cataract 239
Catecholamine 241
- metabolism 60
Catheterisation 76, 183, 187
Caudally positioned umbilicus 20
Cavography 214
Cefotaxime 140
Cephtacidine 143
CE-VUS 75
Chemotherapy 239
Chimeric antiganglioside antibody
  ch 14.18 241
Chloral hydrate 79
Cholecalciferol 124
Chorda urachii 23

Chromium-51-ethylene diamine
    tetraacetate (s. also ^{51}Cr-EDTA) 95
Chromosome 9
Chronic
– obstruction 52
– vesicoureteral reflux 7
Chwalla's membrane 3
CIC 23
Classification 30
– of nephroblastoma 57
– of the posterior urethral valves 25
Clinical
– evaluation 7, 32, 36
– management 53
– presentation 28, 36
– studies in reflux 110
Clitoris 5
Cloaca 1
Cloacal
– exstrophy 22
– membrane 3, 20
Cobra head phenomenon 19
Cohen 46, 209
– cross-trigonal technique 46
Colour Doppler 69, 73, 74
Combined upper and lower tract
    approach 19
Comparative imaging
– of pyelonephritis 105
– of renal scarring 107
Compensatory growth of the
    contralateral side 42
Complete
– obstruction 52
– ureteral duplication 15
Complications 47
Computed tomography
    (s. also CT) 69, 73, 79, 214
Congenital
– bilateral megaureter 176
– cyanotic heart diseases 228
– malformations 13
– obstructive uropathy 52
– stenosis 3
– ureteral stenosis 17
– urethral diverticula 27
Contralateral renal agenesis 54
Contrast medium 78, 79
Contrast-enhanced grey-scale
    voiding urosonography
    (s. also CE-VUS) 75
Corpora cavernosa 4
Cortical
– defects 105
– echogenicity 71
– necrosis 73
– scintigraphy 140
Corticomedullary differentiation 71,
    124, 126, 237
Cowper's glands (s. also glandulae
    bulbourethrales) 5
Creatinine 140
– clearance 206
^{51}Cr-EDTA 95
Crohn's disease 36

Crossed
– ectopia 11
– fused renal ectopia 103
– renal ectopia with or without fusion
    11
Crosstrigonal reimplantation 183
CRP 140, 143, 209
Cryptorchidism 30, 167
Crystallization 34
CT 73, 79, 239
– angiography 81
– scan 241
Cuboidal epithelium 9
Cutaneous depigmentation 216
Cyclic examination 77
Cystic
– disease 6
– – of the kidney 8
– dysplasia 6, 212
– fibrosis 35
– real disease 216
Cystine 36
– stones 36
Cystinuria 36, 38, 231
Cystitis 30
Cystoscopy 181, 223
Cysto-urethrography 176
Cysts of Cowper's glands 27

Dactinomycin 59
Deflux 45
Dehydration 228
Deletion of 11p12 239
Denis-Drash syndrome 239
Detrusor muscle, functional
    disorder 26
Development
– of the Bladder 3
– of the bladder neck 3
– of the female geniatalia 5
– of the genital ducts 4
– of the kidney 1
– of the male genitalia 4
– of the sinus urogenitalis 3
– of the ureter 3
– of the ureteral musculature 3
Dextranomers 44
Diabetes mellitus 49
Diagnostic laparotomy 214
Diaphragmatic hernia 130
Dibasic amino acids 231
2,8-Dihydroxy-adenine 36
Dilatation 51
Direct
– radionuclide cystography 108, 194
– voiding scintigraphy 126, 190,
    200
Disc kidney 11
Dismembered
– pyeloplasty 55
– techniques 55
Diuresis
– renography 71
– scintigraphy 96
– sonography 70, 71

Diuretic
– IVU 78
– scintigraphy 156, 190
Diverticulum of the bladder 22
Documentation of UTI 41
Doppler sonography 74, 228, 237
D-penicillamine-cysteine
    complex 38
Drainage phase 92
Dribbling of urine 181
Drugs 113
Duct 1
Ductus deferens 16
Dumbbell-shaped tumour 60
Duplex
– kidney 196
– system 187, 194
– anomalies 70
– Doppler 74
Duplication 103
– of the bladder 22
– of the urethra 27
Dynamic
– imaging 82
– renal scintigraphy 92
– scintigraphy 187
Dysplasia 6, 171, 181, 190, 200
Dysplastic
– kidney 54, 130, 200
– multicystic kidney 212
– renal pelvis 221

Eagle-Barrett syndrome 28
Ectopic
– megaureter 187
– ostium 187
– ureter 16, 79, 181
– ureteroceles 18
– kidney 103
Effective
– dose 78
– renal plasma flow (s. also ERPF)
    89
Ejaculatory duct 5
Elevation
– of CRP/ESR 105
– of the intravesical pressure 40
Endoscopic
– destruction of the valves 26
– evaluation 29
– incision 20
– treatment 39, 44
Enuresis 79, 196
Epicardia 21
Epididymitis 5, 17, 33
Epididymo-orchitis 33
ERPF 89
Escherichia coli 30, 140, 209
ESR 143, 209
ESWL 38
Etoposide 59
External sphincter 16, 181
– mechanism 5
Extracorporeal
– lithotripsy 231

– shock-wave lithotripsy
  (s. also ESWL) 38
Extrarenalization of the renal pelvis 14
Extravesical approach 45
Extrinsic subpelvic stenosis 152, 163
Extrinsic UPJ obstruction 54

F-15 renogram 101
Failure to thrive 221
Fallopian tubes 6
Fallot's tetralogy 28
Febrile urinary tract infection 183, 194
Female geniatalia, development 5
Fetal
– ascites 28
– kidney 70
Fever 105
– of unknown origin (s. also FUO) 196
First-line investigation 183
Flap techniques 56
Flap-using pyeloplasty 56
Fluoroscopic 41
Follow-up 47
Foreshortened hindgut 22
Fossa navicularis 5
Fowler-Stevens technique 30
Fravesical obstruction 217
Frenulum 5
– study 159, 163
Functional scintigraphic imaging 123
FUO 196

Gadolinium 81
Gadopentetate dimeglumine 163
Gartner's ducts 6
Genital ducts, development 4
Genital tubercle 4
GFR 209
Glandulae
– bulbourethrales 5
– paraurethrales 5
Glandular groove 5
Glomerular disease 71
Glomerulonephritis 163
Glomerulosclerosis 52
Glycerinate-dehydrogenase 35
Gonadal exposure 76
Gradient recalled echo sequences
  (s. also GRE) 81
Grading 42
GRE 81
Greyscale US 69
Gross haematuria 31
Group B β-haemolytic streptococci
  171
Growth factors 52
Growth retardation 124
Gubernaculum testis 5

Haemangiomas 82
Haematogenous pattern of infection
  30
Haematuria 9, 10, 163, 228, 235, 237
Haemoglobin 237
Haemorrhages 82

Haemorrhagic cystitis 32
H-antigen 31
Harmartomas 216
HASTE 82
Helical CT 79
Hemibladders 22
Hemihypertrophy 57
Heminephrectomy 181, 187, 190
Hemiphalluses 22
Hemizygosity 231
Hepatic fibrosis 8
Hepatosplenomegaly 8
Hereditary resorptive hypercalciuria
  235
Heritable cystic lesion 8
High-grade
– dilating reflux 126
– hydronephrosis 159
– reflux 196
– VUR 200, 212
High-risk protocol NB97 241
Hip dysplasia 28
Hippel-Lindau syndrome 8
homovanillic acid 60
Homozygosis 231
Horner's syndrome 60
Horseshoe kidney 12, 103, 134, 136
β-Human-chorionic gonadotropin
  (βHCG) 62
Hutches'diverticulum 171
Hydrocalycosis 14
Hydronephrosis 13, 70, 77, 136, 140,
  147, 152, 156, 159, 163, 167, 176, 200,
  206, 241
Hydroureter 167
Hymen 6
Hypercalciuria 35
– absorptive form 35
Hyperoxaluria 35
Hyperparathyroidism 235
Hyperplastic epithelium 9
Hyperpoliglobulia 228
Hyperreflexia
– of the detrusor muscle 24
– of the sphincter mechanism 24
Hyperresorptive Hypercalciuria 235
Hypertension 7–10, 124, 209
Hypertrophic nephrons 7
Hypertrophy of the bladder wall 25
Hypodysplastic kidneys 7
Hypoplasia 6
– of the bladder 22
Hypoplastic 11
– kidney 103, 124
Hypospadias 13, 163
Hypoxanthine-guanine-phorphoribo-
  syl transferase (s. also Lesch-Nyhan
  syndrome) 36

Ifosfamide 59
Iliac 10
131I-meta-iodobenzylguanidine
  (131I-MIBG) 60
123I-MIBG scan 241
– in Neuroblastoma 113

131I-MIBG therapy 115, 241
– radiobiology 115
– contraindications 115
– indications 115
– in neuroblastoma 115
131I-MIBG 60
Impaired muscular development of the
  ureter 48
Imperforate anus 16
Incontinence 181
Indirect radionuclide cystography
  110
Infantile polycystic kidney disease 8
Infarctions 82
Infectious Stones 34
Infertility 17
Infravesical obstruction 212, 223
Inhibitors of growth and aggregation
  34
Insipidus 49
Insufficiency of the bladder neck 17
Intermittent
– catheterization 167
– colics 163
– renal colics 152
Internal genitalia 16
Interstitial fibrosis 52
Intestinal malrotation 28
Intrarenal reflux 217
Intrathoracic mass 11
Intravesical Approach 46
Intrinsic UPJ Obstruction 54
Introitus 5
Iodine-123 (123I) 89
Ipsilateral multicystic renal
  degeneration 212
Irradiation 76
IRS 63
Isthmus 12

K-antigen 31
Kidney
– development 1
– size 70
Kinking 200
Klebsiella 31

Labia
– majora 6
– minora 6
Laser lithotripsy 39
Lateralization of the orifice 40
Lesch-Nyhan syndrome 36
Leucocytosis 140
– cortical defects 105
Levovist 75
Lich-Gregoir 194
– technique 45
Lipomas 82
Liver 9
Long-term antimicrobial
  prophylaxis 33
Loop ureterostomy 26
Loss of sodium 29
Low bladder capacity 183

Low-dose
- radiation 83
- VCUG 76
Lower
- motoneuron 23
- urinary tract 73
L-shaped kidney 11
Lumbar kidney 10
Lump kidney 11
Lung 9
Lymphadenectomy 239
Lysine 36

Macrohaematuria 163, 235
Magnetic resonance
- imaging 69
- angiography 81
Mainz Pouch II 223
Maldescensus testis 61
Maldevelopment of the bladder 17
Male genitalia
- development 4
Malrotation of the kidney 13, 129
Maturation 43
Medial umbilical ligament 23
Mediation of salt solution 34
Medullary necrosis 73
Megacalycosis 14
Megacolon 28
Megacystis 167
Megalourethra 27
Megameatus urethrae 27
Megaureter 40, 70, 77, 136, 143, 171,
    183, 187
Membranous urethra 5
Mental retardation 216
Mesonephric duct 1, 4
- defect 6
Mesonephros 1
Meta-iodobenzylguanidine in neuro-
    blastoma 112
Metanephrogenic blastema 2
Metanephros 2
Metaphylaxis 38
Metastases 241
Meyer-Weigert law 15
Micturition 77
Midazolam 76
Mild hypertension 214
Modified retroperitoneal
    lymphadenectomy 63
Molecular
- aggregation 34
- genetic methods 123
Monfort's abdominoplasty 29
Monitoring 81
Morphological changes 52
MR angiography (s. also MRA) 81, 123
MR urography (s. also MRU) 81
MRA 81
MRI 123, 181, 241
MRI urography 163
MRU 81
Müllerian
- duct 3–6

- tubercle 4, 6
- vagina 6
Multicystic
- dysplastic kidney 70, 104
- renal degeneration 214
- renal dysplasia 7
Multicystic-dysplastic left kidney 212
Mumps orchitis 33
mutation 231

Nasal obstruction 60
National Wilms' Tumour Study
    (s. also NWTS) 58
Neoadjuvant chemotherapy
    nephrectomy 239
Neonatal
- infection 171
- mortality 25
- sonographic screening 129
Nephrectomy 8, 9, 231, 214
Nephroblastoma 13, 57, 239
- classification 30
Nephroblastomatosis 81
Nephrocalcinosis 72
Nephrolithiasis 72, 231, 235
Nephroliths 163, 231, 235
Nephropyelolithotomy 39
Neuroblastoma 59, 73, 241
- stage-IV 241
- study NB97 60
Neurogenic bladder 181
Neurogenic disorder of lower
    urinary tract 23
Neurogenic voiding disorders 40
Neurospinal dysraphism 23
Newborns 9
N-myc oncogene 59
Nonheritable cystic lesions 8
Nonneurogenic voiding disorders 40
Nonobstructed megaureter 49, 136
Nonrefluxing 49
- megaureter 136
NWTS 58

O-antigen 31
Obstructed Megaureter 48
Obstruction 71, 82
Obstructive
- megaureter 171, 187
- uropathy 51, 190
Occult urinary tract infections 196
Oesophageal atresia 16
OIH 89
Oligohydramnion 6, 8, 26, 70, 221
Omphalocele 22
Open surgery 39
Operative
- exploration 34
- techniques 51
- – in secondary reflux 48
- treatment 44
Orchidectomy 34, 212
Orchitis 33
Ornithine 36
O-serotypes 31

Osteopathy 124
Ovary 6

Paediatric seminoma 62
PAH 89
PAK test 235
Pancake Kidney 129
Pancake-like kidney 129
Pancreas 9
Papin's method 126
Paraaminohippuric acid
    (s. also PAH) 89
Paramesonephric duct
    (s. also Müllerian duct) 3
Paratesticular rhabdomyosarcoma 64
Paraventricular protuberances 216
Parenchymal phase 92
Parenchymatous development 13
Parenteral rehydration 140
Partial obstruction 52
Patent urachus 23
Pathogenesis 30
Pelvic
- floor 5
- kidney 10
- urethra 3
Pelvicaliceal diameters 70
Penile-penile junction 217
Pentaacetic Acid 89
Percutaneous
- endoscopic gastrostomy 221
- nephroscopy 39
- nephrostolithotomy 39
- nephrostomy 39, 55
- puncture 10
- ureterocystostomy 221
Perfusion phase 92
Perirenal haematoma 73, 237
Permanent incontinence 223
Persistence of Chwalle's
    membrane 18
Persistent incontinence 17
Phacoerysis 239
Phallic urethra 3
Phosphate binder 124
Pinhole magnification scintigraphy 91
PKD
- 1 9
- 2 9
Planar scintigraphy 91
Plasma clearance 95
Plicae colliculi 25
Politano-Leadbetter 46, 171
- technique 46
Polycystic kidney disease 82, 104, 214,
    216
Polyps 54
Polytetrafluoroethylene 44
Polyuric nephropathies 49
Portal hypertension 8
Posterior
- commissura 5
- urethra 16
- urethral valves 25, 40, 42, 70, 76
Postnatal US 70

Potassium 29
– phosphate 38
Power Doppler 69, 74
Prenatal sonography 70, 167
Prepuce 5
Primary
– dysplasia 40
– dysplastic kidney 200
– enuresis diurna et nocturna 26
– hyperoxaluria 35
– hyperparathyroidism 35
– malignancy of the left bladder
  plate 21
– nocturnal enuresis 196
– obstructed megaureter 48, 56
– reflux 40
– urinary diversion 21
Primitive
– ducts 7
– phallus 4
– testicle 5
– tigone 3
Processus vaginalis peritonei 5
Prognosis 30
Progressive renal insufficiency 26, 221
Prolapse of the mitral valve 9
Pronephros 1
Prophylactic antibiotic treatment 190
Prostate
– capsule 5
– gland 5
Prostatic urethra 5
Proteinuria 140, 228
Proteus 31
– mirabilis 231
Prune belly syndrome 28, 70, 167
Pseudodiverticulum 22, 217
Pseudomonas aeruginosa 31, 223
Psoas hitch technique 46
Pudendal nerve 23
Pulmonary
– hypoplasia 6, 8, 9, 25, 28
– immaturity 8
– lobe 11
Pulsed fluoroscopy 76
Purine metabolism 36
– disorder 36
Pyelocutaneostomy 29
Pyeloectasia 130
Pyeloneohritis 30, 71, 74, 79, 126, 140,
  143, 190
Pyelonephritogenic nephropathy 32
Pyeloplasty 39, 77
Pyuria 140

Rachitis 206
Radiation Burden of radiolabelled
  MIBG 116
Radiation exposure 78
Radical retroperitoneal lymph-
  adenectomy 59
Radioiodinated o-iodohippurate
  (s. also OIH) 89
Radionuclear 41
Radionuclide

– cystography (s. also RNC) 75, 108
– scan 183
– therapy 241
Radiopharmaceuticals
– for dynamic renal scintigraphy 89
– for statistic renal scintigraphy 90
Radiotherapy 59
Rapid acquisition with relaxation
  enhancement (RARE) 82
Recanalization 3
Recurrent UTI 31
Reduction cystoplasty 29
Reflux 77, 140
– nephropathy 7, 40, 71, 79, 196, 206
Refluxing megaureter 48, 136, 171
Region of interest (s. also ROI) 92
Renal
– abscess 71
– agenesis 6, 126
– aplasia 6
– artery stenosis 73, 74
– biopsy 74
– bruise 237
– cancer 13
– clearance 95
– colic 152, 163, 235
– contusion 80
– cortex 124
– cortical scintigraphy 103
– cystine transporter protein 231
– damage 143
– dimensions 70
– donors 82
– duplication 79, 181, 190, 194
– dysgenesis 6
– dysplasia 6, 15, 78, 130, 217
– dystopia 129
– ectopia 10
– failure 124, 217
– fusion anomalies 69
– hypertension 32, 206, 209
– hypodysplasia 7
– hypoplasia 7, 124
– imaging 69
– insufficiency 124, 206
– – in childhood 7
– length 70
– lesions 140
– loss of phosphate 35
– lymphoma 80
– neoplasms 74
– obstruction 6, 11, 15, 51
– parenchymal or cystic disease 71
– pelvis 176
– plasma flow (s. also RPF) 89
– ptosis 10
– scarring 106
– scarring 32, 40, 71, 140, 143, 206, 209
– transplantation 27, 29, 73, 74, 82,
  221
– tumour 72, 80, 237
– vein thrombosis 74, 228
– volume 70
Renin-angiotensin system 52
Residual urine 167

Resistance 74
Respiratory distress syndrome 228
Response curve to frusemide
– type I 97
– type II 97
– type IIIa 97
– type IIIb 97
– type IV 99
Restriction
– of sodium intake 38
– of the urinary phosphate
  concentration 37
Rete testis 5, 212
Retrograde pyelography 130, 163, 181
Retrovesical space 69
Rhabdomyosarcoma 73
– of the pelvis 63
– of the uterus 64
Rickets 206
Risk of malignancy 8
RNC 75
ROI 92
RPF 89

Sarcoma botryoides 64
Scaphoid variant 27
Scarring 126
Schwarz 206, 209
Scintigraphic grading of reflux 111
Scintigraphy
– with ^{123}I-meta-iodobenzylguanidine
  113
– with ^{131}I-meta-iodobenzylguanidine
  113
Second ureteric bud 181
Second Wilms' tumour gene
  (s. also WT2) 57
Secondary
– bilateral VUR 209
– cancers 59
– obstructive megaureter 49, 56
– reflux 40, 217
– UPJ obstruction 55
– urinary diversion 21
Sedation 70, 79
Seizures 216
Seminal vesicle 5, 16
Sepsis 228
Sertoli cells 5
Serum creatinine 176, 206, 209
Severe VUR 200
Shock wave lithotripsy 79
Sigmoid kidney 11
Significant bacteriuria 209
Simple renal cyst 9
Single ectopic
– kidneys 10
– ureter 183
Single photon emission
  computed tomography
  (s. also SPECT) 91
Single-compartment techniques 95
Sinus urogenitalis
– development 3
SIOP 58

Skene's glands (s. also glandulae paraurethrales) 5
Society International d'Oncologie Pédiatrique (SIOP) 58
Sodium
– cellulose phosphate 38
– phosphate 38
Sonographic screening 124
SPECT 91, 140
Sphincter-detrusor dyssynergia 181
Spinal deformities 28
Spin-echo (SE) sequences 81
Spiral CT 237
Spleen 9
Split
– function 136, 143, 147, 152, 156, 159, 196
– pelvis 223
Spontaneous
– regression 59
– resolution of reflux 43
– rupture 10
Sporadic aniridia 57
S-shaped kidney 11
Staghorn
– calculi 35
– stones 39
Static renal scintigraphy 32
Sterile intermittent (self)-catheterization (CIC) 23
Stone
– formation 11, 13, 34
– – general pathophysiology
– matrix 34
– prevention 37
Streptococcus
– faecalis 143
– pneumoniae 206
Struvite 35
Subarachnoid haemorrhage 9
Subpelvic intrinsic obstruction 130, 147, 152
Subureteric collagen injection 181
Subvesical obstruction 40, 176
Sulphonamides 33
Superalimentation 221
Supermumerary kidney 15
Supersaturation 34
Suprapubic
– catheterization of the bladder 26
– needle aspiration 41
Surgical exploration 10
Symphyseal separation 20
Symptomatic urinary tract infections 134
Syringoceles (s. also cysts of Cowper's glands) 27

T2-weighted sequences 81
Targeted radiation 61
99mTc-DMSA 90, 103, 143, 206, 209, 231
– in the diagnosis of renal scarring 106
– in the diagnosis upper urinary tract infection 104

– scan 126
– SPECT 91
99mTc-DTPA 89
99mTc-GH 91
99mTc-MAG 90
99mTc-MAG3 130, 147, 156, 176, 187, 196, 217, 223, 231
– scan 167
– scintigraphy 143, 152, 171, 183, 190, 200
99mTcO4- 89
99mTc-pertechnetate ($^{99m}TcO_4^-$) 89
Technetium 99m
– diethylene triamine pentaacetic acid 89
– dimercaptosuccinic acid 90
– glucoheptonate 91
– mercaptoacetyltriglycine 90
TER 95
Teratogenic causes 10
Teratoma 62
Terminal Renal Insufficiency 221
Testicles 167
– descends 5
Testicular
– appendix 5
– autotransplantation 30
– dysplasia 212
– tumours 61
Thermodynamic solubility product 34
Thiazide diuretics 37
Third-generation cephalosporins 33
Thoracic Renal Ectopia 11
Time of flight (TOF) sequences 81
Time-activity 147
– curve 92, 93, 136, 156, 159
Tissue-augmenting substance 44
Tract dilatation 71
Transudate 9
Transurethral ureteroscopy 39
Transvesical Approach 46
Triad syndrome 28
Tube current 80
Tuberous sclerosis 214, 216
Tubular
– atrophy 52
– extraction rate (TER) 95
– necrosis 73
Tubules 27
Tumour thrombus 58
Turner's syndrome 12
Two-compartment model 95
Two-hit hypothesis 57

Ultrasonography 10, 69
– technique 69
Ultrasound in the neonate 70
Uncovered bladder plate 20
Undescended testis 13
Unfavourable prognosis 57
Unilateral 159
– agenesis 129
– inferior fusion 11
– superior fusion 11

Unselective proteinuria 214
UPJ 51
– obstruction 54
Upper
– motoneuron 23
– tract approach 19
– urinary tract 71
– – infection 171
Urachal
– cyst 23
– diverticulum 23
– remnants 73
– sinus 23
Urachus 23
Urease 35
Ureter 69, 71
– development 3
Ureteral
– duplication 15
– obliteration 13, 52
– obstruction 13
– reimplantation 29
– stenting 39, 55
– tapering 51
– valves 18, 54
Ureteral musculature
– development 3
Ureterectomy 187, 190
Ureteric
– bud 2, 13, 181
– jets 74
Ureterocele 15, 49, 18, 76, 79, 190
Ureterocystoneostomy 77, 196
Uretero-enterostomy 223
Ureterolithotomy 39
Ureteropelvic junction (UPJ) obstruction 54, 70
Ureteropyelostomy 19
Uretero-ureterostomy 19
Ureterovesical junction 40
– obstruction 70
Urethral
– folds 4
– groove 4, 5
– plate 4
– trauma 78
– value 176
– valve 217, 221
Urethroplasty 27
Urinalysis 32
Urinary
– ascites 25
– culture 32, 140
– diversion 26
– incontinence 183
– tract infection (s. also UTI) 13, 30, 70, 126, 134, 167, 176, 196, 200, 206, 209, 223, 231
Urine
– cultures 196
– flow impairment 70
Urinoma 73, 80
Urodynamics 42
– examination 181

Uroepithelial adherence 31
Urolithiasis 34
– conservative treatment 37
Urorectal septum 3
Uterovaginal primordium 4, 5
Uterus 6
UTI 11, 30, 71
Utriculus prostaticus 5, 16
UVJ 51
– obstruction 56

Vagina 5, 16
Vaginal
– masses 18
– plate 6
– vestibulum 5
Valvotomy 217
Vanillymandelic acid 60
Vas

– deferens 5
– efferens 5
VCUG 75, 76
Ventricular defects 28
Verumontanum 3, 5
Vesical sphincter 181
Vesicoallantoic canal 3
Vesico-amniotic shunt 27
Vesico-renal reflux 105
Vesicostomy 26, 29
Vesico-ureteral reflux (s. also VUR) 7,
  13, 15, 40, 70, 76, 105, 183, 190
Video-urodynamic evaluation 24
Vincristine 59
Vitamin C 36, 38
Vitamin D
– 1,25-(OH)-vitamin D 35
– deficiency 206
– intoxication 235

– therapy 206
Voiding 70
Von Hippel-Lindau's disease 214
VUR 70, 71, 76, 77, 105, 126, 134, 140,
  143, 147, 176, 181, 187, 194, 200, 209,
  212, 217
– grade-III 200, 209
– grade-IV 206
– grade-V 206

WAGR syndrome 57, 239
Wait-and-see strategy 147, 159
Whitacker's test 29
Wilms' Tumour 57, 73, 239
– gene 57, 239
WT1 gene 57
WT2 57

Yolk-sac tumour 62

The manufacturer's authorised representative in the EU is Springer
Nature Customer Service Centre GmbH, Europaplatz 3, 69115 Heidelberg,
Germany. If you have any concerns regarding our products, please
contact ProductSafety@springernature.com

Printed and bound by CPI Group (UK) Ltd, Croydon, CR0 4YY

29/04/2026
02099553-0002